ENVIRONMENTAL TOXINS: PSYCHOLOGICAL, BEHAVIORAL, AND SOCIOCULTURAL ASPECTS, 1973–1989

Cheryl Brown Travis
Barbara E. McLean
Carlotta Ribar
Editors

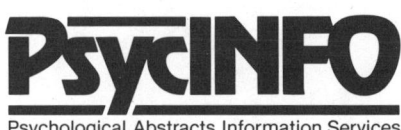

Psychological Abstracts Information Services

Bibliographies in Psychology No. 5

American Psychological Association

Library of Congress Cataloging-in-Publication Data

Environmental toxins: psychological , behavioral, and sociocultural
  aspects, 1973–1989 / Cheryl Brown Travis, Barbara E. McLean, Carlotta Ribar, editors.

p. cm. --(Bibliographies in psychology; no. 5)
         Includes bibliographies and indexes.
           1. Behavioral toxicology--Psychological aspects--Bibliography.
2. Behavioral toxicology--Social aspects--Bibliography.
3. Pollution--Toxicology--Psychological aspects--Bibliography.
4. Pollution--Toxicology--Social aspects--Bibliography.
5. Health behavior--Bibliography.
I. Travis, Cheryl Brown, 1944-   . II. McLean, Barbara E. III. Ribar, Carlotta. IV. Series.
[DNLM: 1. Behavior--drug effects--abstracts. 2. Environmental Pollutants--toxicity--abstracts.
3. Toxins--abstracts.   ZQW 630 E61]
Z7892.B44E58   1989   [RA1224]
016.6159'02--dc20   89-14927
ISBN: 1-55798-063-2

Published by the
American Psychological Association
750 First Street, NE
Washington, DC 20002

Copies may be ordered from:
Order Department
P.O. Box 2710
Hyattsville, MD 20784

Copyright ©1989 by the American Psychological
Association. All rights reserved. Except as permitted
under the United States Copyright Act of 1976, no
part of this publication may be reproduced or
distributed in any form or by any means, or stored
in a data base or retrieval system, without the prior
written permission of the publisher.

Printed in the United States of America.

BIBLIOGRAPHIES IN PSYCHOLOGY SERIES

1. Black Males in the United States: An Annotated Bibliography from 1967 to 1987
2. AIDS: Abstracts of the Psychological and Behavioral Literature, 1983-1988
3. Black Females in the United States: A Bibliography from 1967 to 1987
4. Alzheimer's Disease: Abstracts of the Psychological and Behavioral Literature
5. Environmental Toxins: Psychological, Behavioral, and Sociocultural Aspects, 1973-1989
6. AIDS: Abstracts of the Psychological and Behavioral Literature, 1983-1989, Second Edition

ACKNOWLEDGMENTS

Credit for this bibliography must go to the professional staff of PsycINFO—the coverage selectors, bibliographers, abstractors, editors, and indexers—who have compiled these materials over the years. Special appreciation is due to Alain Dessaint, who managed the project, created the classification system, and devised the search strategy; to Karen Monroe for her professionalism and patience in modifying the computer programs; to James Whitfield for assisting with the search and for downloading and editing the materials; to Gary Broyhill and Jody Kerby for desktop publishing; and to Maurine Jackson for assisting with the programming and photocomposition specifications.

TABLE OF CONTENTS

FOREWORD vii

SECTION I.   SELECTED REFERENCES TO JOURNAL ARTICLES
             AND DISSERTATIONS

        Behavioral Toxicology: General 1
            Human Research 8
            Animal Research 23

        Pesticides 25
            Human Research 26
            Animal Research 27

        Solvents 34
            Human Research 35
            Animal Research 42

        Metallic Elements 47
            Human Research 49
            Animal Research 65

        Food Additives 85
            Human Research 87
            Animal Research 91

        Gases 92
            Human Research 92
            Animal Research 97

SECTION II. CITATIONS TO RECENTLY PUBLISHED JOURNAL ARTICLES 101

SECTION III. SUBJECT INDEX 103

SECTION IV. AUTHOR INDEX 119

APPENDIX: Search Strategy Used to Retrieve References for the Bibliography 125

FOREWORD

Environmental Toxicants: Behavioral and Psychological Dimensions

The Issue

Lead poisoning in children. Links from asbestos to cancer. Industrial chemicals. Just a few obvious reminders of the side effects of progress. What is less obvious is the role of psychology in all this. In fact, psychology has a great deal to say. Neurobehavioral toxicology, the effects of toxic substances on behavior and the nervous system, is one of the more exciting subdisciplines of psychology—and one of the more needed.

Chemicals have become an integral part of our lives. The National Academy of Sciences determined that Americans are now exposed to over 65,000 chemicals. And 1,500 new substances add to the total each year. They are in our food, our workplaces, our homes, our cosmetics, our clothes. Yet, only a relative handful have ever been tested for their effects on behavior. We know something about how chemicals lead to traditionally defined medical illness. We know very little about effects on cognition, memory, perception, speech, or a host of other psychological variables. The NAS concluded: "It is clear that thousands or even tens of thousands of chemicals are legitimate candidates for toxicity testing . . . and that neurobehavioral toxicity evaluation is one of the highest priority toxicity testing needs."

The occupational medicine literature is filled with the effects of *not* testing. The industrial chemical carbon disulfide, used in rayon manufacturing, can produce vision disorder and nerve weakness, increase the incidence of suicide, and eventually cause a raging, raving mania. The "Mad Hatter" of Lewis Carroll's *Alice in Wonderland* was a caricature of the effects of inorganic mercury—social withdrawal, "fidgetiness," memory disorder. Even lead, many of whose toxic effects we have known about for decades, continues to surprise us. Now it seems that levels previously thought safe can still affect the nervous systems of children exposed in utero.

The social and economic effects on individuals and on society of these and other examples are enormous. Even sadder—damage to the human central nervous system is rarely reparable.

The Association's Response

The past few years have seen the American Psychological Association forcefully enter the public policy debate over environmental toxins. Our efforts have been concentrated on strengthening the federal government's position on the issue of behavioral testing of chemicals.

The Federal Insecticide, Fungicide and Rodenticide Act (FIFRA) is the law that regulates pesticides and controls their marketing and testing by the Environmental Protection Agency (EPA). In 1988, APA worked with a coalition of groups to insert provisions into the law that would require neurobehavioral testing of pesticides. The report that accompanies the law now reads: "There is increasing evidence that exposure to pesticides can cause neurotoxic and behavioral effects. EPA currently... does not evaluate a range of effects in the areas of learning ability, memory disruption, and other neurobehavioral functions. In light of the recommendations made by a number of scientific and public health organizations urging expanded neurotoxic and behavioral testing, the [Congressional Oversight] Committee requests that EPA intensify the degree of such testing in its pesticide program." APA was also successful in having similar language added to the report accompanying the FY 1989 EPA appropriations bill.

We have also been active on another front. APA, working with the Center for Science in the Public Interest and other organizations concerned about the neurotoxicity of pesticides, filed a petition with EPA seeking the adoption of more sensitive and appropriate testing methods. In response to this petition, the EPA convened a Science Advisory Panel hearing at which APA testified. As a result, EPA has established an internal working group to begin the process of revising their testing guidelines. To further encourage the agency, APA worked with Senators Patrick Leahy, Chairman of the Senate Agriculture Committee (which has jurisdiction over FIFRA), and Richard Lugar, Ranking Minority Member of that committee, to have a bipartisan letter sent to EPA Administrator William Reilly expressing the Senators' concern over slow progress in this area.

Given the pervasiveness of toxic chemicals in our environment and the poor state of health data in the area, it is not surprising that the public is continually caught off guard. Very recently, APA testified before the Senate Committee on Environment and Public Works on two such public health incidents. One involved worker exposure to what appeared to be highly neurotoxic solvents and resins employed in the aerospace industry for the construction of the Air Force's new Stealth bomber. The other involved public concern over pesticides in the food supply stemming from a report of the Natural Resources Defense Council entitled "Intolerable Risk: Pesticides in our Children's Food." In both instances, the APA described the dangers of neurotoxin insult to the human body and expressed concern over the paucity of test data on pesticides and other potentially neurotoxic substances.

While federal laws have been passed by Congress that provide the basis for federal regulation of potential neurotoxins, the weakness appears to be in the lack of response of the federal agencies. For instance, the Toxic Substances Control Act, enacted in 1976, vests the EPA with the power to monitor, investigate, and regulate chemical substances. The statute states:

> The health and environment effects for which standards for the development of test data may be prescribed include carcinogenesis, mutagenesis, teratogenesis, *behavioral disorders* [italics added], cumulative and synergistic effects, and any other effect which may present an unreasonable risk of injury to health or environment.

Yet, since the passage of TSCA, too little has been accomplished by EPA in exploring the potential health risks, particularly in the area of behavioral disorders, of the vast majority of potentially hazardous chemicals in our environment. What we have presented here has barely scratched the surface of what needs to be done. We will continue our efforts to expand federal activity in this neglected field of health research.

The Contribution of This Bibliography

The psychological and behavioral literature on environmental toxins is expanding in almost direct proportion to the growing concerns of psychologists and behavioral toxicologists. A mini-convention centered on environmental toxins will have a special place at the 1989 APA Annual Convention. As another response to these increasingly serious concerns (and in support of the mini-convention), PsycINFO has compiled this bibliography on the psychological, behavioral, and sociocultural aspects of environmental toxins. The 962 abstracts and citations were drawn from the approximately 1,300 journals regularly covered in the PsycINFO databases.

The bibliography organizes the serial literature into the following broad domains: General Behavioral Toxicology, Pesticides, Solvents, Metallic Elements, Food Additives, and Gases. Each classification is further broken down into Human Research and Animal Research.

Section I includes 918 full abstracts and dissertation citations dating from 1973 to the present and published in *Psychological Abstracts* (*PA*) and the PsycINFO database. Section II contains an additional 44 citations to the most recent journal literature retrieved from the PsycALERT database. A subject index (for Section I) and an author index (for Sections I and II) are also included.

The Appendix contains the search strategy used in retrieving the references in this bibliography. This explanation of the search strategy allows the reader to keep the bibliography continually updated using the online PsycINFO and PsycALERT databases, and it also provides a model for constructing a search tailored to the reader's specific interests.

Alan G. Kraut, PhD, Executive Director
    Science Directorate, APA
Gary R. VandenBos, PhD, Executive Director
    Office of Publications and Communications, APA
Lois W. Granick, Director
    PsycINFO, APA

Section I. Selected References to Journal Articles and Dissertations

This section contains a bibliography of annotated references from the journal literature and citations of the dissertation literature on the psychological, behavioral, and sociocultural aspects of environmental toxins. Documents concerning toxic levels of radiation or noise are included. Those on self-abuse of toxins are omitted. References were retrieved from the PsycINFO database and are organized alphabetically by author within eighteen major and minor categories.

BEHAVIORAL TOXICOLOGY: GENERAL

1. Allen, Gary L. & Morgan, Ben B. (1985). **Assessment of learning abilities using complex experimental learning tasks.** Workshop on Neurotoxicity Testing in Human Populations (1983, Rougemont, North Carolina). *Neurobehavioral Toxicology & Teratology,* 7(4), 355–358.
Discusses complex experimental learning tasks (CELTs), which provide real-time samples of learning, in terms of methodology (hardware and software, learning tasks, and measures of performance on CELTs) and potential applications. Objectives of current studies are the determination of relationships between performance of CELTs and performance on traditional cognitive-abilities tests and the exploration of the predictive value of measures of learning ability for academic performance. After construct and predictive validity are established, this methodology may be applicable to a wide range of assessment situations, including testing for the effects of environmental toxicants on learning abilities. (11 ref).

2. Anger, W. Kent. (1985). **Overview of NIOSH neurobehavioral testing/research.** Workshop on Neurotoxicity Testing in Human Populations (1983, Rougemont, North Carolina). *Neurobehavioral Toxicology & Teratology,* 7(4), 289–290.
Discusses the establishment of the National Institute for Occupational Safety and Health (NIOSH), created by the Department of Health, Education, and Welfare in 1970 and charged with conducting research and recommending standards for assuring safe and healthy workplaces. NIOSH neurobehavioral research includes animal and human laboratory testing and examinations of workers in field studies. NIOSH field or worksite investigations are divided into 2 types: hazard evaluation and industrywide studies. The research that has been conducted by NIOSH on human neurotoxicity testing is outlined. (5 ref).

3. Arezzo, Joseph C.; Simson, Richard & Brennan, Nancy E. (1985). **Evoked potentials in the assessment of neurotoxicity in humans.** Workshop on Neurotoxicity Testing in Human Populations (1983, Rougemont, North Carolina). *Neurobehavioral Toxicology & Teratology,* 7(4), 299–304.
Reviews strengths and weaknesses of evoked potentials (EPs) as an index of toxic insult to the nervous system. EPs are obtained by averaging successive samples of EEG time-locked to the presentation of stimuli. Components of the resulting waveform can be measured for amplitude, latency, and distribution. Normal ranges of these parameters have been characterized for auditory, visual, and somatosensory stimuli. The current lack of standardized recording and analysis techniques has sometimes generated contradictory results, but the evidence thus far supports the ultimate usefulness of EPs as a neurotoxicological screening tool. (31 ref).

4. Baker, Edward L. (1985). **Epidemiologic issues in neurotoxicity research.** Workshop on Neurotoxicity Testing in Human Populations (1983, Rougemont, North Carolina). *Neurobehavioral Toxicology & Teratology,* 7(4), 293–297.
Discusses types of epidemiological studies, phases of epidemiological research, and issues of validity in neurotoxicity research. The stages of execution of an epidemiologic study include problem specification; choice of study type; selection of study population; selection of measures of exposure and effect; specification of relevant confounding factors; and data collection, analysis, and interpretation. Although both case-control and cohort studies have been performed, a deficiency in the number and variety of case-control studies in this area points to a need for future collaborative research. Typical shortcomings of prior research include failure to adequately quantify individual exposure/dose levels, failure to control for relevant confounding factors, and failure to carefully evaluate selection bias. (10 ref).

5. Benignus, Vernon A. (1984). **EEG as a cross species indicator of neurotoxicity.** United States Environmental Protection Agency, Neurotoxicology Division, and the Johns Hopkins University Neurotoxicology Program Conference: Cross species extrapolation in neurotoxicology (1984, Raleigh, North Carolina). *Neurobehavioral Toxicology & Teratology,* 6(6), 473–483.
Discusses quantification schemes for interpreting EEG data and the utility of EEG as a cross-species indicator of neurotoxicity. The relationship of EEG to brain function or brain pathology is not well understood by some standards, perhaps due to poor quantitative methods or erroneous assumptions about brain–behavior relationships. EEG has a similar appearance across species and so has great promise as a cross-species indicator of neurotoxicity. More methods development is needed before the promise of cross-species generality can be realized. (90 ref).

6. Berglund, Birgitta. (1977). **Quantitative approaches in environmental studies.** *International Journal of Psychology,* 12(2), 111–123.
Discusses the application of psychological scaling methods-problems within the realm of environmental hygiene. Methodological issues related to the possibility of obtaining calibrated scales of perceptual variables such as discomfort, annoyance, and unpleasant odors are critical when the scale values are to be entered into a physical pollution index or a perceived environmental quality index, both being applied in the form of norms or recommendations. It is noted that the level of measurement (ordinal, interval, or ratio scale) is related to the question of calibration of scales, and that from a practical point of view, it is important to disguise the effects of observer environment dependence in the scale values. Problems having to do with calibration of scales and with application of knowledge about perceptual processes to the scales are being explored in ongoing research projects (e.g., the measurement of temperature discomfort in different climates and the measurement of annoyance in areas with different noise exposures). Attempts to solve an odorous air pollution problem with psychological measurements are detailed. (French summary) (21 ref).

7. Berglund, Birgitta & Lindvall, Thomas. (1978). **Olfactory evaluation of indoor air quality.** *Reports from the Department of Psychology, U. Stockholm,* 526, 12 p.
Examined indoor and outdoor air pollutants, focusing on volatile organic compounds and on the odor of the air as a whole. Methods for sampling and analysis were developed as well as psychophysical methods for studying sensory reactions. In old buildings 50–75% of volatile organic compounds

BEHAVIORAL TOXICOLOGY: GENERAL

in air were found to be associated with odors. Several pollutants increased in concentration from outdoor to indoor air. The use of heat exchangers that transferred moisture also transferred polar and nonpolar compounds to the inlet air. The air going into a preschool room was found to be contaminated relative to outdoor air. Similarly, the ventilation inlet of a high school classroom was contaminated with bad odors. After 30 min of a class, the room was overloaded with odors when the class size was two-thirds of its nominal capacity. A master scale was developed for obtaining comparable subjective measures of odor strength from different observers as well as objective measures for different odors. On the master scale of odor strength, comparisons were easily made of the odor of classroom air, ventilation inlet air, and kitchen air, obtained from an earlier field study. (10 ref).

8. Brackbill, Yvonne. (1987). **Behavioral teratology comes to the classroom.** *Topics in Early Childhood Special Education,* 6(4), 33–48.
Discusses types of teratogenic agents, behavioral targets, organismic vulnerability during growth spurts, teratogenic routing, exposure, and duration of effects. Some chemical neurotoxins, using lead as a paradigm, that are known to affect cognitive and noncognitive behaviors crucial to learning and appropriate conduct in the classroom are described. Two ways are indicated in which behavioral teratology is particularly important for special education: (1) Behavioral teratology balances the tendency to attribute educational problems exclusively to social or environmental antecedents, and (2) it provides a much needed subject matter for the educational curriculum of junior and senior high schools.

9. Buchanan, Stephen R. (1984). **The most ubiquitous toxin.** *American Psychologist,* 39(11), 1327–1328.
Agrees with B. Weiss's (1983) contention that scientists should consider behavior change as a criterion for judging the safety of a substance to which the public is exposed and that psychologists should cooperate with behavioral toxicologists in developing behavioral tests to assess the effects of toxins on behavior. It is argued that refined sugar should be placed in this category because children who overconsume refined sugar are likely to upset the homeostatic balance necessary for proper metabolism, leading to behavioral changes and clinical symptoms such as hyperkinesis. Factors hindering the recognition of refined sugar as a toxin are discussed. (6 ref).

10. Buckalew, L. W. & Ross, Sherman. (1982). **Behavioral teratology: An interdisciplinary frontier.** *Journal of Alcohol & Drug Education,* 27(3), 34–36.
Discusses a broadened concept of teratogens that includes both negative and positive potential effects and incorporates the traditional perspective of drugs as well as early experiences and environment, hormones, additives, and pollutants. The time frame of concern to behavioral teratology is portrayed as from preconception through weaning. The need for a long-term developmental and behavioral perspective of teratogens is stressed. (9 ref).

11. Buckholtz, Neil S. & Panem, Sandra. (1986). **Regulation and evolving science: Neurobehavioral toxicology.** *Neurobehavioral Toxicology & Teratology,* 8(1), 89–96.
Discusses the relationship of research and development and regulation as they relate to the use of new technical knowledge for chemical regulation. The present discussion derives from the issue of the extent of toxicological testing required for the evaluation of the health and safety aspects of pesticides and other compounds at the US Environmental Protection Agency. The area of neurobehavioral toxicology is used as a case study to address policy and regulatory issues. Scientific issues involved with the selection of test systems are also addressed.

12. Butcher, Richard E. (1985). **An historical perspective on behavioral teratology.** Conference Proceedings of the National Center for Toxicological Research et al: Design considerations in screening for behavioral teratogens: Results of the collaborative behavioral teratology study (1985, Cincinnati, Ohio). *Neurobehavioral Toxicology & Teratology,* 7(6), 537–540.
Comments that the search for useful screening methods for safety evaluation has used 2 basic strategies: (1) having tests chosen by the consensus of experts in the field or through surveys of tests used in behavioral teratology and (2) exploring the utility of test procedures in small, informal interlaboratory reliability studies. It is concluded that neither of these approaches succeeded in identifying appropriate screening methods and that there is a need for research efforts specifically directed at test selection and interlaboratory reliability. (23 ref).

13. Butcher, Richard E. & Nelson, C. J. (1985). **Design and analysis issues in behavioral teratology testing.** Conference Proceedings of the National Center for Toxicological Research et al: Design considerations in screening for behavioral teratogens: Results of the collaborative behavioral teratology study (1985, Cincinnati, Ohio). *Neurobehavioral Toxicology & Teratology,* 7(6), 659.
Outlines several suggestions to increase the utility of behavioral teratology data, including an operational definition of sensitivity, careful control of experiments and increasing the number of Ss to reduce variability, true random selection of litters used in experimentation, and the addition of nonparametric statistics in analysis.

14. Creel, Donnell J. (1984). **Albinism and evoked potentials: Factors in the selection of infrahuman models in predicting the human response to neurotoxic agents.** United States Environmental Protection Agency, Neurotoxicology Division, and the Johns Hopkins University Neurotoxicology Program Conference: Cross species extrapolation in neurotoxicology (1984, Raleigh, North Carolina). *Neurobehavioral Toxicology & Teratology,* 6(6), 447–453.
Outlines pertinent factors that should be considered when using infrahuman models in neurotoxicology research, such as species variation; differential effects on early, middle, and late components of sensory EPs; and the use of albino animals. The experimenter should be cautious of interspecies differences in anatomy and physiology and be aware of intraspecies strain differences, particularly those related to pigmentation, that may restrict one's ability to predict the human response to neurotoxic agents based on data from an infrahuman model. (91 ref).

15. Cuthbertson, Beverley H. (1988). **Emotion and technological disaster: An integrative analysis.** *Dissertation Abstracts International,* 48(7-A), 1885–1886.

16. Cuthbertson, Beverley H. & Nigg, Joanne M. (1987). **Technological disaster and the nontherapeutic community: A question of true victimization.** *Environment & Behavior,* 19(4), 462–483.
Reviews the origin, components, and applications of the therapeutic community concept for natural disaster situations. The question is raised whether such a mechanism emerges in response to environmental hazards other than rapid onset, natural disaster agents. Using case study data from 2 technological events—one involving the aerial application of pesticides and the other the disposal of asbestos tailings—it is concluded that under certain circumstances, the classic therapeutic community is unlikely to develop in technological disasters. The factors mitigating against its development are examined with a primary focus on the question of who are the true victims, the formation of victim clusters, and the emergence of community conflict.

17. Dyer, Robert S. (1984). **Cross species extrapolation and hazard identification in neurotoxicology.** *Neurobehavioral Toxicology & Teratology,* 6(6), 409–411.
Discusses 2 issues in neurotoxicology research: the endpoints to which the "human" or target endpoints can be extrapolated and the endpoints from which the "animal" or source endpoints can be extrapolated. It is argued that other issues, such as predicting an effective dose in one species based on dose–effect data in another, are predicated on understanding the source and target endpoints and the relationship between them. (1 ref).

18. Eckerman, David A. et al. (1985). **An approach to brief field testing for neurotoxicity.** Workshop on Neurotoxicity Testing in Human Populations (1983, Rougemont, North Carolina). *Neurobehavioral Toxicology & Teratology,* 7(4), 387–393.
Describes a microcomputer-based testing system that uses an Apple II microcomputer with the Pascal language and additional hardware resources. Tasks implemented for the system have been selected to broadly sample cognitive functioning and some sensory and motor evaluation as well, including perceptual apprehension, reaction time (RT) and movement, episodic memory readout, and analogical reasoning and algorithmic manipulation. Efforts to evaluate sensitivity, task interrelations, and reliability of measurement are discussed. (8 ref).

19. Evans, Gary W. & Campbell, Joan M. (1983). **Psychological perspectives on air pollution and health.** *Basic & Applied Social Psychology,* 4(2), 137–169.
Reviews representative literature on epidemiological research on air pollution, toxicological research, and attitude research. Gaps and weaknesses in this literature are identified, and a set of psychological and social considerations that previous research has largely neglected are presented. It is argued that conceptually, most previous investigations have focused exclusively on direct, unmediated relationships between air pollution and (typically) catastrophic health outcomes. This approach ignores complex effects on physical and psychological health that are mediated by cognitive processes and sensitive hormonal responses. It also ignores the many variations in contexts that influence exposure to air pollution as well as how pollution is experienced by individuals. In contrast to the limited medical model of disease causation by air pollution, a more complex, dynamic model is proposed that includes contextual and constitutional factors that influence how individuals experience and cope with pollution. It is concluded that understanding what makes pollution stressful will provide clues about what motivates polluting behaviors, and perhaps ultimately point the way to a means of fostering ecologically responsible behaviors. (92 ref).

20. Fein, Greta G.; Schwartz, Pamela M.; Jacobson, Sandra W. & Jacobson, Joseph L. (1983). **Environmental toxins and behavioral development: A new role for psychological research.** *American Psychologist,* 38(11), 1188–1197.
Presents a new multiple-effects model that emphasizes subtle behavioral alteration as an early sign of toxicity and as evidence that a particular chemical agent may produce long-term impairment in susceptible individuals. The permeability of the placenta to a variety of chemical agents and the special sensitivity of the fetus to some of these agents draws attention to prenatal exposure and the need for prospective longitudinal studies of affective, social, and cognitive development in exposed individuals. The multiple-effects model provides a role for the psychologist in teratological diagnosis and research since the measurement of behavioral variation has developed primarily in psychology. Limitations inherent in both experimental animal research and correlational human studies of toxic effects make it necessary for these methodologies to be used in a complementary fashion. The implications of behavioral teratology for the study of human development and the design of protective social policies are discussed. (45 ref).

21. Fisher, Gerald H. (1973). **Current levels of noise in an urban environment.** *Applied Ergonomics,* 4(4), 211-218.
Describes studies made in the UK during 1971 that measured both peak and ambient noise levels prevailing inside and outside residential buildings and that found the levels greatly in excess of those considered tolerable 10 yrs previously. Two methods for reducing noise levels were considered: (a) a barrier designed to reflect rather than absorb noise and (b) a simple form of double-glazing fitted to existing window frames. The barrier succeeded in reducing peak noise levels but failed to influence ambients. The double-glazing attenuated both peak and ambient noise levels significantly. Attention is drawn to the possibility of noise generated within buildings themselves becoming a source of discomfort for occupants and of annoyance to those outside. Data referring to noise levels in the outdoor environment reveal that the upper tolerance limits prescribed by the International Organization of Standardization are now being exceeded by 20 db or more throughout 18 hrs of the day. Findings are discussed in relation to the inevitable limits soon to be reached in adaptation of the human hearing mechanisms to increasing environmental noise.

22. Foster, Harold D. (1988). **The geography of schizophrenia: Possible links with selenium and calcium deficiencies, inadequate exposure to sunlight and industrialization.** *Journal of Orthomolecular Medicine,* 3(3), 135–140.
Data collected by the author (1986) suggest that (1) the presence of selenium in fodder crops and a high rate of sunlight exposure are negatively correlated with prevalence rates of schizophrenia in the US and (2) low selenium/high mercury content in soil, living in industrialized areas, and low exposure to sunshine are positively correlated with schizophrenia rates.

23. Givens, David B. (1982). **From here to eternity: Communicating with the distant future.** *Etc.,* 39(2), 159–179.
Discusses problems of long-term future communication (i.e., of moving detailed, present-day information across several millennia) from the viewpoint of semiotics, information theory, anthropology, and cross-cultural psychology. The following aspects of humanity's *Umwelt* (concepts of the external environment, as defined by sensory data) are discussed: (1) dominance structures, (2) territory, (3) perception and cognition, (4) socioemotional universals, (5) speech, and (6) narratives. (41 ref).

24. Golden, Herbert M. (1973). **The dysfunctional effects of modern technology on the adaptability of the aging.** *Gerontologist,* 13(2), 136-143.
Describes those aspects of technology that adversely affect the elderly, including pollution, mass transportation, the automobile, and health care. It is concluded that societal priorities must be reordered to take into account the psychomotor and cognitive difficulties of the aged. (55 ref).

25. Hammond, E. Cuyler & Selikoff, Irving J. (Eds). (1979). **Public control of environmental health hazards.** *Annals of the New York Academy of Sciences,* 329, 405 p.
Presents the proceedings of a conference held in 1979 covering such topics as environmental hazards and birth defects, neurotoxic effects and distal axonpathy produced by chemical exposure, the validity of extrapolation of results of animal studies to man, and constraints in the rationalization of social response to environmental hazards.

26. Hartlage, Lawrence C. (1986). **The future of behavioral neuropsychology.** *Behavior Therapist,* 9(6), 115–116.

BEHAVIORAL TOXICOLOGY: GENERAL

Discusses the background and emergence of behavioral neuropsychology and 2 trends likely to become more apparent in the future: (1) an increasing focus on behavior as it relates to neurological function and (2) the identification of substances commonly found in the environment that may have potential neurotoxic and neurobehavioral effects.

27. Hartman, David E. (1987). **Neuropsychological toxicology: Identification and assessment of neurotoxic syndromes.** *Archives of Clinical Neuropsychology,* 2(1), 45–65.
Discusses neuropsychological toxicology, which is the study of how naturally or industrially produced nervous system poisons effect neuropsychological functioning. Neuropsychological aftereffects of several representative human neurotoxins are reviewed, including metallic lead, the solvent toluene, organophosphate pesticides, and antihypertensive medication. These substances are exemplars from some of the major classes of potentially neurotoxic substances. Testing procedures sensitive to neurotoxic exposure are also summarized. It is suggested that the neuropsychologist is in a unique position to perform research and clinical evaluations relating to neurotoxic exposure. Neurotoxic effects may be subject to misdiagnosis without knowledge of how to examine for these substances.

28. Ison, James R. (1984). **Reflex modification as an objective test for sensory processing following toxicant exposure.** United States Environmental Protection Agency, Neurotoxicology Division, and the Johns Hopkins University Neurotoxicology Program Conference: Cross species extrapolation in neurotoxicology (1984, Raleigh, North Carolina). *Neurobehavioral Toxicology & Teratology,* 6(6), 437–445.
Describes the development of a sensory test that can be used in animals and in humans and that depends on the phenomenon of reflex modification in which seemingly extraneous psychological events are shown to affect the expression of simple reflex behaviors. It is argued that test batteries for assessing psychological function following toxic exposure should evaluate sensory processes. Sensory function has intrinsic importance as an endpoint measure, and because performance in other behavioral tests typically requires that the organism can detect significant environmental events, its evaluation is necessary to the proper interpretation of other tests. Two parameters of reflex inhibition in several species are detailed, its sensitivity to near threshold stimuli is discussed, and the effects of sensory dysfunction on reflex inhibition are demonstrated. (39 ref).

29. Jewett, D. L.; Heard, G. S. & Chimento, T. C. (1985). **Peripheral neurotoxicity testing by pairs of stimuli.** Workshop on Neurotoxicity Testing in Human Populations (1983, Rougemont, North Carolina). *Neurobehavioral Toxicology & Teratology,* 7(4), 325–328.
Suggests that at the present time, the best electrophysiological test of peripheral nerve function for evaluating neurotoxicity in humans is the analysis of the response to pairs of stimuli. This test is a more sensitive measure of axonal conduction deficit than is the single-action potential of standard clinical technique. While not as sensitive a measure as a train of stimuli at any given frequency of stimulation, the paired stimulus technique has some advantages, including that the interpretation of responses to trains of impulses can be made inaccurate by alternate blocking. The rationale, method, and evaluation of the paired stimulus technique are discussed. (16 ref).

30. Keeney, Ralph L. (1977). **The art of assessing multiattribute utility functions.** *Organizational Behavior & Human Performance,* 19(2), 267–310.
Describes how to use multiattribute utility theory for developing preference models to address value trade-offs among multiple objectives and uncertainty in complex problems. An example, based on energy policy, is presented. Specifically, an 11-attribute utility function over attributes including deaths, pollution, radioactive waste, health effects, and electrical energy generated is assessed. A dialog indicating the procedure used, with comments on why various questions were asked, is presented in detail. The resulting utility function is being used to examine energy policies differing in terms of main fuel (fossil or nuclear) and degree of conservation.

31. Kimmel, Carole A. & Buelke-Sam, Judy. (1985). **Collaborative Behavioral Teratology Study: Background and overview.** Conference Proceedings of the National Center for Toxicological Research et al: Design considerations in screening for behavioral teratogens: Results of the collaborative behavioral teratology study (1985, Cincinnati, Ohio). *Neurobehavioral Toxicology & Teratology,* 7(6), 541–545.
Reviews the organization of the Collaborative Behavioral Teratology Study, which began in 1978 because of concern about potential postnatal dysfunction following developmental chemical exposure. The study design focuses on evaluation of reliability of behavioral testing methods, sensitivity of methods to alterations produced by prenatal chemical exposure, and effects of litter, sex of the animals, and prior testing experience on behavioral responses. The National Center for Toxicological Research served as the pilot testing laboratory, and 5 additional laboratories participated. (18 ref).

32. Kirk, N. S. (1981). **Poison Prevention Packaging Act, 1970: A human factors standard.** *Applied Ergonomics,* 12(4), 195–201.
Outlines US legislation and regulations requiring hazardous pharmaceutical and other household products to be packaged in child-resistant containers. Human factors test procedures and standards, in terms of which child-resistance is defined, are described. The effects of the regulations and of child-resistant containers in reducing mortality and morbidity associated with the ingestion of poisonous substances, particularly aspirin, are described. (10 ref).

33. Kleeman, Walter B. (1988). **The politics of office design.** Special Issue: Political behavior and physical design. *Environment & Behavior,* 20(5), 537–549.
Discusses issues of human discomfort and health hazards related to working in an office environment. Research is reviewed concerning musculoskeletal complaints, possible effects of exposure to radiation from visual display terminals (VDTs), stress symptoms (such as insomnia, irritability, anxiety, and fatigue) in workers using VDTs, vision problems among workers using VDTs, and worker cyberphobia (distrust of computers). Federal occupational safety and health guidelines are presented, and regulations being considered by unions and state legislatures are outlined.

34. Landrigan, Philip J. (1983). **Toxic exposures and psychiatric disease: Lessons from the epidemiology of cancer.** *Acta Psychiatrica Scandinavica,* 67(Suppl 303), 6–15.
Toxic chemicals such as lead, methyl mercury, organic solvents, manganese, kepone, and the organophosphates are known to cause psychiatric disease. Whether such associations are exceptional, or if in fact a high proportion of all psychiatric illnesses are of toxic environmental etiology, and therefore potentially avoidable, is not known. It is contended that the application of epidemiologic techniques to the study of psychiatric illnesses might yield etiologic clues in relation to toxic environmental exposures and may also suggest approaches to disease prevention. (39 ref).

35. Langdon, F. J. (1982). **Monetary evaluation and attitude scaling of environmental disamenity: A different approach or a different problem?** *International Review of Applied Psychology,* 31(2), 237–252.

Discusses the social cost of nuisances (e.g., noise, pollution) and the social benefits derived from eliminating them. Three methods of monetary evaluation are presented, and results obtained by each method are compared. It is concluded that a rating of nuisance derived from an attitude scale is likely to be more practical, even if it cannot be put directly into a cost–benefit equation, than a monetary evaluation that is the outcome of a wide range of circumstantial variations. (28 ref).

36. le Quesne, Pamela M. (1982). **Electrophysiological investigation of toxic neuropathies.** *Acta Neurologica Scandinavica,* 66(Suppl 92), 75–87.
Considers 2 uses of electrophysiological tests relative to toxic neuropathies: establishing a diagnosis in patients with peripheral neuropathy of unknown etiology and determining whether neurotoxic lesions have developed in Ss exposed to potentially neurotoxic substances. For diagnosis, the pattern of electrophysiological abnormality may provide a clue to the cause (e.g., motor or sensory involvement) or degree of peripheral nerve conduction velocity change in relation to clinical severity and duration of disease. (39 ref).

37. Lindström, Kari. (1981). **Käyttäytymistoksikologia: kehittyvä tutkimusalue. / Behavioral toxicology: A developing subject of study.** *Psykologia,* 16(5), 308–312.
Points out that the international psychological study of the damaging effects of industrial chemicals is rather young, but that in Finland, the long-term effects of chemicals have been studied since the beginning of the 1960's. Psychologists at the Institute of Occupational Health are working together with other Nordic psychologists in the field of occupational health, with the National Institute of Occupational Safety and Health in the US, and with corresponding institutes in various Socialist countries. (English abstract).

38. Lindström, Kari. (1977). **Psychological effects of occupational exposure to various chemical agents.** *International Journal of Psychology,* 12(2), 93–97.
Research on the psychological effects of occupational exposure to various chemical agents began at the Institute of Occupational Health in Helsinki in the last half of the 1950's. At first workers occupationally exposed to carbon disulfide in a rayon fiber factory were clinically examined and were submitted to psychological testing because they complained of numerous subjective psychological symptoms. Since then the behavioral effects of occupational exposure to various common solvents and lead have been studied with psychological methods. The earlier projects were either clinical or epidemiologic studies, but now experimental studies with animals have also begun. In all these investigations one of the main objectives has been to develop and find methods sensitive and specific enough to detect adverse behavioral effects. (French summary).

39. Lowensohn, Brent A. (1977). **An investigation of the relation between atmospheric quality and crime rates in the Greater Los Angeles area.** *Dissertation Abstracts International,* 38(5-B), 2432.

40. Madnawat, A. V. & Sinha, S. N. (1987). **Environmental insults and exposure-response relationships: Behavioural assessment.** *Journal of Personality & Clinical Studies,* 3(2), 153–155.
Maintains that effects of human exposure to toxic substances can now be sensitively measured by the assessment of their behavioral effects. Epidemiological pursuits of behavioral symptomatology may prove effective in building a database on representative exposures in the human population.

41. Maurissen, Jacques P. (1985). **Psychophysical testing in human populations exposed to neurotoxicants.** Workshop on Neurotoxicity Testing in Human Populations (1983, Rougemont, North Carolina). *Neurobehavioral Toxicology & Teratology,* 7(4), 309–317.
In a discussion of the psychophysical and electrophysiological approaches to studying human sensory organs, the author notes that even though close parallels have been drawn between these 2 methodologies, discrepancies indicate that they do not measure the same phenomenon. Vibration sensitivity is used to illustrate the role sensory assessment plays in neurotoxicology. Several psychophysical techniques to measure this sensory modality are described. The validity of vibration sensitivity as an indicator of sensory peripheral nerve dysfunction is established through a review of diseases, physical agents, pharmaceuticals, and other neurotoxicants known to alter the morphology and/or the physiology of the peripheral nervous system or sense organs. Factors or conditions affecting vibration detection thresholds, such as age, laterality, gender, and temperature, are also examined. (215 ref).

42. Mayron, Lewis W. (1978). **Ecological factors in learning disabilities.** *Journal of Learning Disabilities,* 11(8), 495–505.
Explored environmental causes of learning and behavior problems, as contrasted with genetic or congenital causes, to alert the learning disabilities (LD) professional to those conditions for which remedial measures may be taken. These environmental causes fall into 5 general categories: chronic anxiety, malnutrition (including vitamin and protein, zinc, magnesium, and calcium deficiencies), toxicity, allergy, and electromagnetic radiation or technical pollution. It is suggested that although remediation procedures will be different for each individual ecologic cause, recognition by the LD professional of ecologic-effected conditions will allow for recommendation and initiation of diagnostic procedures, which in turn could remediate the specific condition. (103 ref).

43. McCunney, Robert J. (1987). **The role of building construction and ventilation in indoor air pollution: Review of a recurring problem.** *New York State Journal of Medicine,* 87(4), 203–209.
Reviews the common types of health effects that can occur from indoor air pollutants in both home and office environments, considers the sources of such contaminants, and the control of these pollutants. Types of building-related health effects discussed are hypersensitivity pneumonitis, infections, humidifier fever, nonspecific reactions, and epidemic psychogenic illness (EPI) also known as mass hysteria. It is suggested that EPI usually occurs in a group of people under some type of physical or emotional stress, with concern usually focusing on an apparent toxic agent. Sources of indoor pollutants that are the major areas of concern include radon; formaldehyde; asbestos; tobacco; indoor combustion; and miscellaneous chemicals found in pesticides, floor cleaners, and detergents. It is concluded that the ideal approach to preventing the adverse effects of indoor pollution is through proper ventilation and preventive maintenance of air handling systems.

44. Otto, David A. & Eckerman, David A. (1985). **Neurotoxicity testing in human populations: Workshop overview.** Workshop on Neurotoxicity Testing in Human Populations (1983, Rougemont, North Carolina). *Neurobehavioral Toxicology & Teratology,* 7(4), 283–285.
Reviews strategies and methods for neurotoxicity testing in human populations. The workshop discussed behavioral and electrophysiological testing methods, with a focus on computerized test batteries. Brief reviews of test methods organized in terms of sensory, motor, and cognitive function were presented, and available test batteries were demonstrated. Chemical exposure scenarios were also presented for group problem solving. The proceedings include critical reviews and technical descriptions of test batteries. (12 ref).

BEHAVIORAL TOXICOLOGY: GENERAL

45. Perry, Ronald W.; Gillespie, David F. & Parker, Howard A. (1976). **Configurations in the analysis of attitudes, importance and social behavior.** *Sociology & Social Research,* 60(2), 135-146.
Reviews the literature on the relationship between overt behavior and verbal attitudes, with an emphasis on synthesis of apparently contradictory findings. The product is a middle-range theory which links attitudes and behavior as mediated by the importance of the attitude object. Evidence is supplied by a secondary analysis of survey data dealing with attitudes and action toward air pollution. It was found that verbal attitudes predict behavior more accurately when attitude object importance is high. When importance is low, the correspondence between attitude and action was more tentative. (26 ref).

46. Proshansky, Harold M. (1973). **The environmental crisis in human dignity.** *Journal of Social Issues,* 29(4), 1-20.
Considers that the environmental crisis in human dignity lies not only in the overuse, misuse, and decay of physical settings, but also in how we conceive of the individual in relation to any such setting. The influences of socioenvironmental values (e.g., scientific-technological progress, urbanism, pseudoprogress-novelty and change) are discussed, and it is concluded that as behavioral scientists pursue systematic studies of human–environment problems, they recognize the need to maintain the contextual reality of these problems as they evolve, develop, and become modified in the time framework of a complex society.

47. Proshansky, Harold M. (1983). **The environmental crisis in human dignity.** *Journal of Social Issues,* 39(4), 207–224. (*The following abstract of the original article appeared in* PA, Vol 52:7477.) Considers that the environmental crisis in human dignity lies not only in the overuse, misuse, and decay of physical settings, but also in how the individual is conceived of in relation to any such setting. The influences of socioenvironmental values (e.g., scientific-technological progress, urbanism, pseudoprogress-novelty, and change) are discussed, and it is concluded that as behavioral scientists pursue systematic studies of human–environment problems, they recognize the need to maintain the contextual reality of these problems as they evolve, develop, and become modified in the time framework of a complex society. (7 ref).

48. Pym, Denis. (1975). **The demise of management and the ritual of employment.** *Human Relations,* 28(8), 675-698.
Discusses the links between the condition of employment and the issues of alienation, the overconsumption of scarce resources, and pollution. A return to the pursuit of emancipation as a primary concern in reexamining the relationship between man, work, and employment is recommended.

49. Rabideau, Gerald F. (1974). **Human, machine, and environment aspects of snowmobile design and utilization.** *Human Factors,* 16(5), 481-494.
Describes and analyzes the major problems—damage and injury-producing accidents, noise pollution, damage to private property, and detrimental effects on natural ecology—associated with the sport of snowmobiling. Examples are given that typify the current state-of-the-art investigations of the problem areas.

50. Rakow, Steven J.; Glenn, Allen D. & Fifer, William E. (1983). **Acid rain: Board game to computer simulation.** *Simulation & Games,* 14(1), 29–46.
Describes the development of a computer simulation designed to help upper elementary students explore some of the basic relationships involved in the problem of acid rain. Several issues involved in making a simulation game an effective learning experience are discussed, such as making it a valid model of the real world so as to be comprehensive to the player, ensuring reliability and predictability of outcomes, and creating utility, so that benefits are worth the cost of time and energy expended. (2 ref).

51. Russell, Roger W. (1981). **Behavior toxicology: Development of a science and a profession.** *Academic Psychology Bulletin,* 3(2), 177–189.
In viewing behavioral toxicology within the perspective of the 1980's, the author discusses basic concepts underlying the discipline, examines roles for behavioral toxicologists, and suggests programs for their education and training. (27 ref).

52. Russell, Roger W. & Singer, George. (1982). **Behavioural toxicology: The emergence of a new discipline in Australian psychology?** *Australian Psychologist,* 17(2), 199–215.
Outlines the basic concepts of behavioral toxicology and suggests roles that behavioral toxicologists can play in the environmental management of Australia's problems. Environmental management always involves trade-offs between biological limitations on the one hand and social cost–benefits on the other. Knowledge about the capability of human and other living organisms to cope behaviorally with potentially toxic conditions of their physical environments can add essential information useful to decision makers and legislators concerned with such matters. It is contended that, in terms of public concern and sophistication in the study of interactions between chemical compounds in the physical environment and behavior, the time is right for the emergence of a new discipline within psychology. (19 ref).

53. Sanes, Jerome N.; Colburn, Theodore R. & Morgan, Newlin T. (1985). **Behavioral motor evaluation for neurotoxicity screening.** Workshop on Neurotoxicity Testing in Human Populations (1983, Rougemont, North Carolina). *Neurobehavioral Toxicology & Teratology,* 7(4), 329–337.
Previous test batteries concerned with behavioral motor function have focused on simple measures of motor performance such as tapping rate, movement times, and reaction times (RTs). These measures, although valuable in certain instances, do not provide a comprehensive description of motor disorders. The present authors describe an alternate approach to evaluating behavioral motor deficits in which simple behaviors are used as initial guides for the study of coordinated movements in more natural and thus more complex situations. The advantages of such an approach may be insights into the central neural correlates of motor disorders caused by toxic agents. Potential limitations of and new approaches to motor psychophysical evaluations are discussed. (27 ref).

54. Schaumburg, Herbert H.; Arezzo, Joseph C.; Otto, David A. & Eckerman, David A. (1985). **Neurotoxic chemical exposure scenarios and suggested solutions.** Workshop on Neurotoxicity Testing in Human Populations (1983, Rougemont, North Carolina). *Neurobehavioral Toxicology & Teratology,* 7(4), 351–353.
Presents 4 exposure scenarios, and their recommended solutions, that represent real-world situations previously encountered by neurologists and epidemiologists. The scenarios involve (1) leaking chemicals from a chemical dump affecting the townspeople; (2) a manufacturing company's dumping of metallic mercury into the ground and creek, possibly contaminating hundreds of the company's workers over a 10-yr period; (3) the contamination of a town's water supply by a pesticide factory's handling of its waste; and (4) the contamination of a small mining community's well water by arsenic and manganese, probably leaked by an adjacent copper mine.

55. Shepherd, Michael. (1974). **Pollution and mental health, with particular reference to the problem of noise.** *Psychiatria Clinica,* 7(4-5), 226-236.

Argues that although the adverse psychological effects of noise as an environmental pollutant are well recognized, much of the relevant work has been focused on the ambiguous concept of "annoyance." A review of the evidence suggests that the relationship between noise and mental illness calls for more direct investigation. In particular, the marked individual variation in reactions to noise requires elucidation. (29 ref).

56. Singh, Jaya; Kumar, P.; Dwivedi, Kamal & Saxena, Vinod B. (1986). **Behavioural toxicology: A developing field in industrial hygiene and occupational health research.** *Journal of Personality & Clinical Studies,* 2(2), 109–116.
Reviews methodologies used in research on the effects of neurotoxic agents on occupationally related behavioral dysfunctions in India. Neurotoxic agents involved in research and their effects and existing and suggested tests of intelligence, memory, and psychomotor abilities are tabulated and discussed. Guidelines for the selection of instruments are outlined; these guidelines address the need to measure functions affected by numerous agents, the use of proven methods with a minimum of error variance, cost-benefit issues, cultural and educational background of Ss, and the motivation of Ss to perform well on tests. Testing issues should be familiar to psychologists, pollution scientists, toxicologists, and government agencies.

57. Slangen, J. L.; Orlebeke, J. F. & Hooisma, J. (1986). **Gedragstoxicologie: Een nieuw veld van toegepaste psychologie. / Behavioral toxicology: A new field of applied psychology.** *Nederlands Tijdschrift voor de Psychologie en haar Grensgebieden,* 41(3), 105–113.
Discusses research on the effects of industrial pollution on psychological processes. Methodologic and practical problems of developing sensitive instruments for the early detection of the harmful effects of (new) chemicals on human and animal behavior are considered. Epidemiologic strategies for assessing neurotoxicity at work sites, widespread pathology, and children's cadmium and lead exposure are outlined. (English abstract).

58. Smirnov, V. K. & Gnelitsky, G. I. (1982). **Psychic disturbances in occupational disease caused by antibiotics (penicillin, streptomycin).** *Zhurnal Nevropatologii i Psikhiatrii,* 82(2), 245–248.
Discusses how occupational diseases caused by antibiotics may be accompanied by polymorphic psychological disturbances that are manifested primarily in the forms of the asthenic, depressive, hallucinatory, and epileptiform syndromes. With the progress of the psychoorganic syndrome in antibiotic-caused diseases, these disturbances become more marked. (English abstract) (10 ref).

59. Smith, Philip J. (1985). **Behavioral toxicology: Evaluating cognitive functions.** Workshop on Neurotoxicity Testing in Human Populations (1983, Rougemont, North Carolina). *Neurobehavioral Toxicology & Teratology,* 7(4), 345–350.
Many substances are known to have effects on cognitive functions such as memory, attention, and perception. Some of the issues that must be addressed when trying to assess these neurotoxic effects on cognition are reviewed, and paradigms that have been explored for use in behavioral toxicology are identified. Some of the issues concerning the assessment of neurotoxic effects on cognition are whether the cognitive tests can detect subtle and subclinical neurotoxic effects and what cognitive function is tested by a particular stage-specific measure such as memory scanning time. Measures are described that are sensitive to language dysfunctions, memory deficits, perceptual disorders, and decrements in attention and vigilance. (38 ref).

60. Steinberg, Marshall. (1987). **The use of traditional toxicologic data in assessing neurobehavioral dysfunction.** Symposium on Predicting Neurotoxicity and Behavioral Dysfunction from Preclinical Toxicologic Data (1985, Bethesda, Maryland). *Neurotoxicology & Teratology,* 9(6), 403–409.
Describes the neurotoxicologic and behavioral information available from traditional toxicologic screens, the collection of study data, the effect of model selection, and the environmental considerations that may affect study outcome. Laboratory observations of factors such as consummatory behavior and motor activity are considered in relation to the evaluation of toxicity. Regulatory guidelines are also discussed.

61. Tilson, Hugh A. (1987). **Behavioral indices of neurotoxicity: What can be measured?** Symposium on Predicting Neurotoxicity and Behavioral Dysfunction from Preclinical Toxicologic Data (1985, Bethesda, Maryland). *Neurotoxicology & Teratology,* 9(6), 427–443.
Examples of neurobehavioral tests used to evaluate the effects of chemicals for toxicity include those that evaluate motor function (e.g., spontaneous motor activity, coordination, weakness, abnormal posture), sensory processes (e.g., reflex modification, instrumental conditioning), learning/memory (nonassociative and associative), instrumental performance (schedules of reinforcement), and naturally occurring responses (consummatory behaviors). Behavioral procedures have also been utilized to study mechanisms of action and to screen for functional dysfunction following exposure during development. Considerations in the use and interpretation of data obtained from behavioral tests are discussed.

62. Valciukas, José A. (1985). **The role of the psychologist in occupational neurotoxicology: Apropos of Huszczo et al.'s "Psychology and organized labor."** *American Psychologist,* 40(9), 1053–1054.
Comments that the views of G. E. Huszczo et al (1984) about labor's needs for psychological services and research are narrow. It is suggested that in occupational neurotoxicology (e.g., of lead, mercury, solvents), close cooperation between psychologists and organized labor can be useful and productive. It is suggested that a reading beyond American Psychological Association journals will reveal many instances of cooperation and contributions between psychologists and organized labor. (11 ref).

63. Vorhees, Charles V. (1987). **Reliability, sensitivity and validity of behavioral indices of neurotoxicity.** Symposium on Predicting Neurotoxicity and Behavioral Dysfunction from Preclinical Toxicologic Data (1985, Bethesda, Maryland). *Neurotoxicology & Teratology,* 9(6), 445–464.
Discusses the validity of measurements in behavioral testing, neuropathologic evaluations, neurochemical tests, and electrophysiological techniques for detecting neurotoxicity. Emphasis is placed on developmental neurobehavioral toxicity, and tests of the effects of compounds such as amphetamine and methylmercury on rats' behavior in procedures including operant conditioning, the water maze, and acoustic startle testing are described.

64. Wasyliw, Orest E. & Golden, Charles J. (1985). **Neuropsychological evaluation in the assessment of personal injury.** *Behavioral Sciences & the Law,* 3(2), 149–164.
Discusses strengths and limitations of neuropsychological testing for personal injury claims, with special attention to applications in the forensic areas of head injury, toxic environments, physical disease, and malpractice. The varieties of cognitive, emotional, and interpersonal damages that may occur with brain injury are described. Issues of neurological malingering, credentialing of the expert, and forensic roles of the neuropsychologist in rehabilitation are discussed. (74 ref).

BEHAVIORAL TOXICOLOGY: GENERAL

65. Weigel, Russell H.; Woolston, Vernon L. & Gendelman, David S. (1977). **Psychological studies of pollution control: An annotated bibliography.** *Catalog of Selected Documents in Psychology,* 7, 71. MS. 1522 (44 pp/paper: $6; fiche: $2).

66. Weiss, Bernard. (1985). **Intersections of psychiatry and toxicology.** *International Journal of Mental Health,* 14(3), 7–25.
Describes the behavioral effects of 3 classes of toxic agents—metals, insecticides, and food additives. The effects of mercury, lead, organic lead compounds, organic tin compounds, and vanadium and the insecticides triorthocresylphosphate, leptophos, and chlordecone are discussed, as is evidence for B. F. Feingold's (1975) hypothesis that some children labeled hyperactive or hyperkinetic were actually displaying a form of behavioral toxicity induced by certain food constituents, notably synthetic colors and flavors. It is concluded that practicing psychiatrists should not ignore toxic chemical etiologies and that vague subjective complaints, unpredictable irritability in children, and other disorders cannot always be ascribed to difficult marriages, deficient self-esteem, inadequate parenting, or other social or behavioral factors. (32 ref).

67. Weiss, Bernard. (1983). **Behavioral toxicology and environmental health science: Opportunity and challenge for psychology.** *American Psychologist,* 38(11), 1174–1187.
Describes the establishment of behavioral toxicology as a component of the environmental health sciences. Behavioral measures are viewed as fulfilling unique roles because (1) many substances act primarily on the nervous system; (2) many poisonings, before they bloom into overt clinical signs, may be heralded by vague, subjective, nonspecific psychological complaints; and (3) there are substances whose actions, although not mediated directly through nervous system mechanisms, produce distinct behavioral reactions. Behavioral toxicology extends across the total spectrum of environmental chemicals, including heavy metals, solvents, fuels, pesticides, air pollutants, and even food additives. Examples are presented of the role psychology can play in resolving critical issues in environmental health science. (76 ref).

Human Research

68. Abueg, Francis R. (1988). **Judgments of risk, behavioral, and emotional sequelae to a toxic chemical contamination: A controlled study of Binghamton State Office Building evacuees and controls.** *Dissertation Abstracts International,* 48(9-B), 2773.

69. Anger, W. Kent. (1985). **Neurobehavioral tests used in NIOSH-supported worksite studies, 1973–1983.** Workshop on Neurotoxicity Testing in Human Populations (1983, Rougemont, North Carolina). *Neurobehavioral Toxicology & Teratology,* 7(4), 359–368.
Reviews the objectives, testing methods, findings, and conclusions of 11 studies published by the National Institute for Occupational Safety and Health (NIOSH) on the neurobehavioral effects of chronic exposure to industrial chemicals among working groups. The studies used a single rationale for selecting tests—tests sensitive to the types of effects reported for the chemical under study were utilized in each case. As a result, different sets of tests were used for different studies. This strategy is distinct from the approach suggested in the other reports that advocate the use of uniform test battery. The wide variety of neurobehavioral effects produced by chemicals found in the environment argues for a rationale of tailoring test selection in many situations. (34 ref).

70. Ansari, Khurshed A. (1986). **Olfactory mucosa, aluminosilicates and Alzheimer's disease.** Special Issue: Controversial topics on Alzheimer's disease: Intersecting crossroads. *Neurobiology of Aging,* 7(6), 575–576.
Comments on the hypothesis by E. Roberts (1986) by noting that age-related degenerative changes in mucosal epithelium may result in decreased barrier function. This change may predispose the adjacent brain areas to invasion by organisms and toxins leading to regional tissue damage as seen in Alzheimer's disease (AD). Age-related decrease in nasal mucosal barrier function, however, would explain some but not all the pathologic changes associated with AD.

71. Árochová, Ol'ga; Kontrová, Jana; Lipková, Valéria & Liška, Jozef. (1988). **Effect of toxic atmosphere emissions on cognitive performance by children.** *Studia Psychologica,* 30(2), 101–114.
96 Czech children (aged 7–8.5 yrs) living in a heavily polluted area were compared with 104 age-matched children living in an unpolluted area on sensory-perceptual and cognitive abilities. Ss' teachers were also interviewed regarding Ss' personality traits, socioeconomic status (SES), and social behavior. Ss' hair was examined for metal residue, including lead and arsenic. Data indicate deficits in hand-eye coordination and memory in heavily pollutant-exposed Ss. (Slovak & Russian abstracts).

72. Avery, Carol E. (1982). **Consumer response to the Tris controversy: A research study.** *Accident Analysis & Prevention,* 14(6), 465–473.
Studied possible long-term effects of the controversy over the flame retardant (FR) finish, Tris, now identified as a potential carcinogen. 269 parents of young children were surveyed. 85% had heard about problems with FR chemicals, 68% remembered that Tris was considered to be a carcinogen, and only 20% reported appropriate changes in their purchasing behavior. Absence of health risk was the primary consideration used in the purchase of children's sleepwear. (15 ref).

73. Baird, Brian N. (1986). **Tolerance for environmental health risks: The influence of knowledge, benefits, voluntariness, and environmental attitudes.** *Risk Analysis,* 6(4), 425–435.
Examined factors affecting risk estimates and tolerance among persons directly exposed to environmental health risks. Data were gathered from questionnaires distributed at public hearings regarding proposed air-pollution standards for an arsenic-emitting copper smelter in Tacoma, Washington. Approximately 80% of the area residents who attended the hearings completed the questionnaires, and the responses of 347 Ss were analyzed. Results indicate that informal risk estimates and risk tolerance were closely associated with judged benefits of the hazard source, acceptance or denial of vulnerability, judgments of exposure voluntariness, and environmental attitudes. Neither factual knowledge of formal risk estimates and proposed standards nor residential distance from the smelter was closely related to risk tolerance or informal risk estimates. Implications are discussed in relation to reactions to risk and risk management policy and practice.

74. Baird, Brian N. (1985). **Estimation and tolerance of an environmental health risk: The influence of risk characteristics, informal judgments, environmental attitudes, and factual knowledge.** *Dissertation Abstracts International,* 45(8-B), 2731.

75. Baker, Edward L. et al. (1985). **A computer-based neurobehavioral evaluation system for occupational and environmental epidemiology: Methodology and validation studies.** Workshop on Neurotoxicity Testing in Human Populations (1983, Rougemont, North Carolina). *Neurobehavioral Toxicology & Teratology,* 7(4), 369–377.

To facilitate the evaluation of populations at risk for nervous-system dysfunction due to environmental agents, the present authors developed a computer-administered neurobehavioral evaluation system. The system includes a set of testing programs, designed to run on a microcomputer, and questionnaires that are used to record symptoms, obtain exposure history, and characterize potential confounding variables. Standard tasks evaluating memory, visual-motor function, vocabulary ability, and mood were selected and adapted for computer presentation. Validation, comparability, and stability studies with 87 20–69 yr old blue-collar workers and university staff and faculty suggested that this approach is a feasible, efficient, acceptable, and sensitive approach to evaluating central nervous system (CNS) function in humans. (33 ref).

76. Baker, H. & Margolis, F. L. (1986). **Deafferentation-induced alterations in olfactory bulb as a model for the etiology of Alzheimers disease.** Special Issue: Controversial topics on Alzheimer's disease: Intersecting crossroads. *Neurobiology of Aging,* 7(6), 568–569.
In response to E. Roberts's (1986) hypothesis, the present author notes that the ability of exogenous agents to enter the brain by way of the olfactory nerve coupled with the early anatomical and behavioral pathology observed in patients has led to the hypothesis that Alzheimer's disease may be of environmental etiology. Studies of the influence of peripheral olfactory deafferentation on the expression of olfactory bulb neuron phenotype suggest that this approach may be a useful model in which to explore the validity of the hypothesis.

77. Bancroft, John et al. (1977). **People who deliberately poison or injure themselves: Their problems and their contacts with helping agencies.** *Psychological Medicine,* 7(2), 289–303.
Interviewed 130 people shortly following self-poisoning or self-injury. Events in the week prior to the attempt and the incidence of various kinds of chronic problems are reported. Events involving key relationships were more common than other kinds. The most important event was a quarrel, particularly in the 48 hrs prior to the attempts and more commonly with female than with male attempters. The possible relevance of quarrels to understanding overdose behavior is discussed. Nearly one-third were receiving nonpsychiatric treatment at the time of the "attempt." Approximately one-quarter were currently receiving psychiatric treatment, and half had received it at some time. A substantial proportion had been admitted to either psychiatric or nonpsychiatric hospitals within the past year. The proportions indicating the need for various kinds of help are reported. Most Ss said they needed "someone to talk to." More than half had been in contact with some form of helping agency during the week prior to the attempt. An attempt was made to look for "syndromes" or groupings of problems. The resulting analysis did not lead to a satisfactory method for classifying individuals. It is concluded that a more satisfactory typology of "attempters" is likely if types of relationship problems are investigated in more detail. (24 ref).

78. Bankovska, R. & Minkova, N. (1985). **Psychophysiological study of tobacco industry workers in dependence on their length of service.** *Psikhologiia (Bulgaria),* 13(2), 33–38.
Studied functional changes in the cardiovascular and nervous systems of 20 female tobacco-industry workers who had been employed for periods ranging from less than 3 yrs to more than 10 yrs. Length of employment was not found to have any effect on the functional state of either system. (English abstract).

79. Barker, M. L. (1974). **Information and complexity: The conceptualization of air pollution by specialist groups.** *Environment & Behavior,* 6(3), 347–377.
Examines how specialists in 5 different professions and disciplines select and organize information about air pollution, and describes the structure and content of their conceptualizations. (26 ref).

80. Bell, Paul A.; Hummel, Carl F. & Fusco, Marc E. (1985). **Effects of high ambient temperature on judgments of air quality.** *Perceptual & Motor Skills,* 60(2), 664.
When 31 male and 33 female undergraduates viewed 40 slides depicting levels of air pollution in urban landscapes in either a cool (73°) or hot (95°) room, temperature effects were found for only 5 slides, suggesting that air quality judgments are independent of ambient temperature. (1 ref).

81. Bergamasco, B. et al. (1976). **Behaviour of CNV during exposure to urban traffic noise.** *Acta Oto-Laryngologica,* 339, 27-29.
Investigated whether road noise modifies cortical responsiveness to psychological and sensory stimuli. 12 21-33 yr old Ss were exposed to flash and click stimuli, and EEG data were gathered to measure the contingent negative variation. No significant effects of road noise were observed on contingent negative variation amplitude or duration. Findings suggest that the effects of environmental noise on psychoattentive functions vary from individual to individual.

82. Bergamasco, B.; Benna, P. & Gilli, M. (1976). **Human sleep modifications induced by urban traffic noise.** *Acta Oto-Laryngologica,* 339, 33-36.
Assessed the effect of up to 90 min of traffic noise on sleep in 5 normal 23–52 yr old Ss. EEG, EKG, and EOG data were obtained. Findings show that noise had marked effects on CNS activity during presleep and actual sleep periods, particularly in the area of sleep regularity. Stage IV sleep was markedly decreased in all Ss; the durations of Stage 2 and REM sleep were essentially the same as in nonnoise conditions, and the duration of Stage 3 was only slightly increased.

83. Bergamasco, B.; Benna, P.; Covacich, A. M. & Gilli, M. (1976). **EEG changes induced by exposure to urban traffic noise and white noise.** *Acta Oto-Laryngologica,* 339, 30-32.
Examined the pattern of EEG activity evoked by road noise (RN) and white noise (WN) in 10 19–33 yr old Ss. A virtual absence of EEG desynchronization produced by both RN and WN in 9 of the 10 Ss was observed, although the desynchronization produced by WN was always much less than that produced by RN, in spite of the former's greater intensity. Administration of the Rorschach and a mental arithmetic task revealed a relationship between basic personality characteristics and noise-induced EEG desynchronization and a possible "tranquilizing" role of RN in Ss with high anxiety levels such that a mental task causes less desynchronization.

84. Bergamasco, B.; Benna, P.; Furlan, P. & Gilli, M. (1976). **Effects of urban traffic noise in relation to basic personality.** *Acta Oto-Laryngologica,* 339, 37-38.
Administered the Rorschach Test to 12 Ss under both road noise and quiet conditions. EEG and Rorschach data indicate the importance of basic personality characteristics in how an individual adjusts to the presence of environmental noise.

85. Bergamasco, B.; Gilli, M. & Rossi, Giovanni. (1976). **Changes in cortical responsivity to multisensorial stimuli during exposure to urban traffic noise.** *Acta Oto-Laryngologica,* 339, 24-26.
Conducted a preliminary study on the effects of traffic noise on cortical responsivity (EEG) to acoustic and visual stimuli. Findings from 20 normal 18-35 yr old Ss exposed to a 10-min road noise tape recording show a striking decrease in evoked auditory potentials but no change in evoked visual potentials.

86. Berglund, Birgitta; Berglund, Ulf; Goldstein, Mikael & Lindvall, Thomas. (1979). **Loudness (or annoyance) summation of combined community noises.** *Reports from the Department of Psychology, U. Stockholm,* 550, 10 p.

BEHAVIORAL TOXICOLOGY: GENERAL

Studied how the loudness (or annoyance) of the constituents in pairs of community noises combined into total loudness (or total annoyance). Three community noises (pile driving, jack hammering, and street traffic) were combined pairwise at different sound levels. Observers (30 undergraduates) judged the total loudness of the combined noises as well as the loudness of each component noise when heard alone. Three models of loudness (or annoyance) summation for noise were tested: a vector summation model, a model assuming that the loudness of the masked constituent noises added arithmetically, and a simple model stating that the total loudness equaled the loudest of the component noises when heard alone. All 3 fitted the data satisfactorily from a statistical point of view. The "loudest component" model was favored because it produced a prediction error of only 14% in the "worst case" and thus could serve as a "rule of thumb" for many practical purposes. (15 ref).

87. Berglund, Birgitta; Berglund, Ulf & Lindvall, Thomas. (1975). **On perceptual interaction of noise and odor.** *Reports from the Department of Psychology, U. Stockholm,* 445, 10 p.
Investigated the possibility of sensory interaction among 7 community noises (e.g., roadway traffic, typewriting, and jet overflight) and a common odorous air pollutant. The loudness of the noises and the perceived odor intensity of the odorant were scaled by a direct scaling method. Eight college students participated. The perceived odor strength of hydrogen sulfide was not influenced by the simultaneous presentation of the noises, and neither was the loudness of the noises influenced by the odorant. Results show that sensory interactions between noise and odor lack practical importance. (12 ref).

88. Berglund, Birgitta; Berglund, Ulf & Engen, Trygg. (1983). **Do "sick buildings" affect human performance? How should one assess them?** *Reports from the Department of Psychology, U. Stockholm,* 609, 13 p.
Describes the "sick building syndrome," which results from contaminated air, and presents findings from an experiment that compared a diagnosed sick with a clean Swedish preschool. 48 previously unexposed 17-46 yr old Ss were exposed to each of the buildings for 2 days; the effect of the exposure was assessed with a battery of physical and psychological measures (e.g., RT, tiredness, short-term memory, vigilance, steadiness). Results show that Ss failed to perceive the 2 indoor environments differently in terms of 14 physical comfort factors (e.g., headaches, eye irritation) and in terms of psychological factors. Findings suggest that only certain people are affected by the sick building syndrome or that the syndrome is the result of an interaction between indoor pollution and certain susceptible individuals. (35 ref).

89. Berglund, Mats; Nielsén, Sören & Risberg, Jarl. (1977). **Regional cerebral blood flow in a case of bromide psychosis.** *Archiv für Psychiatrie und Nervenkrankheiten,* 223(3), 197-201.
Describes the case of a 58-yr-old female with bromide psychosis. A course of repeated measurements of the regional cerebral blood flow (rCBF) was followed, using the irradiated xenon inhalation method. At the first examination, when the serum bromide level was 45 mmol/l, the cerebral blood flow was reduced to about one-third of the normal. The regional flow pattern was also abnormal with low flows in frontal and parieto-occipital regions. Hemodialysis was performed with an overall improvement of the condition and a successive normalization of rCBF. The pronounced decrease of the cerebral blood flow, together with the positive effects of hemodialysis, seems to indicate that bromide psychosis is of a toxic origin and not an abstinence phenomenon. (German summary) (18 ref).

90. Biela, Adam. (1987). **Job stress in foresters employed in a heavily polluted area.** *Polish Psychological Bulletin,* 18(3), 169-175.
Investigated the hypothesis that for nature-related workers the very awareness of the degeneration of their job environment due to industrial pollution becomes a powerful stressing factor. Ss were foresters employed in 2 areas: one heavily and the other only marginally polluted by industry. The Ss were tested for their sense of awareness of the ecological crisis, their sense of alienation in their job and living environment, and their purpose in life. Results indicate that environment degeneration is a major stressing factor in foresters. Those employed in a heavily polluted area revealed a significantly higher sense of alienation and lower sense of purpose in life than did their more fortunate colleagues.

91. Biondi, Massimo. (1986). **Stress e cancro: Il modello di rischio trifattoriale. / Stress and cancer: The 3-factor risk model.** *Rivista di Psichiatria,* 21(4), 299-314.
Proposes a 3-factor risk model for the pathogenesis of human cancer: (1) oncogene risk, outlined in recent studies on cellular genetics of cancer; (2) carcinogen risk, demonstrated by epidemiologic studies; and (3) psychobiological risk, suggested by studies on personality, life events, experimental stress, and the brain-immunity relationship. (English abstract).

92. Bjerke, Tore. (1986). **Miljøgifter, evner og atferd. / Environmental toxins, abilities and behavior.** *Nordisk Psykologi,* 38(4), 273-286.
Discusses recent research on the psychological effects of low-level lead exposure on children. More attention should be paid to other heavy metals, metal-metal interactions, relations between essential trace elements and toxic metals, and better measures of socioeconomic variables. Replacement of the main-effect model with a transactional model is recommended. (English abstract).

93. Bluhm, Louis H. (1974). **Some pollution-related attitudes of high school youth in the United States and Brazil.** *Dissertation Abstracts International,* 34(12-A, Pt 1), 7882.

94. Braithwaite, V. A. & Law, H. G. (1977). **The structure of attitudes to doomsday issues.** *Australian Psychologist,* 12(2), 167-174.
Employed principal components analysis followed by a varimax rotation to investigate the structure of 24 belief statements representing responses to the threats posed by overpopulation, pollution, and nuclear weapons. These items were administered to 170 undergraduates together with the Wilson-Patterson C Scale which was included in the analysis as a marker variable. Little support was found for a general dimension of doomsday consciousness. Of particular interest was the way in which factors of concern and responsibility were orthogonal to factors of support for social action.

95. Branconnier, Roland J. (1985). **Dementia in human populations exposed to neurotoxic agents: A portable microcomputerized dementia screening battery.** Workshop on Neurotoxicity Testing in Human Populations (1983, Rougemont, North Carolina). *Neurobehavioral Toxicology & Teratology,* 7(4), 379-386.
Describes the development, by the present author and D. R. DeVitt (1983), of a microcomputer-based Psychometric Assessment System and Dementia Screening Battery (DSB) with high predictive value for differentiating the normal age-related changes in cognition from those associated with incipient dementia in the aged. The DSB is Diagnostic and Statistical Manual of Mental Disorders (DSM-III) compatible, as it evaluates intellectual deterioration, malignant memory loss, am-

nestic aphasia, and spatial disorientation. A diagnosis of dementia is obtained by findings of intellectual deterioration and malignant memory loss and either amnestic aphasia or spatial deterioration. (67 ref).

96. Brebner, J.; Rump, E. E. & Delin, P. (1976). **A cross-cultural replication of attitudes to the physical environment.** *International Journal of Psychology,* 11(2), 111-118.
Conducted a factor analytic study of attitudes toward the physical environment in Australia which replicated the 1969 study of US attitudes conducted by G. H. Winkel et al. A questionnaire on reactions to the environment was given to 303 South Australian adults, and 3 factors similar to those identified in the US were found. However, the method of factor identification used in the Australian study allowed clearer interpretation and specification of the dimensions, and 3 additional factors reflecting individual attitudes towards the environment were distinguished. (French summary).

97. Bryce-Smith, Derek. (1986). **Environmental chemical influences on behavior, personality, and mentation.** *International Journal of Biosocial Research,* 8(2), 115-150.
Discusses the "2 cultures" problem—the paradox that modern society is controlled by people educated in the humanities but illiterate in science. The present author discusses influences on behavior of involuntary exposure to environmental chemicals. Evidence is presented that nonsensory influences on mental function can and do affect the ways people think and act. It is proposed that neglect of this chemical dimension and its intimate interaction with social influences is at least partly responsible for the widespread failure to understand, remedy, or prevent some social problems of our times such as criminality, and psychiatric disorders such as anorexia nervosa.

98. Burr, Ralph G. & Hoiberg, Anne. (1986). **Health profile of U.S. Navy pilots of electronically modified aircraft.** *US Naval Health Research Center Report,* 85-46, 10 p.
Compared the health profiles of 1,063 pilots of electronically modified aircraft (EMA) with those of 2,126 age-matched controls. Hospitalization rates were significantly higher among controls than EMA Ss in the following diagnostic categories: (1) accidents, poisonings, and violence at ages 21–26 yrs; (2) mental disorders at ages 27–32 yrs; and (3) supplementary classifications at ages 39–44 yrs. Selection and retention standards for EMA pilots were effective in ensuring that healthy pilots were assigned to EMA. Findings also showed that piloting EMA did not pose a unique health risk from radiation effects.

99. Calne, D. B. et al. (1985). **Positron emission tomography after MPTP: Observations relating to the cause of Parkinson's disease.** *Nature,* 317(6034), 246–248.
Used positron emission tomography to determine whether there was destruction of dopamine neurons in 4 asymptomatic Ss exposed to 1-methy-4-phenyl-1,2,3,6-tetrahydropyridine (MPTP). A significant decline in the formation and retention of F-dopamine was found. Results suggest subclinical damage to the nigrostriatal pathway. Findings are discussed in the context of the hypothesis that Parkinson's disease may stem from clinically silent damage to the substantia nigra. (16 ref).

100. Chapko, Michael K. & Solomon, Henry. (1976). **Air pollution and recreational behavior.** *Journal of Social Psychology,* 100(1), 149-150.
Studied daily attendance at 3 recreational sites in New York City: the American Museum of Natural History (July-December, 1972; 1973), the New York Aquarium on Coney Island (1973), and the Central Park Children's Zoo (1972, 1973). Results show that air pollution did have a limited effect on recreational behavior in New York City. The relationship may be moderated by the levels of pollution, the type of recreational site, and the ability of individuals to adapt.

101. Cohen, Randye E. & Anderson, Diane L. (1986). **Botulism: Emotional impact on patient and family.** *Journal of Psychosomatic Research,* 30(3), 321–326.
During the 3rd largest outbreak of botulism reported in the US (October 1983), affective responses of patients and their family members were assessed to examine the emotional distress experienced by the 2 groups during the initial, acute phase of the illness. Ratings of 12 patients (aged 20–74 yrs) and 16 family members indicated that family members were significantly more fearful and depressed than patients during the 1st wk and as fearful and depressed as patients during the 2nd wk of hospitalization/treatment. Anxiety and helplessness decreased significantly in both groups by Week 2. Results illustrate the impact of catastrophic illness on the entire family system and provide support for the utility of family oriented crisis interventions.

102. Corwin, June; Serby, Michael & Rotrosen, John. (1986). **Olfactory deficits in AD: What we know about the nose.** Special Issue: Controversial topics on Alzheimer's disease: Intersecting crossroads. *Neurobiology of Aging,* 7(6), 580–582.
Notes that E. Roberts's (1986) zeolite hypothesis of Alzheimer's disease (AD) rests in part on evidence of olfactory deficits in this disorder. The present authors review this evidence and select evidence for deficits in related disorders and normal aging, stressing gaps in knowledge and problems in assessment. It is concluded that olfactory identification is most likely impaired in AD but that other olfactory functions are poorly characterized at present.

103. Crim, Karen O. (1980). **Using interpretive structural modeling in senior high school environmental studies.** *IEEE Transactions on Systems, Man, & Cybernetics,* 10(9), 581–585.
Results from a controlled experiment with the use of interpretive structural modeling (ISM) indicate that this method can be easily learned by teachers, who can then conduct modeling sessions in their classes. Tested in biology and social studies classes, ISM helped students gain a deeper insight into societal issues involving environmental pollution, energy, and urban affairs. (5 ref).

104. Cripe, Lloyd I. & Dodrill, Carl B. (1988). **Neuropsychological test performances with chronic low-level formaldehyde exposure.** *Clinical Neuropsychologist,* 2(1), 41–48.
13 adults with chronic low-level formaldehyde exposure in domestic environments were administered a comprehensive battery of neuropsychological tests after removal from the environments for several months. The formaldehyde exposure group was group-matched by sex, age, and education with 13 control and 13 mild head-injury Ss, and test results were compared using 1-way analysis of variance (ANOVA) and multivariate analysis of variance (MANOVA). Results indicate that the formaldehyde-exposed group was significantly different from the mild head-injury group and similar to the control group on the neuropsychological measures. Comparisons between the groups on the Minnesota Multiphasic Personality Inventory (MMPI) indicate emotional reactions and somatic concerns for both the formaldehyde and the head-injured groups. Findings suggest that once individuals were removed from a chronic formaldehyde exposure, their neuropsychological performances were within the normal range.

105. Cutter, Susan C. (1981). **Community concern for pollution: Social and environmental influences.** *Environment & Behavior,* 13(1), 105–124.
Determined how community attitudes toward pollution varied among social groups and with levels of pollution. Results from 22 communities in the Chicago area are contrary to the literature. It is suggested that concern about pollution is not

BEHAVIORAL TOXICOLOGY: GENERAL

only a characteristic of the suburban White middle class. High levels of concern were found among other segments of the populace—the minorities and the poor. It is concluded that actual measured levels of pollution do influence concern levels, but both social and environmental measures are necessary to predict community concern. (30 ref).

106. Edelstein, Michael R. (1986). **Toxic exposure and the inversion of the home.** *Journal of Architectural & Planning Research,* 3(3), 237–251.
Interviewed 25 families in an area that had been exposed to toxic chemicals that reached drinking water in the Legler section of Jackson, New Jersey, to determine the impacts on the concept of "home" of such a human-caused disaster. The naturalistic field study, conducted in 1981, used a sample stratified for age of adult members, length of residence, and location of home in relation to the source of contamination. Residential expectations for life in Legler are documented to provide a baseline. Results indicate that, following the disaster, affected residents' views of their homes went through a process of inversion whereby homes once thought of as places of security and identity became places of danger and defilement. The inversion persisted after a new water supply was developed. Implications for the design and planning professions are discussed.

107. Edelstein, Michael R. & Wandersman, Abraham. (1987). **Community dynamics in coping with toxic contaminants.** *Human Behavior & Environment: Advances in Theory & Research,* 9, 69–112.
Discusses how communities respond to toxic contamination and how grass roots organizations help cope with the stresses of living in a community affected by toxic pollution. Topics addressed include environmental turbulence; initial coping efforts; participation in community organizations; environmental, ecological, and social characteristics of the community; individual differences in participation; the effects of participation; the characteristics of community organization; proactive attempts to combat potential hazards; and consensus vs dissensus.

108. Esiri, Margaret M. & Williams, R. J. (1986). **Comments on an olfactory source for an environmental influence and possible involvement of aluminum in the development of Alzheimer's disease.** Special Issue: Controversial topics on Alzheimer's disease: Intersecting crossroads. *Neurobiology of Aging,* 7(6), 582–583.
Comments on 3 aspects of E. Roberts's (1986) review by discussing the proposed toxic effects of aluminosilicates transported from nose to brain; the nature of the deposits of aluminum and silicon in plaques; and the way in which aluminum and silicon, if they were to reach the brain in soluble rather than particulate form, might bring about the pathological changes described in Alzheimer's disease.

109. Evans, Gary W. & Joseph, Stephen V. (1982). **Air pollution and human behavior.** *Managerial Psychology,* 3(1), 1–30.
An organizational structure that demonstrates gaps in the literature on air pollution and human behavior is presented, and an initial conceptual framework derived from attitude-behavior theory is proposed as an alternative framework for organizing this body of literature. Air pollution and human behavior studies should include the cognitive, affective, and conative responses to air pollution. Categories that should be explored include effects of air pollution on human task performance, perception, attention, sensorimotor coordination, memory and problem solving, and work capacity. Social scientists should explore the complexities of psychological mediating factors (such as perceived control, perceived threat, and adaptation) that influence human responses to air pollution. There is also a need for broader multiple measurement strategies of dependent variables that include indices of mental health, irritation, and dissatisfaction. (79 ref).

110. Evans, Gary W.; Jacobs, Stephen V.; Dooley, David & Catalano, Ralph. (1987). **The interaction of stressful life events and chronic strains on community mental health.** *American Journal of Community Psychology,* 15(1), 23–34.
Examined the interplay between major life events and ambient air pollution, using 12 quarterly surveys of 500 households each. Results show that Ss exposed to higher levels of smog, who had also experienced a recent stressful life event, exhibited poorer mental health than those exposed to pollution who had not experienced a recent stressful life event. Results were replicated in both a cross-sectional and a longitudinal study.

111. Evans, Gary W.; Jacobs, Stephen V. & Frager, Neal B. (1982). **Adaptation to air pollution.** *Journal of Environmental Psychology,* 2(2), 99–108.
Examined human adaptation to air pollution by comparing responses to photochemical smog of 19 long-term and 20 recent undergraduate residents of the Los Angeles air basin. Results show that long-term Ss in comparison to recent migrants used a higher response criterion to identify smog in a visual signal detection task. There was no difference in visual sensitivity between the 2 residential groups in detecting the presence of air pollution in photographic slides. Thus, for low levels of visual air pollution, both long-term Ss and new migrants were equally accurate in detecting the presence of smog. Long-term Ss, however, were less likely to decide that smog was present in a scene. This response bias is interpreted in terms of adaptation level theory. Characteristics of the response bias differences between the 2 residential groups are examined using signal detection procedures. (18 ref).

112. Evans, Gary W. & Jacobs, Stephen V. (1981). **Air pollution and human behavior.** *Journal of Social Issues,* 37(1), 95–125.
Reviews the literature on air pollution and behavior and presents an organizational structure that demonstrates gaps in the literature and lays an initial, conceptual framework for future research. Research on the health effects, cognitive, affective, and conative components of air pollution and human response is discussed. In addition, the important roles of mediational constructs, such as controllability of pollutant and adaptation, are presented in detail. (80 ref).

113. Fiedler, Fred E. & Fiedler, Judith. (1975). **Port noise complaints: Verbal and behavioral reactions to airport-related noise.** *Journal of Applied Psychology,* 60(4), 498-506.
Compared the verbal and behavioral reactions of a total of 716 residents living in high-, medium-, and low-noise zones surrounding a major airport, as well as in communities out of the airport's noise range. Results show that the effects of noise were highly complex. While the proportion of those reported to be bothered by noise was correlated with objectively measured noise levels, the intensity and perceived source of the noise were unrelated to reported psychological and physical symptoms, length of residence in the area, or trace measures indicating recreational use of outdoor areas.

114. Flagler, Sally L. & Wright, Logan. (1987). **Recurrent poisoning in children: A review.** *Journal of Pediatric Psychology,* 12(4), 631–641.
Reviews the literature on poisoning accidents or ingestion of toxic substances in children. Special emphasis is given to the phenomenon of recurrent or repeat episodes. Recommendations are made for pediatric psychologists concerning ways to identify children who are at risk for repeat poison episodes and develop methods of intervention to prevent such occurrences. It is noted that passive restraints have been most successful in lowering the mortality of child poisoning vic-

tims, but that is partially because child behavior and parental interaction have not been adequately examined.

115. Fleming, India C. (1986). **The stress reducing functions of specific types of social support for victims of a technological catastrophe.** *Dissertation Abstracts International,* 47(2-B), 848.

116. Franzen, Michael D. & Golden, Charles J. (1984). **Case study: Report of a case of fluoride poisoning.** *International Journal of Clinical Neuropsychology,* 6(4), 264–269.
Neuropsychological evaluation of a woman who was exposed to large concentrations of sodium fluoride included the MMPI, Rorschach, and Luria-Nebraska Neuropsychological Battery. The 1st general class of deficits observed involved those due to fluoride's disruption of normal nerve conduction, namely sensory and motor disturbances. A 2nd class reflected decrements in all cortical functions. However, some of these functions were overlearned and appeared to be relatively intact. Implications of these 2 classes of deficits are discussed. (5 ref).

117. Gilbert, Avery N. (1986). **The neuropsychology of olfaction in Alzheimer's disease.** Special Issue: Controversial topics on Alzheimer's disease: Intersecting crossroads. *Neurobiology of Aging,* 7(6), 578–579.
Contends that E. Roberts's (1986) proposal of a nasal route of entry for an Alzheimer's disease (AD) pathogen leads to a prediction of olfactory dysfunction in AD patients. Recent studies suggesting the presence of olfactory deficits are reviewed, with special attention given to problems in examining olfactory function in demented patients.

118. Guth, Lloyd. (1986). **Commentary on the speculations that Alzheimer's disease may begin in the nose and may be caused by aluminosilicates.** Special Issue: Controversial topics on Alzheimer's disease: Intersecting crossroads. *Neurobiology of Aging,* 7(6), 572.
Critiques E. Roberts's (1986) comprehensive explanation of the pathogenesis of Alzheimer's disease (AD), suggesting that it represents a potentially new principle of neuropathogenesis that can be applied to various neurological disorders. The olfactory cells are considered a likely site for AD to begin because those neurons are deprived of the more extensive physiological protections (e.g., blood-brain barrier) and are vulnerable to toxic substances (e.g., aluminosilicates) in the air.

119. Hänninen, Helena; Nurminen, Markku; Tolonen, Matti & Martelin, Tuija. (1978). **Psychological tests as indicators of excessive exposure to carbon disulfide.** *Scandinavian Journal of Psychology,* 19(2), 163–174.
In order to diagnose cases of carbon disulfide poisoning, 12 psychological tests, including a standardized questionnaire about symptoms, 5 subtests of the WAIS, and the Rorschach, were administered to 206 male viscose rayon workers with long-term exposure to carbon disulfide and to 152 nonexposed men. With the method of multiple discriminant analysis the number of tests was reduced from 12 to 5 and the number of variables from 30 to 7. The variable setting of the obtained discriminant function contained measures of different types of psychomotor performances, emotional behavior, and subjective symptoms. Sensitivity and specificity of the tests and the criteria for a detected effect were evaluated a posteriori. In general, the sensitivity of the method was better than its specificity. Sufficient specificity could be obtained when a higher probability level for belonging to the exposed group was applied as the criterion, but even then, the application of other, reference diagnostic methods seemed necessary to separate the false positive cases. (17 ref).

120. Hardison, Nancy M. & Vanier, Dinoo J. (1976). **Environment and quality of life: Attitudinal measurement and analysis.** *Psychological Reports,* 39(3, Pt 1), 959-965.
Surveyed the attitudes toward pollution and quality of life of 130 men and 153 women from a California city with a highly desirable environment. Ss expressed concern for the environment but were not willing to pay for conservation with higher taxes. There were a few sex differences in the extent of agreement with some of the attitudes surveyed.

121. Harris, C. S. & Johnson, D. L. (1978). **Effects of infrasound on cognitive performance.** *Aviation, Space, & Environmental Medicine,* 49, 565–572.
12 Ss performed a serial search task during 15 min of exposure to each of 4 conditions of background and ambient noise; 12 Ss performed a complex counting task during 30 min of exposure to the same 4 conditions, and 16 Ss performed the counting task for 15 min under each of 4 other conditions of background noise. No performance decrements and no reports of dizziness or disorientation were obtained, contrary to some previous reports. It is concluded that the adverse effects of infrasound have been exaggerated, and the current levels of infrasound components produced by modern jet aircraft are not in themselves a practical problem. (26 ref).

122. Hatcher, Sherry L. (1982). **The psychological experience of nursing mothers upon learning of a toxic substance in their breast milk.** *Psychiatry,* 45(2), 172–181.
97 mothers (mean age 29.5 yrs) with polybrominated biphenyl (PBB) in their breast milk were administered a questionnaire designed to tap their attitudes and affects regarding PBB and breast-feeding. It was hypothesized that (1) the higher the reported level of PBB in the S's milk, the greater would be her denial of the problem and (2) the time when an S learned about PBB contamination would be of importance—Ss in the midst of nursing would exhibit more denial and conflict than those who knew of the PBB issue before they started to breast-feed their babies. Results support the 1st hypothesis but not the 2nd. In addition, Ss in the denial group were less able to allow unconscious conflicts about nursing to surface than were those who used mastery as a coping style. (17 ref).

123. Henderson, Victor W. (1986). **Non-genetic factors in Alzheimer's disease pathogenesis.** Special Issue: Controversial topics on Alzheimer's disease: Intersecting crossroads. *Neurobiology of Aging,* 7(6), 585–587.
Argues that incomplete and insufficient data fail to distinguish between genetic and environmental hypotheses of Alzheimer's disease (AD) pathogenesis. It is suggested that theories such as those proposed by E. Roberts (1986) that implicate aluminosilicates in AD pathogenesis and that emphasize nongenetic mechanisms offer greater opportunity for prevention and cure than do those that assume AD to be genetically determined.

124. Hendrickson, Edward C. (1981). **Primary prevention of accidental poisoning of preschool aged children using labels as deterrents.** *Dissertation Abstracts International,* 41(12-B, Pt 1), 4667.

125. Hepburn, Mary A.; Shrum, John W. & Simpson, Ronald D. (1978). **Effects of coordinated environmental studies in social studies and science on student attitudes toward growth and pollution.** *Theory & Research in Social Education,* 6(3), 71–86.
Used a pre-posttest control group experimental design to assess student environmental attitude changes after study of special social studies and science modules. Two coordinated sets of modules were developed and used with 93 9th and 104 10th graders. These modules were used individually and in combination to detect posttreatment attitude differences toward population growth and pollution among the treatment groups in each grade. Coordinated instruction in both social studies and science classes produced significantly higher mean

BEHAVIORAL TOXICOLOGY: GENERAL

scores on cognitive and affective measures when compared with single treatment and control groups. (14 ref).

126. Hétu, Raymond; Lalonde, Monique & Getty, Louise. (1987). **Psychosocial disadvantages associated with occupational hearing loss as experienced in the family.** *Audiology,* 26(3), 141–152.
Developed a questionnaire to measure awareness of hearing disability, coping strategies, and family response to the consequences of occupational hearing loss (OHL). Answers to the questionnaire were obtained from 54 workers with various degrees of presumed OHL and from 44 normal-hearing workers employed in the same noisy plant. Results show (a) that the family bears several consequences of the noise exposure and of the hearing loss of the worker and (b) that its spontaneous reaction to OHL appears as a psychosocial disadvantage experienced by the worker, inducing feelings in the worker of being inadequate and constraining to others. (French abstract).

127. Hopkins, B. L. et al. (1986). **Behavioral technology for reducing occupational exposures to styrene.** *Journal of Applied Behavior Analysis,* 19(1), 3–11.
Four plastics workers were trained in 9 behaviors selected for potential to reduce their exposures to styrene, a common chemical with multiple toxic effects. Behavioral measures indicated that Ss quickly came to emit most of the behaviors. Measures of air samples indicated that large decreases in exposures to styrene accompanied the changes in behaviors for the 3 Ss who had been selected because they most needed relief from their exposures and because they had opportunities to control their exposures by the ways they behaved. (24 ref).

128. Huebner, Robert B. & Lipsey, Mark W. (1981). **The relationship of three measures of locus of control to environmental activism.** *Basic & Applied Social Psychology,* 2(1), 45–58.
Assessed the adequacy of various locus of control measures for predicting environmental activism and willingness to engage in personal conservation and antipollution activities, examined the modifiability of locus of control under the pressure of a relevant sociopolitical event, and compared unidimensional vs multidimensional and generalized vs situation-specific representations of the locus of control construct. 50 activists, 51 nonactivists, and 53 posttest-only nonactivists were administered Rotter's Internal–External Locus of Control Scale, H. Levenson's (1974) Tridimensional Locus of Control Scale, and the authors' Situation-Specific Internal, Powerful Others, and Chance Scales. Results indicate that locus of control was significantly associated with environmental activism and personal conservation attitudes but that locus of control feelings changed among activists after a disappointing political defeat. The situation-specific, multidimensional locus of control measure was superior to the generalized, unidimensional and generalized, multidimensional measures both in predicting behavior and attitudes and in responding to the sociopolitical event. (32 ref).

129. Hummel, Carl F. (1978). **Effects of induced cognitive sets in viewing air pollution scenes.** *Dissertation Abstracts International,* 38(12-B), 6240.

130. Iwata, Osamu. (1977). **Some attitudinal determinants of environmental concern.** *Journal of Social Psychology,* 103(2), 321–322.
Investigated how conservatism, authoritarianism, masculinity–femininity, approach to environmental problems (Approach), confidence in science and technology, and appreciation of natural beauty (Appreciation) affect environmental concern. Results of data from 118 Japanese female college students show that (a) there was positive environmental concern for higher conservatism and negative for higher authoritarianism; (b) higher femininity was found to contribute to positive environmental concern but was associated with less effort or intention for pollution control; and (c) Approach and Appreciation were very potently and positively related with higher environmental concern.

131. Iwata, Osamu. (1978). **Empirical examination of a model for anti-pollution behavior.** *Japanese Journal of Psychology,* 48(6), 315–320.
Tested a model of antipollution behavior which consisted of 5 independent variables: approach to information on environmental problems, confidence in science and technology, appreciation of natural beauty, awareness of causes of pollution, and insight into the consequences of pollution. Antipollution behavior included purchasing and coping behavior. 189 adults responded to 83 5-point scales. Correlation coefficients were calculated and 6-variable path analyses were performed for purchasing and coping behavior. Results indicate that the approach to information on environmental problems was a moderately strong direct determinant of antipollution behavior but that awareness of the causes of pollution was a weak determinant. Insight into the consequences of pollution had a weak indirect effect on antipollution behavior. (English summary).

132. Iwata, Osamu & Takeda, Tsuneichi. (1976). **A factor-analytic study on the perception of pollution concepts.** *Japanese Journal of Psychology,* 47(4), 211–214.
102 female college students rated 4 pollution concepts (air, water, soil, and noise) on 13 7-point semantic differential scales. Ss also rated a man-made event (traffic) and a natural disaster (typhoon). Data of all concepts were factor analyzed using a correlation matrix based on the 13 scales, yielding the following factors: Psychological Stability, Nature-Artificiality, Predictability, and Polluted Area. Factor analysis of correlation coefficients among the 6 concepts showed that Ss perceived the 4 pollution concepts as man-made events.

133. Jacobs, Abraham H. (1978). **The response of farmers to industrial air pollution in England.** *Dissertation Abstracts International,* 39(3-A), 1835–1836.

134. Jacobs, Stephen V.; Evans, Gary W.; Catalano, Ralph & Dooley, David. (1984). **Air pollution and depressive symptomatology: Exploratory analyses of intervening psychosocial factors.** *Population & Environment: Behavioral & Social Issues,* 7(4), 260–272.
Interviewed 406 English- and Spanish-speaking residents (aged 18 yrs or older) of the Los Angeles metropolitan area to investigate associations of individual perceptions, social factors, and physical components of air pollution with depressive symptomatology. Findings show that Ss who had experienced a recent, undesirable life event and who perceived poor air quality in their neighborhood had greater symptoms of depression. These effects controlled for socioeconomic status (SES) and prior psychological status. It is concluded that perceived air quality is a function of both toxic components of ambient air and individual psychosocial experiences. (34 ref).

135. Jacobson, Joseph L. et al. (1984). **Prenatal exposure to environmental toxin: A test of the multiple effects model.** *Developmental Psychology,* 20(4), 523–532.
The multiple effects model of teratological exposure predicts that neonatal deficits associated with intrauterine exposure to small doses of a potentially teratogenic agent will vary considerably across individuals. This hypothesis was tested in a sample of 242 newborns exposed prenatally to low levels of polychlorinated biphenyls (PCBs) from maternal consumption of contaminated lake fish and 71 control infants whose mothers did not eat these fish. Behavioral outcomes were assessed using the Brazelton Neonatal Behavioral Assessment Scale (NABS). Contaminated fish consumption predicted motoric

immaturity, poorer lability of states, a greater amount of startle, and more abnormally weak (hypoactive) reflexes. The most highly exposed Ss were more likely than controls to be classified as "worrisome" on 3 NBAS clusters. Results from a stepwise regression analysis are consistent with the multiple effects model, indicating that some affected Ss were born small and/or early, whereas others exhibited one or another of the behavioral deficits. The analysis indicated that 12.2% of the variance in contaminated fish consumption was associated with measurable neonatal deficits. (40 ref).

136. Jacobson, Joseph L.; Jacobson, Sandra W. & Fein, Greta G. (1986). **Intrauterine exposure to environmental toxins: The significance of subtle behavioral effects.** Special Issue: Beyond the individual: Environmental approaches and prevention. *Prevention in Human Services,* 4(1–2), 125–137.
Examined the effects associated with exposure to environmental toxins using the case of polychlorinated biphenyls (PCBs), a family of environmental toxins found in moderate concentrations in humans who consume Lake Michigan sports fish. 242 newborns whose mothers had consumed these fish and 71 newborns whose mother had abstained were examined in the immediate postpartum period. Degree of exposure was measured by both maternal contaminated fish consumption and cord serum PCB level. Data suggest that, at the exposure levels found in the present sample, a maternal report may be more sensitive and reliable than a biochemical analysis. While significant effects on birth size, gestational age, and neonatal behavior were observed, the clinical significance of these effects is not yet known since none of the exposed infants weighed less than 1,500 g and criteria for newborn behavioral adequacy have not been established. Research on other toxic substances suggests that subtle neonatal deficits frequently signal the existence of an ongoing toxic process with clinically significant implications for later development. (26 ref).

137. Jacobson, Sandra W. et al. (1985). **The effect of intrauterine PCB exposure on visual recognition memory.** *Child Development,* 56(4), 853–860.
Adverse neonatal outcomes have been associated with intrauterine exposure to polychlorinated biphenyls (PCBs). In a follow-up study of exposed and nonexposed infants, 123 White infants tested at birth were administered a test of visual recognition memory at 7 mo of age. Two measures of prenatal PCB exposure, cord serum PCB level and maternal report of contaminated fish consumption, both predicted less preference for a novel stimulus. Preference for novelty decreased in a dose-dependent fashion with increasing levels of prenatal PCB exposure. Postnatal exposure from nursing was not related to visual recognition memory. The relation between prenatal exposure and visual recognition was not mediated by the neonatal deficits, suggesting that intrauterine PCB exposure may have a delayed effect on CNS functioning. (42 ref).

138. Jaggi, Bikki & Westacott, George. (1975). **Third-world managers' attitudes toward pollution.** *Journal of Applied Psychology,* 60(3), 392–394.
Examined pollution awareness and concern over pollution among 120 Indian managers from several industries. Pollution attitudes were measured by questionnaire responses to the open-ended question, "What is your firm's position in regard to pollution of the environment (in your own words)?" Responses were content analyzed and coded into 3 categories: (a) nonaware (51%), (b) aware-lacking concern (30%), and (c) aware-concerned (19%). Pollution attitudes displayed significant relationships with both individual and organizational variables. It is concluded that although pollution is becoming a serious problem in India, awareness and concern are lagging compared to the more developed countries.

139. Jason, Leonard A. (1979). **Preventive community interventions: Reducing school children's smoking and decreasing smoke exposure.** *Professional Psychology,* 10(5), 744–752.
Preventive interventions directed toward (a) building strengths and competencies in individuals to prevent disorders and (b) modifying environmental irritants predisposing to pathology are high priority needs inherent within a community perspective. The present article reviews projects illustrating these 2 approaches. The 1st project deals with efforts to prevent and reduce rates of smoking in school youngsters. The 2nd series of studies focuses on documenting the extent of exposure to smoke in various naturalistic settings and investigating strategies to reduce this exposure. (24 ref).

140. Jodelet, Francois. (1975). **The social representation of pollution of the environment.** *Bulletin de Psychologie,* 28(9-12), 617-638.
Describes an interview study designed to present and clarify the social representation and attitudes associated with the concept of pollution. Semi-structured interviews were conducted with 16 Ss. The interview protocols were qualitatively summarized under these broad topics: sources and modes of information about pollution available to the public, types of pollution, general aspects of pollution, imputation of causes and responsibilities for pollution, modalities of intervention and possible solution to the problem, and future outlook.

141. Jones, John W. & Bogat, G. Anne. (1978). **Air pollution and human aggression.** *Psychological Reports,* 43(3, Pt 1), 721–722.
Examined the effects of secondary cigarette smoke on human aggression with 24 male and 24 female nonsmoking undergraduates. Ss were first either angered or not angered and then were given a chance to aggress against their provoker in the Buss aggression machine situation. While aggressing, half of the Ss were exposed to secondary cigarette smoke (PSs) and the rest were exposed to clean ambient air (CSs). The aversive stimuli ostensibly administered to the victim were noise bursts ranging in intensity from 1 to 10; the major measure of aggression was the mean loudness score of 20 noise bursts administered to the provoker. As predicted, PSs were significantly more aggressive than were CSs. Angered Ss were significantly more aggressive than were nonangered Ss. (7 ref).

142. Kane, D. N. (1977). **Bad air for children.** *Environment,* 18(9), 26–34.
Review of US and international data suggests that comprehensive protection is required in view of children's special susceptibility to air pollution. This susceptibility is due to children's size, higher breathing rate, greater activity, play activity, mouth breathing, more frequent respiratory tract infections, and pediatric development factors. Maternal-transmitted risks are also present (many chemicals pass the placental barrier). As few as 2 million or as many as 60 million children under 14 yrs of age in the US may be exposed to troublesome levels of pollution, according to American Public Health Association and Environmental Protection Agency data. It is suggested that children are not adequately shielded from air pollution by public health standards that are designed for healthy adults. Especially vulnerable groups are (a) poor under age 14 yrs, (b) Blacks under age 14 yrs, and (c) all urban children under age 5 yrs. Pollution exposure is raised by contaminated indoor air, containing tobacco smoke; aerosal sprays; heating, ventilation, and cooking contaminants; household dust; lead; and asbestos. Developmental effects include retarded bone structure, abnormalities in blood biochemistry, larger than normal tonsils and lymph nodes, depressing effects on athletic activity, and higher incidences of retarded physical development, childhood cancer, and mental illness.

BEHAVIORAL TOXICOLOGY: GENERAL

143. Kennedy, R. S.; Wilkes, R. L.; Dunlap, W. P. & Kuntz, L. A. (1987). **Development of an automated performance test system for environmental and behavioral toxicology studies.** *Perceptual & Motor Skills,* 65(3), 947–962.
25 university students were tested repeatedly with 11 tests previously identified as good candidates for repeated-measures research in paper-and-pencil versions. The 11 tests were administered concurrently in their traditional paper-and-pencil modes and in newly implemented microcomputer-based versions, along with the Wechsler Adult Intelligence Scale (WAIS). Nine of the 11 microcomputer-based tests achieved stability, and reliabilities were generally high. Cross-correlations of microbased tests with traditional paper-and-pencil versions suggested equivalency between the test constructs in the different media. Correlations between 6 of the microbased subtests and the WAIS identified common variance, and these might comprise an efficient short battery of tests.

144. Knave, Bengt; Mindus, Per & Struwe, Göran. (1979). **Neurasthenic symptoms in workers occupationally exposed to jet fuel.** *Acta Psychiatrica Scandinavica,* 60(1), 39–49.
Standardized medical interviews showed a higher occurrence of neurasthenic symptoms (e.g., anxiety and mood changes) in 30 workers exposed to jet fuel as compared with 60 nonexposed matched controls. Exposed workers also scored higher than the controls on a modified Comprehensive Psychopathological Rating Scale, particularly regarding the neurasthenic symptoms. (18 ref).

145. Korgeski, Gregory P. (1982). **Psychological, neuropsychological and medical correlates of self-reported and objective ratings of herbicide exposure among Vietnam veterans.** *Dissertation Abstracts International,* 42(12-B, Pt 1), 4933.

146. Kronus, Carol L. (1977). **Mobilizing voluntary associations into a social movement: The case of environmental quality.** *Sociological Quarterly,* 18(2), 267–283.
Studied the mobilization behavior of voluntary associations in a community to explain why some organizations were successfully recruited into the environmental quality movement and others were not. Analysis of a random sample of 209 community organizations in a midwest urban area showed that approximately half were mobilized into supporting the environmental quality movement. Hypotheses on the effects of goal overlap, organizational resources, and position in the multi-organizational field were tested. The significant factors were the size of the manpower base, the leader's personal mobilization into the environmental quality movement, and the allocation of social responsibility among community groups for solving local pollution problems. The last factor—the acceptance or rejection of group responsibility for working for the collective good—emerged as the most important explanatory factor; it explained 31% of the variance in the mobilization of organizational interest and 22% of the variance in the mobilization of group activity. (17 ref).

147. Kurlychek, Robert T. (1987). **Neuropsychological evaluation of workers exposed to industrial neurotoxins.** *American Journal of Forensic Psychology,* 5(4), 55–66.
Presents an overview of research and information on the neuropsychological evaluation of industrial workers exposed to neurotoxins. Early indicators of industrial neurotoxicity and potentially problematic worksites are identified. The neurotoxic effects of exposure to pesticides, solvents, metals (e.g., lead), and gases (e.g., carbon monoxide) are considered. Solvents that can affect central nervous system (CNS) functions are identified, and acute and chronic syndromes associated with solvent exposure are discussed. Journals on behavioral toxicology, assessment techniques, and confusion of subjective and functional symptoms are also considered. Implications for forensic psychology are noted.

148. Landrigan, Philip J. (1985). **The uses of epidemiology in the study of neurotoxic pollutants: Lessons from the workplace.** *International Journal of Mental Health,* 14(3), 44–63.
Presents 3 occupational medicine examples of neurologic and psychiatric syndromes that have been found through a 3-stage process (clinical recognition, epidemiologic assessment, and toxicologic corroboration) to be of chemical origin. These case histories, involving workers primarily under 30 yrs of age, illustrate that chemical etiology is not uncommon and should be considered when evaluating neurological and mental disorders. (39 ref).

149. Lawson, Billie Z. (1987). **Work-related post-traumatic stress reactions: The hidden dimension.** *Health & Social Work,* 12(4), 250–258.
Identifies individual and workplace factors that can place employees at high risk for developing posttraumatic stress responses. These assessment guidelines, developed in the course of working with 18 toxic exposure patients, can be adapted to evaluate employee reactions to different types of occupational injury. The author considers the following issues in evaluating clinical patients: life-threatening experience, betrayal by the employer, ability to change jobs or vocation, patient's explanatory model of injury outcome, and patient's mental and psychosocial status. Interventions are discussed.

150. Lazar, Alexandru. (1988). **The comparative action of the effect of hexavalent chromium and fibrotizing dust on personality dimensions.** *Studia Psychologica,* 30(1), 57–64.
Investigated the effects of exposure to noxious chemicals on personality dimensions, using 74 adult patients intoxicated with hexavalent chromium, with silicosis, or with polycythemia vera; 115 Ss exposed to hexavalent chromium or silicogen risk; and 104 nonexposed adults. Ss were administered the Eysenck Personality Inventory, the Taylor Manifest Anxiety Scale, and the Freiburger Personality Inventory. Neuroticism, anxiety, and depression were higher in exposed Ss; and Ss exposed to chromium exhibited more aggressivity, depression, irritability, inhibition, neuroticism, anxiety, and psychoticism. The toxic effect of hexavalent chromium showed a correlation with Extraversion and Neuroticism scores. (Russian & Slovak abstracts).

151. Lester, David. (1987). **Suicide and homicide rates and fluoride.** *Psychological Reports,* 61(3), 802.
The author failed to find a positive relationship between the percentage of each state's population drinking fluoridated water and suicide and homicide rates for each state.

152. Levenson, Hanna. (1973). **Perception of environmental modifiability and involvement in antipollution activities.** *Journal of Psychology,* 84(2), 237–239.
Hypothesized that people who were involved in antipollution activities would have expectations that something positive could be done to ameliorate environmental conditions. Ss were 32 adult members of a local antipollution group and 64 nonmembers. All Ss completed a self-report measure (the author's Environmental Modifiability Test) to assess their attitudes concerning the possibilities of eliminating pollution. Contrary to expectation, members were significantly less optimistic about the possibilities of cleaning up the environment than nonmembers. An examination of the content of the test items indicated that members were less in favor of technological means to lessen pollution and believed restoration of the environment would be difficult.

153. Levenson, Hanna. (1974). **Involvement in antipollution activities and perceived negative consequences from pollution.** *Perceptual & Motor Skills,* 38(3, Pt 2), 1105–1106.
Administered an involvement activities checklist and a measure of the perceived importance of the issue of pollution to 96 male and female members and nonmembers of an antipollution group. Members considered pollution a significantly

higher priority problem and believed to a greater degree that they would be negatively affected by pollution than did nonmembers.

154. Levenson, Hanna. (1974). **Participation in antipollution activities and complexity of judgments about environmental degradation.** *Journal of Social Psychology,* 94(1), 147-148.
In 2 studies with 77 sociology students and 96 other adult Ss, C. Hovland and M. Sherif's research (1953) was replicated in investigating the hypotheses that (a) when given a fixed number of categories, people who are more involved in antipollution activities will concentrate their placement of items concerning pollution into a small number of categories and will be highly discriminating in accepting terms at their own end of the scale, and (b) when given an unrestricted number of categories, people who are more involved will sort issue statements into significantly fewer piles than less involved people. Results indicate that Ss spaced their items more evenly over the 11 categories and placed more items in the extreme categories; the 2nd hypothesis was not confirmed.

155. Mackay, Colin. (1987). **The alleged reproductive hazards of VDUs.** *Work & Stress,* 1(1), 49–57.
Reviews the available evidence on the alleged reproductive hazards of video display units (VDUs). It is concluded that it is unlikely that any threat is posed by irradiation. Poor design of the work station and job-related stress may pose a problem for some users.

156. Maggiotto, Michael A. & Bowman, Ann. (1982). **Policy orientations and environmental regulation: A case study of Florida's legislators.** *Environment & Behavior,* 14(2), 155–170.
Explored the manner in which perception and definition shape legislative environmental attitudes. A survey of 43 state legislators revealed 2 competing formulations of air pollution: One saw pollution as a question of economics; the 2nd saw it as a health and environmental issue. Ss scoring high on the health and environmental dimension (1) were less receptive to environmental deterioration, (2) found present controls less adequate, (3) saw a wider and more beneficial scope of social outcomes, (4) prosecuted their claims more vigorously, and (5) advocated an expanded governmental approach to the problem. Ss with an economic orientation functioned as polar opposites in each instance. It was found that air pollution stances were not easily transferable to other environmental issues. (17 ref).

157. Markowitz, Jeffrey S.; Gutterman, Elane M.; Link, Bruce & Rivera, Maria. (1987). **Psychological response of firefighters to a chemical fire.** *Journal of Human Stress,* 13(2), 84–93.
80 firefighter Ss involved in a polyvinyl chloride (PVC) fire and a comparison group of 15 firefighters not involved were compared on a number of postincident psychological distress measures. Using a structured, self-administered questionnaire, PVC Ss were more psychologically distressed on demoralization, specific emotional distress, and perceived threat to physical health. After controlling for baseline characteristics on which Ss and the comparison group differed, these between-group effects remained significant.

158. Maugh, Thomas H. (1984). **Acid rain's effects on people assessed.** *Science,* 226(4681), 1408–1410.
Discusses the effects of acid rain on human health and suggests that, although available evidence remains inconclusive, acidic pollutants create health problems. Studies implicating acidic pollutants in human health problems (e.g., learning impairments and CNS toxicity in children exposed to abnormal concentrations of lead; dialysis encephalopathy, senile dementia, and amyotrophic lateral sclerosis with severe dementia due to excessive concentrations of aluminum in the brain) are reviewed.

159. Mayron, Lewis M. & Kaplan, Ervin. (1976). **Bioeffects of fluorescent lighting.** *Academic Therapy,* 12(1), 75-90.
Bean seeds were grown in a classroom under fluorescent lamps. Germination time; root, stem, and leaf growth; and negative tropism were negatively influenced by the lamps especially when the plant was located near the electrode ends of the lamps. Toxic effects of tryptophan degradation, thought to be produced by emission of short-wave ultraviolet rays, is regarded as an explanation of the phenomenon. These effects are less marked when grounded aluminum screening is used as a shield. This study corroborates and further extends an earlier experiment by L. Mayron, J. Ott, R. Nations, and E. Mayron (1974), in which the use of full-spectrum fluorescent lighting and radiation shielding, over a period of 6 mo, decreased the hyperactive behavior of 1st-grade students in classrooms lighted previously by cool-white fluorescent lighting. The academic achievements of these Ss also appeared to be favorably influenced by these new conditions.

160. Mayton, Daniel M. (1986). **The structure of attitudes to doomsday issues: A replication.** *Australian Psychologist,* 21(3), 395–403.
V. A. Braithwaite and H. G. Law (1977) developed a doomsday issues questionnaire and administered it to an Australian sample. The study was replicated, using 169 American undergraduates; also investigated was the underlying structure of the doomsday belief statements. The present Ss also completed a liberalism-conservatism scale. Analyses retained 5 components: (1) a general component primarily concerned with ineffectiveness of actions taken by individuals and humanity; (2) a general component concerning personal and societal commitment to action; (3) a nuclear war component referencing societal concerns; (4) an overpopulation component concerning effectiveness of personal actions with a high liberalism-conservatism loading; and (5) a general pollution-overpopulation component.

161. Mazis, Michael B. (1975). **Antipollution measures and psychological reactance theory: A field experiment.** *Journal of Personality & Social Psychology,* 31(4), 654-660.
Conducted a field experiment with 121 housewives in middle-income areas to determine whether hypotheses derived from psychological reactance theory could explain response to the implementation of an antiphosphate ordinance. Ss deprived of phosphates expressed more positive attitudes toward the eliminated alternative than did control Ss, thereby supporting reactance theory predictions. Within the experimental group, Ss were divided into 2 groups based on their degree of choice deprivation. As predicted, Ss forced to switch from their preferred detergent brand expressed less favorable attitudes about the effectiveness of no-phosphate vs phosphate detergent than Ss who could maintain brand continuity. Reduced attractiveness of forced alternative rather than enhancement of forbidden alternative was the principal mode of response resulting from psychological reactance.

162. Mazis, Michael B.; Settle, Robert B. & Leslie, Dennis C. (1973). **Elimination of phosphate detergents and psychological reactance.** *Journal of Marketing Research,* 10(4), 390-395.
Administered a questionnaire about attitudes toward laundry detergents, laws regulating the use of phosphates, and demographic characteristics to 76 housewives in Miami, Florida, and to 45 Ss in Tampa (control). Based on reactance theory, it was hypothesized that Miami consumers, who were prohibited by law from buying products containing phosphates, would have more positive attitudes toward the effectiveness of phosphate detergents than consumers living in an area where phosphates were for sale (Tampa housewives), and that Miami consumers would have more negative attitudes toward governmental water pollution measures and laws against phosphate detergents than the consumers unaffected by the phosphate ban. Findings support the hypotheses and also show that Ss forced to switch from their favorite detergent

BEHAVIORAL TOXICOLOGY: GENERAL

were less favorable about the effectiveness and cost of the no-phosphate vs phosphate detergents than were consumers who were able to maintain brand continuity.

163. McLeod, W. R. (1975). **Merphos poisoning or mass panic?** *Australian & New Zealand Journal of Psychiatry,* 9(4), 225-229.
Describes events which led to the evacuation of 6,000 individuals because of a Merphos contamination scare in a New Zealand city. It is argued that while the compound was found to be unharmful to humans, the belief that it was toxic precipitated panic reactions in city officials, the press, and residents of the area.

164. Miller, Bruce L. (1986). **Aluminum in Alzheimer's disease: A testable hypothesis.** Special Issue: Controversial topics on Alzheimer's disease: Intersecting crossroads. *Neurobiology of Aging,* 7(6), 570-571.
Comments on the article by E. Roberts (1986), which suggests that Alzheimer's disease (AD) might be caused by the entrance of aluminosilicates into the aging nasal mucosa. The present author argues that while the article is speculative it offers a testable hypothesis with experiments that could be carried out to prove or disprove the theory.

165. Moser, G. (1984). **Water quality perception, a dynamic evaluation.** *Journal of Environmental Education,* 4(3), 201-210.
In a dynamic evaluation of individuals' perceptions of water quality, 76 regular, adult users of a camp ground along the River Loing (France) participated in semidirective interviews concerning their perceptions of water pollution levels of the river. Results of the interviews were analyzed in conjunction with objective water-pollution data supplied by the water quality monitoring authority. While there was some relationship between Ss' estimates and objective quality classifications, Ss appeared to be tolerant of water pollution. Quality estimates were not affected by the specific water-related activities of Ss. (9 ref).

166. Navarro, P. Larrain; Simpson-Housley, P. & de Man, A. F. (1987). **Anxiety, locus of control and appraisal of air pollution.** *Perceptual & Motor Skills,* 64(3, Pt 1), 811-814.
Studied the relationship among locus of control (LOC [Rotter's Internal-External Locus of Control Scale]), trait anxiety (TA [Speilberger State-Trait Anxiety Inventory]), and perception of air pollution in 100 17-65 yr old residents of Santiago de Chile. Concern over the problem of atmospheric pollution and number of antipollution measures taken were related to TA. LOC was associated with variation in awareness of pollution hazard.

167. Nelkin, Dorothy. (1983). **Workers at risk.** *Science,* 222(4620), 125.
Interviews with workers routinely exposed to hazardous chemicals showed how perceptions of and responses to risk were related to social relationships, attitudes about work, choices, and the extent of their control over working conditions. Many Ss conveyed a sense of isolation fostered by persistent anxiety and fear that complaining would jeopardize their jobs. Ss also expressed a feeling of powerlessness related to the uncertainty of long-term effects on health, an inability to use what information they received, and the burden of choosing between work and health.

168. Okasha, Ahmed; Bishry, Z.; Osman, N. M. & Kamel, M. (1976). **A psychosocial study of accidental poisoning in Egyptian children.** *British Journal of Psychiatry,* 129, 539-543.
Compared 127 accidentally poisoned children (ages 1-6 yrs) who had been treated at a university hospital with an equal number of controls. The highest age incidence for both sexes in poisoned Ss was 36 mo. Males outnumbered females at a ratio of 3:2. Behavioral problems such as hyperactivity, temper tantrums, aggression, stubbornness, nocturnal enuresis, and impulsiveness occurred more often in poisoned Ss than in controls and more often in 24 Ss referred with accidental poisoning on more than one occasion. The families of poisoned Ss differed significantly from the controls in their large size, low level of education, disturbed home atmosphere, and the accessiblitiy to the child of the poisonous substance.

169. Orr, Robert H. (1974). **The additive and interactive effects of powerlessness and anomie in predicting opposition to pollution control.** *Rural Sociology,* 39(4), 471-486.
Attempted to determine the additive and interactive effects of different aspects of alienation on attitudes toward pollution control for 213 residents of a midwestern community that was concerned with a sewage treatment issue. Ss were administered questionnaires during May 1971. Powerlessness and anomie, while not additive, were found to act interactively to explain opposition to pollution control. Furthermore, this relationship was characterized by a "saturation" or diminishing return effect. Alienation produced negativism toward the issue up to a certain point, with a subsequent increase serving to lessen the issue opposition. The interaction effect was found to exist, controlling for respondent socioeconomic and demographic characteristics.

170. Orr, Robert H. (1973). **Community alienation and pollution control.** *Dissertation Abstracts International,* 34(2-A), 874.

171. Otto, David A.; Baumann, Stephan & Robinson, George. (1985). **Application of a portable microprocessor-based system for electrophysiological field testing of neurotoxicity.** Workshop on Neurotoxicity Testing in Human Populations (1983, Rougemont, North Carolina). *Neurobehavioral Toxicology & Teratology,* 7(4), 409-414.
Describes a portable microprocessor-based system designated PEARL II (Portable Environmental Assessment and Research Laboratory), developed by E. B. Heffley et al (1983) for neurotoxicity testing in human populations. PEARL II provides a flexible and powerful data acquisition capability to record sensory evoked potentials (auditory, visual, and somatosensory), event-related slow potentials (contingent negative variation and the P300), and behavioral measures. PEARL II was used to collect neurobehavioral data from different cohorts of children at risk for lead poisoning. Results show that PEARL II is a reliable and effective system for the neurotoxicity field-testing of humans. (20 ref).

172. Pallak, Michael S. & Kleinhesselink, Randall R. (1976). **Polarization of attitudes: Belief inference from consonant behavior.** *Personality & Social Psychology Bulletin,* 2(1), 55-58.
Investigated the conditions under which shifts to more extreme attitudes may result from attitude-consistent behavior. 56 male undergraduates agreed to deliver arguments favoring stricter controls on water pollution (a consonant position) either to passersby on a street corner (proselytizing act) or to a tape-recorder for research use. Half the time a confederate agreed to perform the same act (about a different issue) either because he believed in the issue (belief-relevant cue) or because he wanted to help the study along (belief-irrelevant cue). Ss in the proselytize-belief relevant condition adopted a more extreme attitude favoring controls on water pollution relative to Ss in the remaining conditions.

173. Parker, Donald C. (1975). **An analysis of environmental attitudes as measured by a modified semantic differential instrument.** *Dissertation Abstracts International,* 35(11-A), 7142.

174. Parker, Howard A.; Perry, Ronald W. & Gillespie, David F. (1974). **Prolegomenon to a theory of attitude-behavior relationships.** *Pakistan Journal of Psychology,* 7(3-4), 21-39.

To resolve the discrepancy between attitude and behavior, it is theorized that a number of intervening variables need to be considered, such as importance of an attitude object, perceived consequences of not taking action, the history of an individual's involvement, and the number of issues evaluated. Survey data of 221 households provided support for the hypothesis that action against air pollution is related to the degree of importance of the air pollution issue. A composite index of the importance included the individual's ranking of air pollution as well as the extent of agreement among his or her friends and workmates. Air pollution behavior was scaled in terms of commitments: signing a petition, circulating a petition, or giving money. (31 ref).

175. Pedersen, Darhl M. (1979). **Changing beliefs concerning the causes of pollution.** *Journal of Social Psychology,* 107(2), 295–296.
Investigated the effects of 2 kinds of persuasive communications on beliefs regarding the causes of pollution. Results from 60 undergraduates confirm the hypothesis that a "man as polluter" article would increase existing beliefs about humans as the responsible agents and a "nature as polluter" article would produce a decrease in existing beliefs. (3 ref).

176. Peterson, Rebecca L. (1975). **Levels of air pollution and attendance in recreation behavior settings in the Los Angeles Basin.** *Dissertation Abstracts International,* 36(3-B), 1416-1417.

177. Preston, Valerie; Taylor, S. Martin & Hodge, David C. (1983). **Adjustment to natural and technological hazards: A study of an urban residential community.** *Environment & Behavior,* 15(2), 143–164.
Human adjustments to natural and technological hazards were examined using questionnaire data provided by 75 residents on the Beach Strip in Hamilton, Ontario. This area is exposed to 5 hazards: flooding, severe storms, air pollution, water pollution, and noise pollution. It was hypothesized that residents made cognitive and/or behavioral adjustments to these problems. Results indicate that behavioral adjustments were widespread but did not reduce the perceived severity of environmental problems. It appears that many residents remain in the area because of low-cost housing and a closely knit community structure. (25 ref).

178. Protess, David L.; Cook, Fay L.; Curtin, Thomas R.; Gordon, Margaret T. et al. (1987). **The impact of investigative reporting on public opinion and policymaking: Targeting toxic waste.** *Public Opinion Quarterly,* 51(2), 166–185.
Investigated the public opinion and policymaking impact of news media investigative journalism concerning the toxic waste disposal practices of a major Chicago university. Results from 395 telephone survey respondents show that the media disclosures in this field experiment had limited effects on the general public but were influential in changing the attitudes of surveyed policymakers. Results also indicate how changes in public policymaking resulted from collaboration between journalists and government officials. The present authors develop an exploratory model for specifying the conditions under which media investigations influence public attitudes and agendas.

179. Prusiner, Stanley & McKinley, Michael P. (1986). **Relationship of aluminosilicates to CNS degenerative disorders.** Special Issue: Controversial topics on Alzheimer's disease: Intersecting crossroads. *Neurobiology of Aging,* 7(6), 573.
Comments on E. Roberts's (1986) hypothesis, by noting that the ubiquity of aluminum and silicon makes the study of these elements in Alzheimer's disease all the more difficult. Research is cited indicating that aluminosilicates may play a central role in the pathogenesis of a variety of central nervous system (CNS) degenerative disorders (e.g., amyotrophic lateral sclerosis, Parkinson's disease).

180. Roberts, Eugene. (1986). **Alzheimer's disease may begin in the nose and may be caused by aluminosilicates.** Special Issue: Controversial topics on Alzheimer's disease: Intersecting crossroads. *Neurobiology of Aging,* 7(6), 561–567.
Suggests that genetic factors may interact with aging changes in the nasal mucociliary apparatus to increase the probability that ubiquitously occurring aluminosilicates may enter sensory neurons of the olfactory epithelium and spread transneuronally to several olfactory-related areas of the brain, thereby initiating changes that eventually result in neuronal damage typical of Alzheimer's disease. A speculative sequence of events is suggested by which neuronally contained aluminosilicates might cleave or otherwise alter a normal cellular protein in such a manner that aggregates would arise that could interfere with cellular function and that also could act in a pseudoinfective manner, relaxing translational and transcriptional controls in the synthesis of the native protein. Some relevant experiments and potential therapies arising from the hypothesis presented are discussed.

181. Rodriguez, Gary P. (1987). **Changes in acoustic reflex activity following two hours of industrial noise exposure in normal hearing subjects.** *Dissertation Abstracts International,* 47(11-B), 4458.

182. Rossi, Giovanni; Magliano, C. & Scevola, M. (1976). **Changes in the time of reaction to light and sound signals in the presence of urban traffic noise.** *Acta Oto-Laryngologica,* 339, 19-23.
Investigated changes in the reaction time required for the performance of a simple and a complicated movement following a light or an acoustic stimulus presented at the same time as road noise. Findings from 10 20-25 yr old Ss with normal hearing show that less time was required to execute either a simple or complicated movement in response to an acoustic stimulus, and that exposure to road noise and an acoustic signal produced a 24% increase in reaction time for both types of movements.

183. Rotton, James et al. (1979). **The air pollution experience and physical aggression.** *Journal of Applied Social Psychology,* 9(5), 397–412.
60 undergraduate males delivered electric shocks to 1 of 6 confederates as punishment for making errors on a learning task. Half did so after being exposed to an aggressive model, whereas the other half did so without being exposed. Shocks were delivered from a room whose atmosphere was either unpolluted or contaminated by a moderately unpleasant odor (ethyl mercaptan) or an extremely obnoxious stench (ammonium sulfide). As hypothesized, the moderately unpleasant pollutant facilitated higher levels of aggression than either the extremely obnoxious one or the absence of pollution; however, pollution facilitated aggression only in the model's absence. Since the former finding supports and extends the affect–aggression model from heat research, it is suggested that the latter resulted either from a ceiling effect or from malodor distracting attention from the aggressive cues of the model. (39 ref).

184. Rotton, James. (1983). **Affective and cognitive consequences of malodorous pollution.** *Basic & Applied Social Psychology,* 4(2), 171–191.
In Exp I, 24 male and 24 female undergraduates evaluated paintings, peers in photographs, and persons described by adjectives while breathing air that was either unpolluted or polluted by ethyl mercaptan. As predicted, evaluations of unfamiliar neutral, but not extreme stimuli were lowered by pollution. In Exp II, 40 male and 40 female undergraduates were exposed to 1 of 4 15-min sequences of odor and no-odor while they worked on simple (arithmetic) and complex (proofreading) tasks. Half of these Ss were led to believe that they could avoid exposure, and the other half were led to believe that exposure was uncontrollable. As hypothesized, the mal-

BEHAVIORAL TOXICOLOGY: GENERAL

odor impaired performances on complex but not simple tasks, and exposure produced behavioral aftereffects in the form of lowered tolerance for frustration when Ss had been deprived of control. Under conditions of low control, aftereffects were greatest when Ss were exposed to the malodor for relatively long periods of time and were tested immediately after exposure. It is concluded that malodorous pollution exerts effects similar to ones produced by noise, density, and other stressors. (48 ref).

185. Rotton, James; Barry, Timothy; Frey, James & Soler, Edgardo. (1978). **Air pollution and interpersonal attraction.** *Journal of Applied Social Psychology,* 8(1), 57–71.
Tested the prediction that negative affect associated with one component of air pollution (malodor) reduces attraction toward both similar and dissimilar strangers. In 1 experiment, 27 undergraduates rated attitudinally similar or dissimilar strangers while confined in a room whose atmosphere was ambient (no-odor control) or polluted by ammonium sulfide. Contrary to predictions, similar strangers elicited greatest liking in the polluted atmosphere. It is suggested that air pollution increased attraction for another who might be experiencing the same disagreeable situation (i.e., "shared stress"). In a 2nd experiment, this suggestion was examined by assuring Ss (60 undergraduates) that they were alone and would not meet the similar or dissimilar person they rated. As predicted, exposure to either ammonium sulfide or butyric acid combined additively with attitudinal dissimilarity to depress liking, mood-affect, time spent in the setting, and ratings of the environment. Results are consistent with the reinforcement–affect model of attraction, but it is cautioned that the effects of air pollution may depend on social factors, such as shared stress and dosage level of the pollutant. (43 ref).

186. Rotton, James & Frey, James. (1984). **Psychological costs of air pollution: Atmospheric conditions, seasonal trends, and psychiatric emergencies.** *Population & Environment: Behavioral & Social Issues,* 7(1), 3–16.
Assessed and controlled for seasonal and secular differences in psychiatric emergencies using analysis of covariance (ANCOVA) and stepwise regression on data obtained from the Dayton, Ohio police department. During a 731-day period, dispatchers logged 1,535 phone calls as mental cases. During the same time period, the county environmental protection agency obtained 24-hr averages for photochemical oxidants on 722 days, carbon monoxide on 575 days, sulfur dioxide on 459 days, and suspended particulates of 712 days. Five continuous and 4 dichotomous measures of meteorological conditions were obtained from the US Weather Bureau. Results show that, as anticipated, more psychiatric emergencies were reported to police when oxidant and sulfur dioxide levels were high than when they were low. Positive relationships between oxidants and emergencies emerged after weather and temporal variables were partialled out. (41 ref).

187. Ryan, Christopher M.; Morrow, Lisa A.; Bromet, Evelyn J. & Parkinson, David K. (1987). **Assessment of neuropsychological dysfunction in the workplace: Normative data from the Pittsburgh Occupational Exposures Test Battery.** *Journal of Clinical & Experimental Neuropsychology,* 9(6), 665–679.
Describes the development of the Pittsburgh Occupational Exposures Test Battery, which is comprised of a collection of tests including subtests from the Wechsler Adult Intelligence Scale—Revised (WAIS—R) and Wechsler Memory Scale, and a number of learning, memory, visuospatial, and visuomotor tests sensitive in detecting impairments in neurobehavioral functioning that are associated with exposure to toxic substances. The procedures used to collect appropriate age-scaled norms from 182 blue-collar males are detailed and the factor structure of the test battery delineated. The interrelationships among test scores and certain demographic variables are examined, and the epidemiologic and clinical relevance of these data are discussed. Revised scoring criteria for visual reproduction are appended.

188. Sauter, Diana L. (1981). **The development and application of a battery for the exploratory screening for neuropsychological deficits in children exposed to formaldehyde.** *Dissertation Abstracts International,* 42(4-A), 1559.

189. Schiffman, Susan S. (1986). **The nose as a port of entry for aluminosilicates and other pollutants: Possible role in Alzheimer's disease.** Special Issue: Controversial topics on Alzheimer's disease: Intersecting crossroads. *Neurobiology of Aging,* 7(6), 576–578.
Contends that considerably more research is necessary to evaluate the possible role of aluminosilicates in the brain pathology of Alzheimer's disease (AD) and that other environmental pollutants could be equally responsible for the neurodegeneration and olfactory deficits reviewed by E. Roberts (1986). Animal studies could be useful in determining which chemicals might actually invade the central nervous system (CNS) through the nose and produce the pattern of neurodegeneration characteristic of AD.

190. Schneider, Kenneth C. (1977). **Prevention of accidental poisoning through package and label design.** *Journal of Consumer Research,* 4(2), 67–74.
Reports findings of a study which investigated the possibility of controlling accidental childhood poisoning by designing packages and labels to reduce children's attraction toward these products. Data from 81 42–66 mo old children in 3 nursery schools support the conclusion that such an approach to poison control is feasible. (18 ref).

191. Schoental, R. (1985). **Fusarial mycotoxins and behaviour: Possible implications for psychiatric disorder.** *British Journal of Psychiatry,* 146, 115–119.
Notes that humans and animals are sporadically exposed to mycotoxins (the secondary metabolites of molds), which include those produced in damp and cool environment by the almost ubiquitous soil-microfungi, the *Fusaria*. Humans may be exposed through the consumption of contaminated food products. Perinatal exposure to the mycotoxins may cause damage to many organs, including the CNS and those that are targets for estrogenic agents. Depending on the levels of the mycotoxins and the time of their action, the effects may manifest themselves as neonatal abnormalities, or as neurological and behavioral anomalies and chronic disorders later in life. It is concluded that the relationship between the anatomical and behavioral development of individuals and their perinatal exposure to fusarial mycotoxins requires further investigation. (43 ref).

192. Shaffer, Howard J. & Costikyan, Nancy S. (1988). **Cocaine psychosis and AIDS: A contemporary diagnostic dilemma.** *Journal of Substance Abuse Treatment,* 5(1), 9–12.
Examines the differential diagnostic considerations associated with the interaction between advanced cocaine psychosis and the neuropsychiatric manifestations of acquired immune deficiency syndrome (AIDS)-spectrum disorders by reviewing the concerns associated with cocaine abuse and the psychiatric aspects of AIDS. A clinical case of a 36-yr-old female illustrates the potential for institutional countertransference in the treatment of substance abusing patients. The role of a multidimensional hypothesis testing model in cocaine-related cases is discussed.

193. Shield, Lloyd K.; Coleman, Timothy L. & Markesberry, William R. (1977). **Methyl bromide intoxication: Neurologic features, including simulation of Reye syndrome.** *Neurology,* 27(10), 959–962.
Three family members (a 42-yr-old man, his 41-yr-old wife, and their 6-yr-old grandson) intoxicated with methyl bromide presented with a variety of neuropsychiatric manifestations including coma, severe status epilepticus, hyporeflexia, and

acute psychosis. The simulation of Reye syndrome in the child emphasizes the need for careful toxicologic screening of all children presenting with this syndrome. (28 ref).

194. Shor, Ronald E. & Williams, Daniel C. (1978). **A brief survey of beliefs about the effects of tobacco smoke pollution on intellectual performance in college classrooms.** *Psychological Reports,* 43(3, Pt 2), 1047–1050.
A subset of 4 questions was selected from a longer questionnaire to survey beliefs about the effects of tobacco smoke pollution on intellectual performance in college classrooms. Sizable majorities of both the 246 nonsmokers and 61 smokers believed that nonsmoking students with smoke-aversive handicaps suffer discriminatory treatment because of smoke pollution. (11 ref).

195. Smith, Michael J. (1987). **Mental and physical strain at VDT workstations.** *Behaviour & Information Technology,* 6(3), 243–255.
Discusses health complaints that have been associated with the use of video display terminals (VDT), including visual and musculoskeletal discomfort and psychological distress, fears about radiation from VDTs, and concerns about adverse reproductive effects. A review of current research literature indicates that stress may be the most significant issue in terms of VDT work, but this is due to the way in which computers change the work activity.

196. Snyder, Solomon H. & D'Amato, Robert J. (1985). **Predicting Parkinson's disease.** *Nature,* 317(6034), 198–199.
Discusses recent studies of N-methyl-4-phenyl-tetrahydropyridine (MPTP), a simple phenylpyridine derivative that elicits parkinsonism, that have stimulated speculation that specific environmental toxins may underlie most cases of Parkinson's disease. The present authors present the main points of a study by D. B. Calne et al (1985), which has found a significant decline in the formation and retention of F-dopamine in 4 Ss exposed to MPTP, although not as great as in the Ss with severe idiopathic Parkinson's disease. Other environmental toxins that are likely factors in the etiology of idiopathic Parkinson's disease are also discussed. (29 ref).

197. Steinberg, William. (1981). **Residual neuropsychological effects following exposure to trichloroethylene (TCE): A case study.** *Clinical Neuropsychology,* 3(3), 1–4.
TCE is a neurotoxic compound commonly used at industrial sites. The present case report details the events surrounding 1 incident of intoxication and its chronic aftereffects in a 62-yr-old male who was hospitalized at age 56. The S, tested 5½ yrs following the accident using the Luria-Nebraska Neuropsychological Battery, WAIS, and Aphasia Screening Test, continued to show significant neurobehavioral deficits.

198. Stewart, Thomas R.; Middleton, Paulette & Ely, Daniel. (1983). **Urban visual air quality judgments: Reliability and validity.** *Journal of Environmental Psychology,* 3(2), 129–145.
A procedure based on judgments of human observers for measuring visual air quality in urban areas is described, and its reliability and validity are examined using the results of several studies conducted in a metropolitan area. Data from 8 observers indicate that the procedure provides a measure that is sufficiently reliable and valid to warrant its use in studies of the causes and consequences of changes in visual air quality. (19 ref).

199. Stone, Jimmy D.; Breidenbach, Steven T. & Heimstra, Norman W. (1979). **Annoyance response of nonsmokers to cigarette smoke.** *Perceptual & Motor Skills,* 49(3), 907–916.
In 3 experiments, a total of 160 18–29 yr old nonsmoking Ss rated their annoyance by task environments while either exposed or not exposed to ambient tobacco smoke. In Exps I and II, Ss rated annoyance with the environment while exposed to 3 intensities of noise, and in Exp III, Ss rated annoyance while performing multiplication problems under conditions of high and low task motivation. The source of the ambient smoke in Exp I was a smoke pump. For Exps II and III, the source of the smoke was confederate Ss. No differences in annoyance were obtained in Exps I and II as a function of exposure to smoke. Exp III showed that nonsmokers' annoyance to a task environment is dependent upon task motivation and exposure to ambient smoke. In Exp III, nonsmokers exposed to smoke were more annoyed than those not exposed under low motivating conditions. When Ss were highly motivated in the task environment, those exposed to smoke were significantly less annoyed than those not exposed. (8 ref).

200. Stone, Russell A. & Levine, Adeline G. (1986). **Reactions to collective stress: Correlates of active citizen participation at Love Canal.** Special Issue: Beyond the individual: Environmental approaches and prevention. *Prevention in Human Services,* 4(1–2), 153–177.
Describes events related to the chemical accident in the spring of 1978 at Love Canal as an environmental crisis leading to acute collective stress. As the crisis unfolded, Love Canal residents' perceptions of the situation, and the actions they took, were monitored through interviews with 58 families in the fall of 1978. Of these, 39 were reinterviewed the following spring. Among interviewed families, 24 had at least one activist member who became personally involved in a community organization formed to help resolve the crisis. The social characteristics, Love Canal-related problems, sources of help, and general views of the impacts on personal lives and interpersonal relations of activist and nonactivist families are compared. Activists relied on government and crisis-related organizations for help, while nonactivists had more family support. Neither group utilized the mental health services provided by the community's crisis center. Activists felt better about themselves and had a stronger feeling of personal efficacy in affecting government decisions. They perceived that the crisis had brought about positive personal and interpersonal changes. (15 ref).

201. Struwe, Göran; Knave, Bengt & Mindus, Per. (1983). **Neuropsychiatric symptoms in workers occupationally exposed to jet fuel: A combined epidemiological and casuistic study.** *Acta Psychiatrica Scandinavica,* 67(Suppl 303), 55–67.
30 27–66 yr old workers exposed to jet fuel (about 250 mg/m^3) for 4–32 yrs were compared with 2 matched control groups (30 Ss each) of nonexposed workers. Standardized interviews and examination of medical records showed that exposed Ss had, after their employment, more often sought medical advice because of emotional dysfunctions, such as depression and anxiety, than had controls. When mental symptoms, indicative of brain lesion, were rated later by psychiatrists, exposed Ss scored higher than controls. 14 Ss showing most symptoms were selected for neuropsychiatric clinical investigation comprising psychosocial inquiries, psychological testing, personality assessment, and neurological/neurophysiological examinations. Seven Ss were judged to suffer from mild organic brain syndrome. Ss had all undergone a slow but steady personality change over the years, starting from an ordinary strength without neurotic traits and moving toward an asthenic state with fatigue, anxiety, and vegetative hyperreactivity. It is concluded that personality changes and emotional dysfunctions are the foremost effects of long-term exposure to petroleum products. (23 ref).

202. Summers, David M. (1980). **Clinical electrophysiological investigation of a sleep disorder related to a suspected neurotoxin: A field study on Michigan residents exposed to PBB.** *Dissertation Abstracts International,* 41(4-B), 1299.

203. Suzuki, Tatsuzo; Ohsumi, Noboru & Takahashi, Kazuko. (1977). **Attitudes toward environmental problems.** *Proceedings of the Institute of Statistical Mathematics,* 24(2), 95–127.

BEHAVIORAL TOXICOLOGY: GENERAL

Examined the relationship between residents' subjective assessments of air pollution and pollutant data obtained by observatories. Questionnaires were completed by the residents of the southwest section of Chiba City, where 19 observatories obtained data on SO_2, O_2, NO, NO_2, CO, HC, HF, tape dust, digital dust, wind direction, wind velocity, temperature, and humidity. Data for November 1974 to April 1975 were analyzed by the use of a multidimensional scaling method. The subjective assessments of pollution by residents living very near the observatories and the pollutant data obtained by the observatories themselves were highly correlated, but there was no correlation between the observatory data and the subjective assessments of residents who lived farther away from the observatories. Results also indicate that the residents' subjective assessments were clearly influenced by the physical conditions of their environment (e.g., population density, weather, and noise pollution). (English summary).

204. Tapia, C. (1978). **Environment and odours.** *International Review of Applied Psychology,* 27(1), 39–51.
Interviewed 171 townspeople, chosen on the basis of their distance from or relationship with a local factory, to determine their attitudes toward pollution caused by odors. No correlation was found between the actual concentration of the odorous pollution and the sensitivity of the people to it. Sensitivity varied as a function of psychological, situational, and sociological factors; e.g., the age of those interviewed, and the Ss' opinions about the factory's influence on the community, influenced their estimates of the discomfort they experienced. (English summary).

205. Taylor, Eric. (1979). **Food additives, allergy and hyperkinesis.** *Journal of Child Psychology & Psychiatry & Allied Disciplines,* 20(4), 357–363.
A review of the literature indicates that there is no persuasive evidence that intolerance of food additives is a major cause of hyperactivity. Evidence from challenge studies and from clinical anecdotes suggests that eliminating additives from the diet might prove to have helpful effects for a minority of children (especially those under 6 yrs). Research should aim not only to replicate the design of existing studies, but also to include more objective measures of change, more evidence of allergy, and more attention to the possibility of predicting change. (30 ref).

206. Tedeschi, Richard G.; Cann, Arnie & Siegfried, William D. (1982). **Participation in voluntary auto emissions inspection.** *Journal of Social Psychology,* 117(2), 309–310.
43 drivers attending a voluntary auto emissions inspection and 63 randomly selected drivers responded to a study on environmental problems. Those attending the inspection reported perceiving that pollution had a direct effect on their lives more than did those in the random sample. The 2 groups did not differ on measures of environmental concern, knowledge, and control or in their assignment of responsibility for pollution and its control. Heightening awareness of the direct effects on pollution may be more effective in enhancing personal responsibility for pollution than efforts to change attitudes, knowledge, or personality variables.

207. Terry, Robert D. (1986). **Does Alzheimer's disease spread, and is it causally related to aluminum?** Special Issue: Controversial topics on Alzheimer's disease: Intersecting crossroads. *Neurobiology of Aging,* 7(6), 570.
Questions views expressed by E. Roberts (1986) concerning lesions in the olfactory cortex associated with Alzheimer's disease (AD), which Roberts believes is an indication of the early involvement of this area, with subsequent spread. The present author contends that degenerative diseases probably do not spread, but rather affect the nervous system according to local vulnerability.

208. Thatcher, R. W.; McAlaster, R.; Lester, M. L. & Cantor, D. S. (1984). **Comparisons among EEG, hair minerals and diet predictions of reading performance in children.** *Annals of the New York Academy of Sciences,* 433, 87–96.
Examined the relationship between nutrition (focusing on refined carbohydrate intake, hair trace elements, and electrophysiological measures) and reading ability as the 1st step in developing a causal model of ecological factors that play a role in child development and reading ability. 184 children (aged 5–16) completed a dietary assessment, psychometric measures (including either the WISC or the WPPSI and the Wide Range Achievement Test), a hair analysis, and electrophysiological data analyses. Results indicate that EEG measures of relative power and interhemispheric coherence, hair mineral concentrations, and refined carbohydrate intake were significantly related to reading achievement. Partial correlation coefficients showed that relative EEG power in the delta band in the temporal region and the concentration of cadmium were negatively correlated with reading achievement, while frontal coherence and the concentration of zinc were positively associated with reading achievement. (19 ref).

209. Trigg, Linda J.; Perlman, Daniel; Perry, Raymond P. & Janisse, Michel P. (1976). **Anti-pollution behavior: A function of perceived outcome and locus of control.** *Environment & Behavior,* 8(2), 307–313.
Examined the moderating effects of perceived outcome on the relationship between activism in the form of antipollution behavior and internal-external (I-E) locus of control. A representative sample of the adult population of Winnipeg, Manitoba (433 Ss) was interviewed. As predicted, among people optimistic about future levels of pollution, internally oriented individuals engaged in more antipollution activities. Among pessimistic respondents there was virtually no relationship between I-E and social actions. Internals also had more accurate information about environmental pollution.

210. Tvedt, Bjørn. (1984). **Nevropsykologisk testing ved løsemiddelskader. / Neuropsychological testing by chronic toxic encephalopathy.** *Tidsskrift for Norsk Psykologforening,* 21(10), 500–505.
Administered psychological testing to 95 patients between 1980 and 1983. 25 Ss had test results considered compatible with chronic toxic encephalopathy; 20 Ss had results indicating other causes; and 36 Ss had normal results. 14 Ss had results that could not be accurately interpreted. A case of encephalopathy in a car painter exemplified the method used. It is probable that only a few of the total number of cases are reported. (English abstract) (27 ref).

211. Valentine, John H.; Ebert, John; Oakey, Richard & Ernst, Karl. (1975). **Human crises and the human environment.** *Man-Environment Systems,* 5(1), 23–28.
Studied the relationships between 3 classes of environmental events (13 weather factors, 5 pollution measures, news events) and human crises and their resolution (29 dependent variables, including psychiatric diagnoses and the nature of death). The multiple regression analysis was based on 849 psychiatric contacts at one municipal hospital, and 1,513 deaths, city wide, all in Philadelphia, over a 92-day period June to September 1970. As proposed by R. W. Moos (unpublished APA task force report), the relationship between environmental events and human crises was polyfactorial, summative, and differential. That is, the summation of the 3 classes of environmental events accounted for significant amounts of the variability in patient flow (patient sex, age, marital status; type of hospital contact; hospital shift) and psychiatric diagnoses. Moreover different environmental variables summated to account for different dependent variables. As a group, weather variables were the most important factors; news events, as a class, showed the least linkage. The potential effects on human crises of manipulating news headlines and pollution are explored. The usefulness of a regional

fingerprint, formulating environment-behavior patterns across regions varying in earth-meteorological and topographic features, is noted. (27 ref)

212. Vasilescu, I. P. (1984). **Danger evaluation.** *Revue Roumaine des Sciences Sociales - Série de Psychologie,* 28(1), 43–50.
Studied differences of subjective danger evaluation of 83 industry workers concerning 2 situations: accident danger and industrial illness (illness related to exposure to toxic industrial agents). It was found that the subjective probability and the perceived importance of loss were not the only factors that interfered in danger evaluation. The subjective importance of loss often influenced and was influenced by the subjective probability of the dangerous event. Implications of these results for the classical model of perceived magnitude of danger are discussed.

213. Wall, Geoffrey. (1973). **Public response to air pollution in South Yorkshire, England.** *Environment & Behavior,* 5(2), 219–248.
Compared a survey of 40 residents in each of 3 areas of South Yorkshire, conducted in March 1972, with results of an earlier survey in Sheffield. Topics included perceptions of air pollution and attitudes toward alternative adjustments to air pollution. Responses in the 2 surveys tended to be similar. Different rates of adoption of smoke control zones were attributed to group processes involving decision makers and/or interest groups who put pressure on decision makers. It is concluded that the household interview may not be the most appropriate research instrument for studying this process.

214. Ward, Christopher D. (1986). **Commentary on "Alzheimer's disease may begin in the nose and may be caused by aluminosilicates."** Special Issue: Controversial topics on Alzheimer's disease: Intersecting crossroads. *Neurobiology of Aging,* 7(6), 574–575.
Argues that E. Roberts's (1986) suggestion that the nose is the portal of entry for aluminosilicates is implausible but readily testable. The proposed mode of action of aluminosilicates in triggering changes in the structure and function of cerebral proteins is considered plausible but lacking in convincing data supporting the model.

215. White, Mary C.; Baker, Edward L.; Larson, Marilyn B. & Wolford, Rodney. (1988). **The role of personal beliefs and social influences as determinants of respirator use among construction painters.** *Scandinavian Journal of Work, Environment & Health,* 14(4), 239–245.
169 male spray painters were questioned about their beliefs concerning the consequences of wearing cartridge respirators, as well as about the perceived attitudes of others in the workplace toward respirators. Intended respirator use was more strongly associated with beliefs than was past use. The most important beliefs concerned discomfort or inconvenience. Other determinants associated with respirator use were respirator availability, cigarette smoking, and social influences.

216. Wimer, Richard E. (1986). **Two topics for further exploration.** Special Issue: Controversial topics on Alzheimer's disease: Intersecting crossroads. *Neurobiology of Aging,* 7(6), 584.
Comments on E. Roberts's (1986) hypothesis by arguing that information concerning brain regions selectively affected in Alzheimer's disease is still incomplete, and the unique involvement of olfactory regions remains to be demonstrated conclusively. The very high incidence of Alzheimer neuropathology in aging humans with Down's syndrome raises issues concerning the role of aluminosilicates.

217. Wolpert, Edward A. (1977). **Nontoxic hyperlithemia in impending mania.** *American Journal of Psychiatry,* 134(5), 580–582.
Presents the case report of a 26-yr-old woman with prodromal symptoms of mania that led her to take large amounts of lithium, reaching a maximum serum level of 4.5 mEq/liter, without experiencing any psychological, physiological, or electrolyte abnormalities. It is hypothesized that the presence of prodromal symptoms indicates a state in which lithium transport is interfered with temporarily, and high serum lithium levels can occur without lithium entering cells where toxic effects would occur.

218. Wright, I. & Simon, F. (1976). **Effects of data classification on mind set of grade six students.** *Alberta Journal of Educational Research,* 22(4), 297–304.
Researched the purported effects of reduction of "mind set" and achievement of greater consistency in data classification when using F. Simon's (1970) problem-solving approach. The presence of "mind set" relating to the desirability and feasibility of further controlling water pollution in Canada was identified in a pretest administered to 248 6th graders in 4 schools. Within each school, 4 random groups were formed, and a posttest, consisting of an article that pointed to the undesirability and unfeasibility of further controlling water pollution, was administered. Group 1 read the article; Group 2 classified the data with feasibility criteria specified; Group 3 was given desirability criteria also; and Group 4 was trained in classification procedures. Trained Ss scored significantly more correct classifications than did untrained Ss and achieved significantly more correct conclusions, indicating that "mind set" could be partially reduced through the classification procedures.

219. Zeidner, Moshe & Shechter, Mordechai. (1988). **Psychological responses to air pollution: Some personality and demographic correlates.** *Journal of Environmental Psychology,* 8(3), 191–208.
Examined affective reactions toward air pollution, and personality and demographic correlates of these reactions, by means of a survey of 923 households around Haifa, Israel. Data on trait anger and anxiety and perceptions and attitudes with respect to air pollution were also compiled. It was found that perceived level of pollution was a stronger predictor of affective reaction and willingness to pay to reduce pollution than was objective level of pollution. Findings suggest that Ss who were more emotionally aroused with respect to a polluted environment were more prone to put in time and more willing to allocate financial resources toward pollution abatement. Age, perceptions of tax inadequacy, and personality variables were implicated as correlates of negative affect and willingness to pay.

Animal Research

220. Adams, J.; Oglesby, D. M.; Ozemek, H. S.; Rath, J. et al. (1985). **Collaborative Behavioral Teratology Study: Programmed data entry and automated test systems.** Conference Proceedings of the National Center for Toxicological Research et al: Design considerations in screening for behavioral teratogens: Results of the collaborative behavioral teratology study (1985, Cincinnati, Ohio). *Neurobehavioral Toxicology & Teratology,* 7(6), 547–554.
Describes 2 microcomputer systems developed for use in J. Buelke-Sam and colleagues' (1985) Collaborative Behavioral Teratology Study. System 1 was designed to control stimulus delivery to and record behavioral responses from rats during a visual discrimination learning task and to accept data from physical landmark, negative geotaxis, and olfactory discrimination evaluations. System 2 controlled stimulus delivery and recorded behavioral responses from rats during an auditory startle habituation task and recorded rodent activity levels in figure 8 mazes for periods of 1, 4, or 23 hrs.

BEHAVIORAL TOXICOLOGY: GENERAL

221. Berman, Mark S. (1981). **The feeding behavior of the calanoid copepods of Narragansett Bay, Rhode Island.** *Dissertation Abstracts International,* 41(8-B), 2853.

222. Cohen, Gerald & Mytilineou, Catherine. (1985). **Studies on the mechanism of action of 1-methyl-4-phenyl-1,2,3,6-tetrahydropyridine (MPTP).** Meeting of the American Society for Pharmacology & Experimental Therapeutics: Pharmacological features of the dopaminergic neurotoxin MPTP (1984, Indianapolis, Indiana). *Life Sciences,* 36(3), 237–242.
Established explant cultures of embryonic rat substantia nigra that were sensitive to MPTP at concentrations approximating the doses given in vivo to monkeys. Fluorescence microscopy and ^{3}H-dopamine uptake measurements revealed that the toxicity is selective for dopamine neurons, whereas other neurons and cells in the culture appear normal by phase contrast microscopy. Results implicate monoamine oxidase (MAO) in the mechanism of action of MPTP. Two possible mechanisms for protection by MAO are discussed. (23 ref).

223. Correa Cruz, Manuel. (1984). **Physiological short-term indicators of chronic stress on the dragonfly *Somatochlora cingulata* (de Selys) (Odonata: Anisoptera).** *Dissertation Abstracts International,* 45(6-B), 1719.

224. Evans, G. W.; Lyes, M. & Lockwood, A. P. (1977). **Some effects of oil dispersants on the feeding behaviour of the brown shrimp, *Crangon crangon*.** *Marine Behavior & Physiology,* 4(3), 171–181.
Concentrations in the range 1–100 ppm of 2 commercial oil dispersants BP 1100X and Slickgone LT2, and an emulsifier, Tween 80, in sea water were shown to decrease both the food consumption of the shrimp and the ability of the animal to select the arm of a Y-maze that contained food extract. The ability to locate food was largely recovered within 4 hrs of return of the animals to clean sea water after prior exposure to 10 ppm Tween 80, 10 ppm BP 1100X, or 10 ppm Slickgone LT2.

225. Fries, Cara R. (1977). **Effects of phenol on the defense system of *Mercenaria mercenaria*.** *Dissertation Abstracts International,* 38(4-B), 1604.

226. Gerber, Gary J. & O'Shaughnessy, Donald. (1986). **Comparison of the behavioral effects of neurotoxic and systemically toxic agents: How discriminatory are behavioral tests of neurotoxicity?** *Neurobehavioral Toxicology & Teratology,* 8(6), 703–710.
Studied the specificity of behavioral measures of neurotoxicity by determining the extent to which behavioral measures were affected by organ toxicity or reduction of food and water intake using 4 groups with 10 male Sprague-Dawley rats in each. Liver damage produced by carbon tetrachloride, reduction of plasma glucose produced by insulin, or reduction of food and water intake for 1 wk caused effects similar to those of the neurotoxicants triethyltin, acrylamide, and 2,5-hexanedione; and the neuroleptic haloperidol. Among behavioral tests of activity and motor function, grip strength was best in distinguishing neurotoxicant and neuroactive agents. It is suggested that the function of nonneural tissues should be evaluated along with behavioral function in neurotoxicity evaluation.

227. Johannessen, Jan N. et al. (1985). **In vitro oxidation of MPTP by primate neural tissue: A potential model of MPTP neurotoxicity.** *Neurochemistry International,* 7(1), 169–176.
Examined the brain tissue of an adult rhesus monkey to determine mechanisms behind the neural metabolism of 1-methyl-1-4-phenyl-1,2,3,6-tetrahydropyridine (MPTP) in primates. Results indicate that the metabolism of MPTP occurred in the brain tissue in vitro. A model of MPTP neurotoxicity that incorporates findings to date is presented. It is proposed that since the toxicity of MPTP is metabolism dependent, the in vitro metabolism of MPTP by brain tissue should provide a useful model for studying selected aspects of MPTP neurotoxicity. (13 ref).

228. Karns, Daryl R. (1985). **Toxic bog water in northern Minnesota peatlands: Ecological and evolutionary consequences for breeding amphibians.** *Dissertation Abstracts International,* 45(9-B), 2794–2795.

229. Lewis, Stephen J. & Malecki, Richard A. (1984). **Effects of egg oiling on larid productivity and population dynamics.** *Auk,* 101(3), 584–592.
Conducted a study in which oil was applied to naturally incubated great black-backed gull (*Larus marinus*) and herring gull (*L. argentatus*) eggs and assessed its effects on reproductive success. Embryo survival was inversely proportional to the quantity of petroleum applied to eggshell surfaces. Dose responses were dependent on embryonic age at the time of treatment. Fuel oil weathered outdoors for several weeks was as toxic as fresh oil to larid embryos. (60 ref).

230. Nowak, Robert T. (1984). **The importance of pharmacologically active skin agents of the newt *Taricha granulosa* including the behavioral toxicology of tetrodotoxin.** *Dissertation Abstracts International,* 44(12-B), 3684.

231. Parker, Howard B. (1981). **Inclusive fitness and optimal poisoning-prevention strategies: A perspective on food-aversion learning.** *Dissertation Abstracts International,* 42(3-B), 1227.

232. Poje, Gerald V. (1981). **Responses of *Gammarus tigrinus* to short-term exposure at elevated temperatures and chlorine-produced oxidant stress.** *Dissertation Abstracts International,* 42(3-B), 878–879.

233. Revusky, Sam; Parker, Linda A. & Coombes, Shannon. (1977). **Flavor aversion learning: Extinction of the aversion to an interfering flavor after conditioning does not affect the aversion to the reference flavor.** *Behavioral & Neural Biology,* 19(4), 503–508.
In 2 experiments, male Sprague-Dawley rats consumed 2 flavored solutions prior to the same instance of toxicosis. One solution was called the reference solution because the study was concerned with the subsequent aversion to it, while the other solution was called the interfering solution. It is known that if the interfering flavored solution has been made familiar to the rat prior to toxicosis training, the aversion to the reference solution will be stronger than if the interfering solution is novel. It is as though the S considers it unlikely on the basis of prior experience that the familiar solution could have produced the toxicosis and, hence, decides that the reference solution must have been responsible. However, by similar logic, Ss ought to have equally strong aversions to the reference solution if the interfering solution is made familiar after toxicosis training but before testing. Results show, however, that this did not occur.

234. Salzinger, Kurt; Fairhurst, Stephen P.; Freimark, Steven J. & Wolkoff, F. Dmitri. (1973). **Behavior of the goldfish as an early warning system for the presence of pollutants in water.** *Journal of Environmental Systems,* 3(1), 27–40.
Reviews toxicity and behavioral studies of the effects of pollutants on fish and presents results of an experiment on the effects of 2 levels of polluted water on the behavior of 12 goldfish. Ss were trained to press a lever on FI, FR, extinction, and discrimination schedules of reinforcement. Three Ss from each condition were then placed in water with high and low concentrations of mercury (.01 and .006 ppm) or in unpolluted water. All Ss placed in highly polluted water showed the largest percentage drop in response rate, and all but 1 S in the low pollution water showed the 2nd largest

decrease in response rate. Results suggest that goldfish may be used as monitors of pollution. (31 ref).

235. Silbergeld, Ellen K. (1985). **The relevance of animal models for neurotoxic disease states.** *International Journal of Mental Health,* 14(3), 26–43.
Discusses the use of animal models to develop preclinical markers of exposure and effects for neuropsychiatric disorders associated with exposure to environmental pollutants. Animal models can be used to provide the basic data for establishing exposure markers under conditions in which external or environmental exposure can be controlled and quantitated and various tissues or fluids can be sampled during or after exposure. Animal models, however, usually reflect human disease states in terms of exposure rather than effect. In the absence of agreement on the relationship between certain well-described human mental illnesses and behavioral states in animals, fundamental behavioral states in animals such as locomotor activity, active and passive avoidance, and simple maze learning are likely to be most useful for determining neurotoxic effects. The need to increase communication between clinical and experimental toxicologists is stressed. (43 ref).

236. Silverman, A. Paul. (1988). **An ethologist's approach to behavioural toxicology.** *Neurotoxicology & Teratology,* 10(2), 85–92.
Describes the application of 2 ethological methods that may provide a basis for solving behavioral toxicology problems. The 1st method involves objective observation of rat behavior in social situations to detect chemically induced changes at low doses. Such changes were specific and repeatable in long-term experiments: Effects of nicotine at a smoking dose or trichloroethylene at the threshold limit value were reversible; limited tolerance developed to methyl mercury dicyandiamide. The 2nd, exploration-thirst method is simple enough for use as a screen. It was compared with conventional toxicological methods for 30 compounds in routine screening (20 acute ip, 10 subacute inhalation). Both ethological methods were sensitive enough to estimate no-effect doses and distinguish nonspecific toxic effects (consistent with the animal's equivalent of "feeling ill") from more specific central nervous system (CNS) effects comparable to those of human experience.

237. Sutterlin, A. M. (1974). **Pollutants and the chemical senses of aquatic animals: Perspective and review.** *Chemical Senses & Flavor,* 1(2), 167–178.
Reviews experimental research from the literature on (a) the importance of chemical communication in aquatic animals, (b) possible types of interactions between pollutants and chemosensory systems resulting in disturbances in behavior patterns, (c) methods used in studying some of these interactions, and (d) pollution types. Results indicate that fish under laboratory testing conditions avoid a variety of pollutants at sublethal levels; however, only in a few instances has similar behavior been observed in the field. The degree of toxicity and the avoidance level of many pollutants do not seem to be related, and many pollutants are not avoided at concentrations exceeding the lethal level. In fact, some instances of attraction by lethal concentrations are reported. Attempts to extend laboratory avoidance levels to field conditions where other variables, such as gradient steepness and the presence of other motivational factors, should be done with caution. Analogies to human senses and environments are noted. (3 p ref).

238. Tamaki, Yoshitaka & Inouye, Minoru. (1988). **Go/no-go discriminated avoidance learning in prenatally x-irradiated rats.** *Neurotoxicology & Teratology,* 10(1), 35–38.
Exposed male rats to x-irradiation on Day 17 of gestation and tested them at age 10–13 wks in a go/no-go (active-passive) discriminated avoidance conditioning paradigm. During the 1st conditioning session, Ss learned only active avoidance responses to 2 different warning signals. During the 2nd and 3rd sessions, Ss learned active and passive avoidance responses in response to 1 warning signal. Ss made more active avoidance responses than controls to both warning signals in the 1st session. In the early training phase of the go/no-go task, Ss performed more active and fewer passive avoidance responses than controls. Ss established a strong tendency to respond actively to the no-go signal but eventually learned the associated passive response.

239. Young, Robert W. (1979). **Prediction of the relative toxicity of environmental toxins as a function of behavioral and non-behavioral endpoints.** *Dissertation Abstracts International,* 40(4-B), 1937.

PESTICIDES

240. Blackburn, Archie B. (1983). **Review of the effects of Agent Orange: A psychiatric perspective on the controversy.** *Military Medicine,* 148(4), 333–340.
Discusses research on the harmful effects of exposure to Agent Orange, a defoliant used in Vietnam to destroy jungle vegetation that provided cover for guerilla warfare and destroyed enemy food crops. It is concluded that regardless of whether or not Vietnam veterans suffer from Agent Orange toxicity, many who present with complaints or fears of Agent Orange effects are significantly psychiatrically disordered. It is suggested that the term "Agent Orange pseudo-toxicity" be used to represent a possible presentation of veterans with posttraumatic stress disorder or other mental disorders.

241. Burchfiel, James L. & Duffy, Frank H. (1982). **Organophosphate neurotoxicity: Chronic effects of sarin on the electroencephalogram of monkey and man.** *Neurobehavioral Toxicology & Teratology,* 4(6), 767–778.
Rhesus monkeys were injected with sarin according to 1 of 2 schedules: (1) a single "large dose" (5 µg/kg) that produced overt signs of acute toxicity or (2) a series of 10 "small doses" (1 µg/kg at 1-wk intervals) that did not produce any major clinical signs. EEGs were recorded before sarin injection and at 24 hrs and 1 yr postdrug. Both large- and small-dose sarin injections resulted in significant and persistent increases in the relative amount of high frequency beta activity (13–50 Hz) in comparison with controls injected with vehicle only. In Study 2, waking and sleep EEGs were obtained from 125 industrial workers exposed or not exposed to sarin. Exposed Ss showed increases in beta activity and REM sleep. Attempts to derive classification rules were inconclusive, but suggested that the EEGs of some workers exposed to sarin were not affected and that there is a threshold for this type of sarin neurotoxicity. Results are discussed in terms of previous studies indicating that organophosphates were responsible for schizophrenia and depressive reactions, memory deficits, and difficulties in maintaining attention. (42 ref).

242. Cawte, John. (1985). **Psychiatric sequelae of manganese exposure in the adult, foetal and neonatal nervous systems.** *Australian & New Zealand Journal of Psychiatry,* 19(3), 211–217.
Discusses the effects of manganese on the fetal, neonatal, and adult nervous systems; the eco-toxicology of manganese and its effects on brain amines; variations in individual susceptibility; and difficulties in clinical testing. It is noted that the manganese content of infant formulas may be related to the development of learning disabilities and hyperkinesis, and that manganese can lead to a progressive syndrome in adults that includes symptoms of mania, memory deficits, and motor disturbances.

PESTICIDES

243. Hall, Wayne & MacPhee, Donald. (1985). **Do Vietnam veterans suffer from toxic neurasthenia?** *Australian & New Zealand Journal of Psychiatry,* 19(1), 19–29.
Discusses the case for and against toxic neurasthenia in Australian troops exposed to pesticides while serving in Vietnam who subsequently developed psychiatric disorders. The case for has been made mainly by C. Van Tiggelen (1982) who cited evidence that occupational exposure to chemicals can produce a neurasthenic syndrome and asserted that toxic neurasthenia can be distinguished from neurasthenia due to other causes by the presence of the linguomental reflex. The case against includes data from controlled studies, the pattern of exposure in veterans vs workers, a difference in natural history, and the known psychiatric consequences of war. It is suggested that the hidden agenda of much of the argument is the issue of compensation. It is concluded that the psychiatric disorders among Vietnam veterans are connected to war service but are not the result of chemical exposure. (56 ref).

244. Lewin, Roger. (1985). **Parkinson's disease: An environmental cause?** *Science,* 229(4710), 257–258.
Examines the developmental/environmental controversy over the etiology of Parkinson's disease by contrasting findings presented at a National Institutes of Health meeting regarding behavioral correlates of Parkinson's disease with Canadian findings that correlated disease incidence with pesticide use. It is suggested that the delayed onset of symptoms in Ss exposed to 1-methyl-4-phenyl-1,2,3-tetrahydropyridine (MPTP) might be a result of MPTP conversion to the major stable metabolite 1-methyl-4-phenylpyridinium ion (MPP+) in glia, followed by selective uptake by dopaminergic neurons; however, it is asserted that many etiological questions remain unanswered. (3 ref).

245. Miller, Diane B. (1982). **Neurotoxicity of the pesticidal carbamates.** *Neurobehavioral Toxicology & Teratology,* 4(6), 779–787.
Reviews research on the neurotoxicity of carbamate compounds, as characterized by behavioral, neurochemical, electrophysiological, and neuropathological indices. Acute administration of cholinesterase-inhibiting carbamates decreases activity and schedule-controlled behavior, interferes with avoidance and escape performance, and decreases the amplitude of a variety of electrophysiological measures. Evidence that these compounds interfere with learning and memory is equivocal, and there is no adequate data that they produce neurobehavioral consequences following exposure during gestation or the early postnatal period. High doses of dithiocarbamates have produced hyperactivity and ataxia, followed by a decrease in muscle tone, decreased activity, and clonic convulsions. Certain compounds have been shown to produce nerve degeneration, hindlimb paralysis, and EEG abnormalities. Certain compounds have also been implicated in developmental deficits in open-field activity, passive avoidance, and decreases in brain weight and norepinephrine levels. (135 ref).

Human Research

246. Bonithon-Kopp, Claire; Huel, Guy; Moreau, Thierry & Wendling, Robert. (1986). **Prenatal exposure to lead and cadmium and psychomotor development of the child at 6 years.** *Neurobehavioral Toxicology & Teratology,* 8(3), 307–310.
In 1977, a hair sample was taken from 26 newborn babies and their mothers and analyzed for lead and cadmium. Each child was given a psychometric test (McCarthy Scales of Children's Abilities) 6 yrs later. Statistical analysis showed a significant negative relationship between the degree of in utero exposure to cadmium and lead and the child's motor and perceptual abilities. Effects on memory or verbal skills were not significant. Allowing for the confounding variables did not consistently affect the results.

247. Carlson, Shally L. (1983). **The effectiveness of fear appeals as a measure of persuasion in the acceptance of pesticide protective garments.** *Dissertation Abstracts International,* 43(9-A), 3096.

248. Davis, Kenneth L.; Yesavage, Jerome A. & Berger, Philip A. (1978). **Possible organophosphate-induced parkinsonism.** *Journal of Nervous & Mental Disease,* 166(3), 222–225.
Presents a case of possible organophosphate-induced parkinsonism in a 53-yr-old male crop duster who had had numerous episodes of acute organophosphate intoxication and chronic organophosphate exposure. A possible relationship between chronic organophosphate exposure and alterations in central cholinergic or dopaminergic activity is suggested.

249. Green, Lois M. (1987). **Suicide and exposure to phenoxy acid herbicides.** *Scandinavian Journal of Work, Environment & Health,* 13(5), 460.
When a cohort mortality study was carried out on 1,222 male workers employed 6 mo or more in forestry work and exposed to phenoxy acid herbicides, an excess number of deaths due to suicide were revealed. Reports citing associations between neurological toxicity and exposure to phenoxy acid herbicides are discussed.

250. Hawkes, Glenn R.; Pilisuk, Marc; Stiles, Martha C. & Acredolo, Curt. (1984). **Assessing risk: A public analysis of the Medfly eradication program.** *Public Opinion Quarterly,* 48(2), 443–451.
Examined the cases of 126 15–74 yr old residents from a metropolitan area who, during the 1981–1982 Mediterranean fruitfly crisis, were undergoing exposure to aerial spraying with a pesticide. Four dependent variables were measured: degree of perceived health risk, degree of perceived environmental risk, number of precautions taken, and degree of acceptability. Results exemplify the politicization of risk; this perception was influenced by perceived benefit, political affiliation, and confidence in experts. (17 ref).

251. Hoffman, Jeanne S. (1986). **The effects of prenatal heptachlor exposure on infant development.** *Dissertation Abstracts International,* 46(7-B), 2474.

252. Korgeski, Gregory P. & Leon, Gloria R. (1983). **Correlates of self-reported and objectively determined exposure to Agent Orange.** *American Journal of Psychiatry,* 140(11), 1443–1449.
Examined the relationship between 100 27–59 yr old Vietnam veterans' self-reported and objectively determined exposure to the herbicide Agent Orange and the relationship between self- or objective ratings and self-reported psychological and medical problems. Ss who believed they had been exposed reported more psychological and medical problems than the other Ss but did not differ on "success at living" indices; the medical problems many reported suggested psychosomatic etiologies. Grouped according to objective ratings of herbicide exposure, Ss did not show such differences in psychological or medical problems. No differences on neuropsychological testing appeared, regardless of how Ss were grouped. (14 ref).

253. Levin, Harvey S.; Rodnitzky, Robert L. & Mick, David L. (1976). **Anxiety associated with exposure to organophosphate compounds.** *Archives of General Psychiatry,* 33(2), 225–228.
24 commerical pesticide sprayers and farmers recently exposed to organophosphate agents were compared to 24 controls (mean ages, 39.17 and 38.83 yrs, respectively) on the Taylor Manifest Anxiety Scale, Beck Depression Inventory, a structured interview, and cholinesterase level. The commercial sprayers but not the exposed farmers showed elevated levels of anxiety and lower plasma cholinesterase than control Ss. Assessment of other behavioral manifestations and red blood cell cholinesterase failed to disclose other group differ-

ences. Findings tentatively point to the possibility that organophosphate compounds may produce subtle defects in workers who are not obviously toxic. (24 ref).

254. Levy, Charles J. (1988). **Agent Orange exposure and posttraumatic stress disorder.** *Journal of Nervous & Mental Disease,* 176(4), 242-245.
Evidence of organic psychological deficits in Vietnam veterans exposed to the herbicide Agent Orange was established through a neuropsychological battery. The 6 exposed Ss, in contrast to a matched control group of 25 veterans, showed a significantly higher rate of posttraumatic stress disorder (PTSD) and its associated features: depression, anxiety, and increased aggression. The latter was subdivided into uncontrollable pressures, verbal violence, violence against objects, assaults, and suicidal thoughts. Active cases of chloracne, a medical indicator, were used to determine Agent Orange exposure.

255. Rodnitzky, Robert L.; Levin, Harvey S. & Morgan, Donald P. (1978). **Effects of ingested parathion on neurobehavioral functions.** *Clinical Toxicology,* 13(3), 347-359.
Gave 2 healthy male volunteers (aged 53 and 62 yrs) small doses of parathion over 4 5-day periods separated by 1-8 wks. At prescribed intervals, Ss were subjected to a battery of neurobehavioral tests. Using Ss' preexposure performance as a control, data analysis showed that the pesticide had no significant effects on cognitive, psychomotor, or emotive functions. (26 ref).

256. Sadovnikova, L. D. & Churkin, E. A. (1982). **Clinical picture of acute poisonings with organophosphorus compounds: Follow-up data.** *Zhurnal Nevropatologii i Psikhiatrii,* 82(4), 595-597.
Examined 59 patients who had suffered acute poisoning with organophosphorus insecticides. The main psychopathological disorders in the late period after the poisoning manifested in the forms of asthenic or hypochondriacal syndromes of varying degree. These symptom complexes were related to the psychopathological structure of the acute intoxication period. A group of patients showing no psychic disorders in the late postintoxication period was revealed. (English abstract) (9 ref).

257. Săndulescu, Georgeta et al. (1982). **Aspecte ale encefalopatiei toxice profesionale cu clorură de etil-mercur. / Aspects of occupational toxic encephalopathy following intoxication with mercury-ethyl chloride.** *Neurologie, Psihiatrie, Neurochirurgie,* 27(4), 271-276.
Studied the clinical manifestations in 20 patients hospitalized for chronic or subacute intoxication with mercury-ethyl chloride (Cryptodyl), a pesticide. In order of predominance, neurological changes consisted of headache, vertigo, asthenia, sleep disturbances, and behavioral changes consisting of agitation or increased impulsivity, memory disturbances, or a confusional state. Some Ss also had paresthesia (especially in the upper limbs), trembling of the fingers or head, and speech disturbances (slight dysarthria and slowness or slurring of speech). All of these changes coexisted with other clinical manifestations (e.g., digestive or kidney disturbances). Toxicological tests were strongly positive. Therapy with chelating agents and removal of Ss from the toxic environment produced progressive attenuation of symptoms only in some cases. A case study is presented. (English & Russian abstracts).

258. Schum, Timothy R. & Lachman, Barry S. (1982). **Effect of packaging and appearance on childhood poisoning: Vacor Rat Poison.** *Clinical Pediatrics,* 21(5), 282-285.
Reviewed the records of 14 10-mo-old to 6.5-yr-old patients hospitalized for rodenticide ingestions over a 13-mo period. 10 Ss had ingested Vacor Rat Poison (N-3-pyridylmethyl N'-p-nitrophenyl urea). It is argued that small children could easily mistake Vacor, which resembles corn meal, for breakfast cereal. To intervene for safer packaging of toxic substances, pediatricians need to be aware of the health hazard posed to children by attractive packaging. (14 ref).

259. Senewiratne, B. & Thambipillai, Shanthi. (1974). **Pattern of poisoning in a developing agricultural country.** *British Journal of Preventive & Social Medicine,* 28(1), 32-36.
Reports data from 472 cases of poisoning during a 2-yr period in Ceylon. The overall mortality rate was 23.7%. The pattern of poisoning was different from that observed in Western countries (49.8% were due to insecticides and only 10.7% due to drugs). Age, sex, and hospitalization data are presented.

260. Sterman, Arnold & Varma, Andre. (1983). **Evaluating human neurotoxicity of the pesticide aldicarb: When man becomes the experimental animal.** *Neurobehavioral Toxicology & Teratology,* 5(5), 493-495.
Assessed aldicarb-induced neurobehavioral/neurologic syndromes by means of a questionnaire sent to 25 families who had been exposed to the pesticide in well water. Results are presented in terms of the need for further study since they indicate, but do not prove, a significant association between the number of neurological symptoms reported and increasing aldicarb exposure. (15 ref).

261. Weisman, Joan M. (1986). **The effects of exposure to Agent Orange on the intellectual functioning, academic achievement, visual-motor skills, and activity level of the offspring of Vietnam war veterans.** *Dissertation Abstracts International,* 47(3-B), 1300.

Animal Research

262. Abou-Donia, Mohamed B. (1978). **Role of acid phosphatase in delayed neurotoxicity induced by leptophos in hens.** *Biochemical Pharmacology,* 27(16), 2055-2058.
Studied leptophos, an insecticide which causes neurological damage, in 21 adult female chickens that received doses of 0.0, 0.5, 1.0, 2.5, 5, 10, and 20 mg/kg/day for up to 129 days. Onset of ataxia and paralysis and histological changes in nerve tissues (myelin and axons) were related to the dosage levels, as were decreased plasma cholinesterase and increased acid phosphatase activity. Possible explanations for the results are discussed, along with their relevance for encephalomyelitis and multiple sclerosis research and for the detection of overexposure to such chemicals. (25 ref).

263. Adams, Jane; Buelke-Sam, Judy; Kimmel, Carole A.; Nelson, C. J. et al. (1985). **Collaborative Behavioral Teratology Study: Preliminary research.** Conference Proceedings of the National Center for Toxicological Research et al: Design considerations in screening for behavioral teratogens: Results of the collaborative behavioral teratology study (1985, Cincinnati, Ohio). *Neurobehavioral Toxicology & Teratology,* 7(6), 555-578.
Reviews preliminary experiments conducted prior to the beginning of J. Buelke-Sam and colleagues' (1985) Collaborative Behavioral Teratology Study (CBTS) to permit the selection and verification of dosage levels of dextroamphetamine sulfate and methylmercuric chloride to be used in the CBTS. The studies included evaluations of any teratogenic effects on rats produced by selected concentrations of the chemicals, the potential pathology produced in the dams and offspring, and the postnatal behavioral consequences of the prenatal exposures. It is noted that this preliminary research allowed the determination of the most appropriate experimental design for the CBTS, verified the practicality of the schedule of work, specified all necessary procedural details, and provided a database for the determination of the appropriate statistical techniques for the analyses of the data.

PESTICIDES

264. Akkermans, Louis M.; Van den Bercken, Joep & Van der Zalm, Johan M. (1975). **Effects of aldrin-transdiol on neuromuscular facilitation and depression.** *European Journal of Pharmacology,* 31(2), 166-175.

265. Albright, Michael E. & Simmel, Edward C. (1979). **Behavioral effects of the cholinesterase inhibitor and insecticide carbaryl (*Sevin*).** *Journal of Biological Psychology,* 21(1), 25-31.
16 male Long-Evans hooded rats received 8 adaptation trials in a white translucent Plexiglas box placed on a Selective Activity Meter. Ss received no injection before the 1st 6 trials. 30 min before the 7th and 8th trials, Ss received 1 cc/kg polyethylene glycol 200, sc. Then Ss were divided into drug and control groups. The drug group received 10 mg/kg carbaryl dissolved in polyethylene glycol 200, and the control group received polyethylene glycol 200. All injections were sc into the abdominal region and were given 30 min before the trials. Ss then received 2 more trials in the box. Ss received, 1 wk later, the same injections and were placed into a novel exploratory chamber containing 2 stimulus cards. After carbaryl injections there was a significant increase in activity in the familiar situation. In the novel situation, carbaryl decreased the number of approaches to the novel stimuli, decreased exploration of the exploratory box, and increased habituation. (29 ref).

266. Al-Hachim, Ghazi M. (1973). **Effects of chlordane on conditioned avoidance response, brain seizure threshold and open-field performance of prenatally-treated mice.** *British Journal of Pharmacology,* 49(2), 311-316.
Gave 3 groups of 6 pregnant albino mice daily oral doses of chlordane (1 or 2.5 mg/kg) or olive oil (10 ml/kg) for 7 consecutive days. Three 3 groups of 10 young Ss, progeny of treated mothers, were tested for conditioned avoidance response, electroshock seizure threshold, and open-field performance. Results indicate significant differences between chlordane-treated and olive oil-treated offspring in the following respects: Chlordane seems to diminish avoidance learning, to raise brain seizure threshold, and to increase exploratory activity.

267. Ali, S. Fatehyab; Chandra, Om & Hasan, Mahdi. (1980). **Effects of an organophosphate (Dichlorvos) on open field behavior and locomotor activity: Correlation with regional brain monoamine levels.** *Psychopharmacology,* 68(1), 37-42.
Dichlorvos, which is used as both a contact and systemic insecticide, was administered ip (3 mg/kg) daily for 10 days to male albino Charles Foster rats. Open-field behavior was significantly depressed below the mean of the control group. On Day 7, ambulation was reduced to 24% of the mean but recovered to 60% on Day 10. Rearing responses were decreased on Day 7 and showed a fast recovery on Day 10, but preening responses further declined on Day 10. Defecation was not suppressed on Day 7 and showed complete recovery on Day 10. Motor activity showed significant depression, and fine movements were reduced more than gross movements. Dopamine was significantly decreased in Days 5 and 7 but showed a 13% recovery in the brain stem on Day 10. Norepinephrine was significantly reduced in the cerebral hemisphere, while serotonin was decreased both in the cerebral hemisphere and brain stem. Neither of these 2 amines showed significant recovery on Day 10. (20 ref).

268. Arunachalam, S. & Palanichamy, S. (1982). **Sublethal effects of carbaryl on surfacing behaviour and food utilization in the air-breathing fish, *Macropodus cupanus*.** *Physiology & Behavior,* 29(1), 23-27.
25 *M. cupanus* were reared individually in pesticide-free water or 4 sublethal concentrations of carbaryl (1-2.5 ppm). Ss exhibited increased surfacing with the increased concentration of carbaryl, possibly as the result of stress exerted by the toxicant. Food intake did not vary significantly across conditions, while growth decreased with increased concentrations of carbaryl. It is suggested that these effects are due to excessive expenditure of energy on metabolism that otherwise could have been channelled into growth. (17 ref).

269. Baker, Thomas & Lowndes, Herbert E. (1980). **Muscle spindle function in organophosphorus neuropathy.** *Brain Research,* 185(1), 77-84.
Reports that impairment of both sensory and motor functions contributes to the neurological signs (a peculiar high-step gait and a sluggish response to noxious stimuli) of organophosphorus neuropathy in cats. (19 ref).

270. Barbeau, A. et al. (1985). **Comparative behavioral, biochemical and pigmentary effects of MTPP, MPP$^+$ and Paraquat in *Rana pipiens*.** *Life Sciences,* 37(16), 1529-1538.
Examined the effects of 1-methyl-4-phenyl-1,2,3,6-tetrahydropyridine (MPTP), 1-methyl-4-phenyl-pyridinium ion (MPP$^+$), and the herbicide Paraquat (PQ$^+$) in 343 *Rana pipiens* frogs. Selected findings indicate that all 3 substances produced the main symptoms of parkinsonism (rigidity, akinesia, and tremor) as well as a drop in brain dopamine concentrations. These reactions varied in intensity and rapidity. Simultaneous administration of the monoamine oxidase (MAO) inhibitor pargyline blocked the behavioral and biochemical reactions to MPTP, potentiated the behavioral reaction to MPP$^+$ and PQ$^+$, and had no effect on the biochemical reaction to MPP$^+$ and PQ$^+$. It is suggested that the toxic process of PQ$^+$ may be a new model for the study of Parkinson's disease. (14 ref).

271. Bechard, Marc J. (1980). **Factors affecting nest productivity of Swainson's Hawk (*Buteo swainsoni*) in southeastern Washington.** *Dissertation Abstracts International,* 41(5-B), 1675.

272. Biggs, James D. (1977). **The effects of malathion on behavior in the European house cricket, *Acheta domesticus*.** *Dissertation Abstracts International,* 38(4-B), 1542.

273. Bloom, Alan S.; Staatz, Christina G. & Dieringer, Therese. (1983). **Pyrethroid effects on operant responding and feeding.** *Neurobehavioral Toxicology & Teratology,* 5(3), 321-324.
Examined the effects of permethrin, its cis and trans isomers, and deltamethrin on operant behavior and food intake. Male Sprague-Dawley rats were trained to respond on a VI 20-sec schedule of food reinforcement. Ss were injected ip with pyrethroids or their Emulphor vehicle 20 min prior to testing. Technical grade permethrin (15-60 mg/kg) produced a dose-related decrease in operant response rate. The 60 mg/kg dose decreased rates by 60%. Lower doses of cis-permethrin (30 mg/kg) and deltamethrin (2 mg/kg) also produced significant decreases in response rate. A 30 mg/kg dose of trans-permethrin was without effect. Food intake was measured for 1.5 and 24-hr periods after tech-permethrin treatment. Food intake decreased over both intervals with the 60 mg/kg dose. Results indicate that subconvulsive doses of pyrethroid insecticides can have significant effects on learned behavior and food intake. (22 ref).

274. Bracy, Odie L. et al. (1979). **Effects of methomyl and ethanol on behavior in the Sprague-Dawley rat.** *Pharmacology, Biochemistry & Behavior,* 10(1), 21-25.
Emotional behavior and activity levels were studied in 32 male Sprague-Dawley rats after administration of ethanol and/or a carbamate pesticide, methomyl, via a ground chow diet. Acetylcholinesterase (AChE) levels were lowered following the experimental diets. The group having the greatest reduction in AChE, the methomyl group, showed less evidence for habituation in an open-field test. No differences relative to control Ss were noted on handling and muricide tests. (22 ref).

275. Burbacher, Thomas M.; Grant, Kimberly S. & Mottet, N. Karle. (1986). **Retarded object permanence development in methylmercury exposed *Macaca fascicularis* infants.** *Developmental Psychology,* 22(6), 771–776.
Mothers of 12 full-term, normal birth-weight macaques received methylmercury (MeHg) hydroxide orally in apple juice at 50 µg/kg/day for 4 mo to 2 yrs before conception and at individual doses during pregnancy. Mothers of 12 control infants received apple juice without MeHg. Infants were separated from their mothers on delivery and were laboratory reared. Beginning at 14 days of age, infants were tested for object permanence development using a plain reach task and hiding tasks. Results indicate that the performance of the MeHg-exposed infants on the full hiding task was significantly retarded compared with controls. On average, exposed infants required nearly twice as many sessions and were over 1 mo older than control infants when they would retrieve the fully hidden object. Although not all of the MeHg-exposed infants who exhibited retarded object permanence development showed signs of attentional problems, it is suggested that for some infants, these attentional problems may be an early precursor to later cognitive deficits. (26 ref).

276. Busbee, Everette L. (1977). **The effects of dieldrin on the behavior of young loggerhead shrikes.** *Auk,* 94(1), 28-35.
60 loggerhead shrikes were divided into 5 groups, and 1 day after hatching, they were given daily doses of either 0, 1, 2, 4, or 8 mg/kg of dieldrin. Mean ages at death were 78.25, 36.75, 21.33, and 16.75 days for the 1-, 2-, 4-, and 8-mg groups, respectively. When the shrikes in the 0- and 1-mg groups were 25 days old, a cricket and mouse were presented daily, and behavior was recorded. The 2 groups showed no significant difference in their ontogeny of cricket killing, but the ontogeny of mouse killing was significantly prolonged in the treated birds. This study is the first to determine the chronic toxicity of an organochloride insecticide to an insectivorous passerine, and the first to demonstrate an insecticide-induced change in a complex behavioral ontogeny. (23 ref).

277. Carlson, Jeffrey N. & Rosellini, Robert A. (1987). **Exposure to low doses of the environmental chemical dieldrin causes behavioral deficits in animals prevented from coping with stress.** *Psychopharmacology,* 91(1), 122–126.
Conducted 2 experiments to assess the effects of low doses of an environmental contaminant in conjunction with various forms of stress. Male Sprague-Dawley albino rats were given acute doses (0, 0.5, 1.5, or 4.5 mg/kg) of dieldrin and subsequently exposed to a series of 40 escapable shocks, identical inescapable shocks, or no shock in an operant chamber. Eight hours later, Ss were re-exposed to escapable footshock. Escape deficits related to the size of the dieldrin dose were found in the inescapable shock group only. Data suggest that experience with the lack of control over stress is critical in determining the behavioral effects of the agent and that the behavioral effects caused by uncontrollable stress may be exacerbated by concurrent exposure to such compounds. The response to uncontrollable stress and the common neuronal systems that may be involved are discussed.

278. Carricaburu, Pierre & Lacroix, Roger. (1973). **Effect of parathion on the electroretinogram of the white mouse.** *Vision Research,* 13(4), 793-796.
Recorded the electroretinograms of pentobarbital anesthetized white mice. Intoxication by parathion resulted in a rapid cancelling of c-wave. At the same time, the latency of b-wave increased and its height decreased until it vanished. The a-wave disappeared last. Those modifications can be explained by synaptic sections. (German & Russian summaries).

279. Colvin, Bruce A. (1985). **Barn owl foraging behavior and secondary poisoning hazard from rodenticide use on farms.** *Dissertation Abstracts International,* 46(2-B), 405.

280. Custer, Thomas W.; Hensler, Gary L. & Kaiser, T. Earl. (1983). **Clutch size, reproductive success, and organochlorine contaminants in Atlantic coast Black-crowned Night-Herons.** *Auk,* 100(3), 699–710.
Presents information gathered in 1979 on the relationship of clutch size, reproductive success, and organochlorine contaminants among Atlantic Coast colonies of black-crowned night-herons (*Nycticorax nycticorax*) nesting in 3 New England and 2 North Carolina colonies. Latitudinal differences in clutch initiation were not evident. Mean clutch size was larger in the New England than in the North Carolina colonies. Nest success was greater in 2 New England colonies than in 1 North Carolina colony. Within-season differences in nest success occurred but were inconsistent among colonies. In the 4 instances where statistical comparisons could be made, larger clutches were more successful than smaller ones in 2 colonies; large and small clutches had similar success in 2 other colonies. One egg was collected from each of several nests in each colony for organochlorine contaminant analysis, and the fate of the remaining eggs was recorded. Concentrations of DDE and PCBs did not differ with clutch size; concentrations of PCBs were lower, however, in eggs laid late in the season. Although the data suggest an effect of DDE on hatching success in the northern more contaminated colonies, the impact of environmental contaminants on overall reproductive success appears to be minimal. (53 ref).

281. Galindo, Janine C.; Kendall, Ronald J.; Driver, Crystal J. & Lacher, Thomas E. (1985). **The effect of methyl parathion on susceptibility of bobwhite quail (*Colinus virginianus*) to domestic cat predation.** *Behavioral & Neural Biology,* 43(1), 21–36.
Five-week-old bobwhite quail (*Colinus virginianus*) that received either 0, 2, 4, or 8 mg/kg methyl parathion (*O,O*-dimethyl *o-p*-nitrophenyl phosphorothioate [MP]) treatment were investigated with regard to their susceptibility to predation by a cat. Four hours after receiving MP, physical activity levels were monitored in Ss and included the number of seconds spent still, walking, running, or flying before and after a cat was introduced into the experimental arena. The cholinesterase (ChE) activity for each S during the experiment was determined. Ss that were captured exhibited significantly greater inhibition of brain ChE activity and spent significantly more time being still than noncaptured Ss. Ss receiving MP at 8 mg/kg spent more seconds being still than those in other treatment groups, with ChE activity reduced to 42.8% of normal activity. There was a tendency for quail at increasing treatment levels to be more susceptible to capture by the cat. The ecological ramifications of the neurological and behavioral effects of MP are discussed. (41 ref).

282. Gause, E. M.; Hartmann, Roy J.; Leal, B. Z. & Geller, I. (1985). **Neurobehavioral effects of repeated sublethal soman in primates.** *Pharmacology, Biochemistry & Behavior,* 23(6), 1003–1012.
Six juvenile male baboons (*Papio cynocephalus*) were trained to perform a match-to-sample discrimination task, and the effects of repeated sublethal exposure to the organophosphate nerve gas soman (SO [3–5 µg/kg]) on task performance were explored. Both acute and subchronic exposure schedules were used; SO potency was verified by assay of SO-induced inhibition of acetylcholinesterase activity in whole blood, plasma, and erythrocytes. A characteristic profile of behavioral effects was observed. Immediate dose-related effects of SO included increases in mean session response time, increases in errors, and decreases in extra responses. Seizures were observed at the highest dose (5 µg/kg). The increase in mean session response time was due to intermittent lapses in responding to stimuli (attentional deficits). Both the attentional deficits and intermittent generalized seizures were persistent effects, with both occurring randomly after acute exposure to 5 µg/kg of SO. It is suggested that the occurrence of attentional deficits

PESTICIDES

may have been associated with generalized and/or focal seizures and that these effects may reflect irreversible lesions that become more threatening with increasing time. An additional, delayed effect was a sudden marked increase in the incidence of extra inconsequential responses that occurred several weeks after cessation of SO exposures. The persistent attentional deficits observed may represent an operant behavioral analog of the mental confusion defined as attention lapses for humans exposed occupationally to organophosphorus insecticides.

283. Giardini, Valerio et al. (1982). **Behaviorally augmented tolerance during chronic cholinesterase reduction by paraoxon.** *Neurobehavioral Toxicology & Teratology,* 4(3), 335–345.
Repeated injection of paraoxon (.125 mg/kg daily, sc) to 152 pretrained male Wistar rats 2 hrs before avoidance sessions, at a dose causing intoxication symptoms and reduction of brain acetylcholinesterase, induced marked performance depression followed by progressive development of tolerance. Additional groups of Ss ($N = 72$), treated either after each session (i.e., 23.5 hrs before each subsequent session) or treated and not tested, showed a substantial depression when shifted to treatment 2 hrs before sessions after achievement of tolerance by the Ss tested from the beginning of the experiment at the time of maximal paraoxon effect. Findings indicate that chronic paraoxon tolerance cannot be ascribed entirely to metabolic and/or physiological changes occurring as a consequence of repeated treatment per se, but must be explained at least in part by postulating a behaviorally augmented (or "learned") component. In an additional experiment, 34 chronic paraoxon (.1 mg/kg, sc) Ss were indistinguishable from 4 control Ss with respect to acquisition of light/go, noise-light/no go discrimination, i.e., of an active-passive avoidance task known to be highly sensitive to the disrupting effect of antimuscarinics. It is concluded that the enhanced sensitivity to antimuscarinics in organophosphate tolerant rats, which is usually ascribed to cholinergic receptor changes, does not appear to be associated with a spontaneous antimuscarinic-like syndrome. (34 ref).

284. Glowa, John R. (1986). **Acute and sub-acute effects of deltamethrin and chlordimeform on schedule-controlled responding in the mouse.** *Neurobehavioral Toxicology & Teratology,* 8(1), 97–102.
Compared the effects of 2 pesticides, deltamethrin (DN [0.03–3 mg/kg]) and chlordimeform (CDM [0.3–56 mg/kg]), on schedule-controlled responding in 31 male Charles River CD-1 mice. The response (interruption of a photocell beam) was maintained under an FI 60-sec schedule of milk delivery. Acute doses of DN larger than 0.1 mg/kg decreased responding in a dose-related manner. Acute doses of CDM larger than 10 mg/kg decreased responding in all Ss, but in Ss not previously receiving drugs lower doses had a greater rate-decreasing effect. The behavioral toxicity of both CDM and DN was augmented by repeated administration. Results suggest that the behavioral effects of some pesticides can depend on the schedule of reinforcement controlling responding.

285. Grant, Corbert V. (1978). **Studies of conditioned aversion in starlings.** *Dissertation Abstracts International,* 39(5-B), 2033–2034.

286. Hanse, S.; Köhler, Ch.; Goldstein, M. & Steinbusch, H. V. (1982). **Effects of ibotenic acid-induced neuronal degeneration in the medial preoptic area and the lateral hypothalamic area on sexual behavior in the male rat.** *Brain Research,* 239(1), 213–232.
Results of a study of male Wistar rats indicate that bilateral infusions of the neurotoxin ibotenic acid in the medial preoptic area (MPOA) were as effective as electrolytic lesions in eliminating copulation. Data suggest that (1) the functional integrity of MPOA nerve cell bodies is necessary for the expression of sexual behavior and (2) disruption of mating produced by electrolytic lateral hypothalamic area lesions is due to disruption of medial forebrain bundle fiber systems. (85 ref).

287. Heise, George A. & Hudson, Jeffrey D. (1985). **Effects of pesticides and drugs on working memory in rats: Continuous delayed response.** *Pharmacology, Biochemistry & Behavior,* 23(4), 591–598.
Conducted 3 experiments in which the effects of 4 pesticides (carbaryl, propoxur, chlordimeform, and deltamethrin) and 4 reference drugs (physostigmine, scopolamine, methscopolamine, and chlordiazepoxide) were measured in 2 delayed response, working memory procedures: go/no-go alternation in which 28 male Sprague-Dawley rats initiated their own trials, and spatial reversal. Four compounds (carbaryl, propoxur, physostigmine, and scopolamine) were also tested in a go/no-go alternation procedure in which Ss did not initiate their trials. The pesticides and physostigmine did not selectively affect working memory in any of the procedures: Low doses only moderately decreased response accuracy; higher doses suppressed responding indiscriminately. The pesticides and physostigmine had similar effects on go/no-go alternation (i.e., working memory) and analogous go/no-go discrimination performance. Effects on go/no-go alternation performance did not depend on whether the Ss initiated their own trials. Scopolamine, in contrast, appeared to disrupt working memory. It profoundly disrupted accuracy at doses that only moderately decreased overall responding and impaired go/no-go alternation accuracy much more than discrimination accuracy. (19 ref).

288. Heise, George A. & Hudson, Jeffrey D. (1985). **Effects of pesticides and drugs on working memory in rats: Continuous non-match.** *Pharmacology, Biochemistry & Behavior,* 23(4), 599–605.
Measured the effects of 4 pesticides (carbaryl, propoxur, chlordimeform, and deltamethrin) and 2 reference drugs, physostigmine and chlordiazepoxide, on the performance of 16 male Sprague-Dawley rats trained on a continuous nonmatch (CNM) delayed comparison, working memory procedure. These compounds were also tested in analogous, large and small stimulus difference discrimination (i.e., non-working-memory) procedures. The effects of the pesticides and physostigmine on CNM were qualitatively similar and also similar to their effects on discrimination performance. As dosage of these compounds increased, only small effects on accuracy were observed, followed at still larger doses by an abrupt and nonselective decrease in all responding. The pesticides and physostigmine did not selectively affect working memory: The magnitude of their effects did not increase with intertrial interval, and the compounds were equally effective in disrupting discrimination and CNM. Effects of chlordiazepoxide on performance in CNM and discrimination control procedures differed qualitatively from those of the pesticides and physostigmine. (23 ref).

289. Herr, D. W.; Gallus, J. A. & Tilson, H. A. (1987). **Pharmacological modification of tremor and enhanced acoustic startle by chlordecone and *p,p'*-DDT.** *Psychopharmacology,* 91(3), 320–325.
Studied the effects of pretreatment with phenoxybenzamine (5 mg/kg) on the neurobehavioral effects of chlordecone (60 mg/kg) and 1,1,1,-trichloro-2,2-*bis*(parachlorophenyl)ethane (DDT [75 mg/kg]) in male, Fischer 344 rats and examined the consequence of increasing the extraneural calcium concentration on the peak tremor magnitude caused by administration of DDT or chlordecone. DDT and chlordecone both produced a characteristic tremor and increased startle reactivity.

290. Hollingworth, Robert M. & Murdock, Larry L. (1980). **Formamidine pesticides: Octopamine-like actions in a firefly.** *Science,* 208(4439), 74–76.
The effectiveness of formamidine pesticides in plant and animal protection results, at least in part, from the induction of abnormal behavior in the pest rather than by direct lethality. Reduced feeding, dispersal from plants, erratic mating behavior, and detachment of ticks from their host are typical of these behavioral effects.

291. Hopper, David L. (1977). **Delayed matching to sample performance and parathion toxicity in the squirrel monkey (*Saimiri sciureus*).** *Dissertation Abstracts International,* 37(11-B), 5856–5857.

292. Hrdina, Pavel D.; Peters, David A. & Singhal, Radhey L. (1974). **Role of noradrenaline, 5-hydroxytryptamine and acetylcholine in the hypothermic and convulsive effects of alpha-chlordane in rats.** *European Journal of Pharmacology,* 26(2), 306–312.
Reports that alpha-chlordane (ACD), an organochlorine insecticide from the cyclodiene group, administered orally to male Wistar rats in doses of 200 or 300 mg/kg produced slight tremor, hindleg paralysis, convulsive episodes, and a dose-dependent decrease in rectal temperature. Time-course study of the changes in brain amines revealed a gradual alpha- or beta-adrenergic and striatal acetylcholine (ACh) decrease, with concomitant enhancement in the activity of ACh esterase. The hypothermic response to ACD coincided with a marked decrease in brain-stem noradrenaline (NA) and was followed by a rise in the levels of 5-hydroxyindoleactic acid, while 5-hydroxytryptamine remained unaltered. Concurrent treatment with alpha-methylparatyrosine, but not with 6-fluorotryptophan, partially antagonized the hypothermic effect of ACD without influencing the other neurotoxic symptoms. It is suggested that decrease in brain ACh is related to convulsive episodes, while increased release and use of NA may be involved in the hypothermic effect of ACD. (25 ref).

293. Jarrell, Theodore W.; Romanski, Lizabeth M.; Gentile, Christopher G.; McCabe, Philip M. et al. (1986). **Ibotenic acid lesions in the medial geniculate region prevent the acquisition of differential Pavlovian conditioning of bradycardia to acoustic stimuli in rabbits.** *Brain Research,* 382(1), 199–203.
Examined the effect of ibotenic acid lesions in the medial portion of the medial geniculate nucleus (mMGN) on differential heart rate (HR) conditioning to acoustic stimuli in 18 New Zealand albino rabbits. Lesions in mMGN prevented the acquisition of differential HR conditioned responses but not bradycardiac responses to the conditioned stimuli. Data suggest that cells in this region play an important role in the discriminative component of HR conditioning.

294. Jellestad, Finn K.; Markowska, Alicja; Bakke, Hans K. & Walther, Bernt. (1986). **Behavioral effects after ibotenic acid, 6-OHDA and electrolytic lesions in the central amygdala nucleus of the rat.** *Physiology & Behavior,* 37(6), 855–862.
In a study using 46 Wistar rats, selective lesions of central amygdaloid neurons with ibotenic acid and electrolytic destruction of the nucleus both led to marked increases in open field activity and activity during passive avoidance conditioning. However, electrolytic lesions of both neurons and fibers resulted in the most pronounced passive avoidance impairments. The 6-hydroxydopamine (6-OHDA) lesions resulted in no significant changes in the behavioral parameters under investigation or in plasma corticosterone levels. It is concluded that the lack of reduced corticosterone levels in any of the lesioned groups does not indicate that general fear arousal is critically dependent on intact central amygdala neurons in the rat. The behavioral data are, however, compatible with a hypothesis of a temporary reduction in fear arousal during the initial phase of the passive avoidance conditioning.

295. Joy, R. M. (1974). **Alteration of sensory and motor evoked responses by dieldrin.** *Neuropharmacology,* 13(2), 93–110.
Compared the responses evoked by stimulating peripheral and central pathways in 53 male cats treated with dieldrin and metrazol, and attempted to determine the mechanism of dieldrin's action in the CNS. The close similarities observed between dieldrin and metrazol strengthen the hypothesis that they share either a common mechanism or final common pathways responsible for electrophysiological events. (51 ref).

296. Joy, Robert M. (1982). **Mode of action of lindane, dieldrin and related insecticides in the central nervous system.** *Neurobehavioral Toxicology & Teratology,* 4(6), 813–823.
Evidence suggests that chlorinated hydrocarbon insecticides act on neurons in a global manner. Their primary target is the synapse, where they intensify activity by enhancing transmitter release from the presynaptic terminal. It is proposed that the modifications that occur in behavior, such as decreased maze and operant performance in the rat, are based on this same mode of action. A simplified model of brain plasticity, the kindled seizure model, is described as a potential tool for further investigation. (54 ref).

297. Keith, James O. (1978). **Synergistic effects of DDE and food stress on reproduction in brown pelicans and ringdoves.** *Dissertation Abstracts International,* 39(2-B), 598.

298. Kessler, Josef & Markowitsch, Hans J. (1982). **Behavioral effects of systemic injection of ibotenic acid manifested without neuromorphological correlates.** *Brain Research Bulletin,* 8(4), 439–442.
Ibotenic acid (IBO; 20–120 mg/kg, ip) led to a number of marked behavioral disturbances (e.g., reduced activity, respiratory changes, gait disturbances, and exophthalmus) that ultimately resulted in the death of 6 of 13 IBO-treated F_2 hybrid rats. Despite marked changes in behavior, no morphological changes could be detected in the brain tissue of surviving Ss. (32 ref).

299. Kurtz, Perry J. (1977). **Behavioral and biochemical effects of the carbamate insecticide, MOBAM.** *Pharmacology, Biochemistry & Behavior,* 6(3), 303–310.
In 4 experiments with a total of 300 male Sprague-Dawley albino (Wistar-derived) and 40 male Long-Evans hooded rats, decreases in rat plasma, erythrocyte, and brain cholinesterase levels after the ip injection of 1–5 mg/kg of 4-benzothienyl-N-methylcarbamate (MOBAM) were compared with decrements in both spontaneous motor activity and conditioned avoidance performance produced by this compound. Significant effects were observed with all 5 measured phenomena at dosages producing no obvious clinical signs. In albino rats, a dosage of 2 mg/kg significantly depressed plasma and erythrocyte cholinesterase activity and decreased motor activity 15 min after injection, but only higher dosages (3 and 5 mg/kg) significantly depressed brain cholinesterase activity and avoidance performance. In Long-Evans rats, both brain cholinesterase activity and avoidance performance were significantly reduced by the lower (2 mg/kg) dosage. The avoidance impairments observed after 3 mg/kg could be prevented by prior injection with atropine sulfate. It is suggested that both central and peripheral cholinesterase changes are important in determining the nature of the behavioral effects observed after exposure to this compound. (23 ref).

300. Lehotzky, Kornelia. (1982). **Effect of pesticides on central and peripheral nervous system function in rats.** *Neurobehavioral Toxicology & Teratology,* 4(6), 665–669.
The neurobehavioral toxicity of 3 organophosphate pesticides was evaluated in rats using measures of open-field activity, rotorod performance, conditioned escape from shock, and nerve conduction velocity. These measures were correlated with blood and brain cholinesterase level determinations. All

PESTICIDES

3 chemicals disrupted behavior ranging from transient disruptions accompanied by alterations in nerve conduction to disruption throughout the exposure. Even in the case of prolonged behavioral disruption, however, some recovery of performance occurred. Cholinesterase in both blood and brain decreased with initial dosing and remained low with continued dosing regardless of changes in the behavioral measures. Results are discussed in terms of the necessity of using mammalian behavioral tests to determine the toxicity of organophosphorous compounds in order to safeguard the health of the human population. (18 ref).

301. Lehotzky, Kornelia et al. (1982). **Effects of prenatal triphenyl-tin exposure on the development of behavior and conditioned learning in rat pups.** *Neurobehavioral Toxicology & Teratology,* 4(2), 247–250.
Examined the neurotoxic effects of the fungicide triphenyl-tin acetate in 264 rat pups of mothers treated perorally on Days 7–15 of gestation. The gait and development of motor coordination did not differ from those of controls in spite of the high mortality rate of controls during the nursing period. Spontaneous locomotor activity of treated Ss at the age of 23 and 36 days was increased; however, by the age of 90 days, activity returned to control levels. Conditioned avoidance was acquired more rapidly but was also extinguished sooner in Ss born from and nursed by poisoned mothers than in controls. (30 ref).

302. Mactutus, Charles F. & Tilson, Hugh A. (1984). **Neonatal chlordecone exposure impairs early learning and retention of active avoidance in the rat.** *Neurobehavioral Toxicology & Teratology,* 6(1), 75–83.
40 male and 40 female Fischer-344 rats were administered 1 mg of chlordecone (sc) on Postnatal Day 4. Body weights were slightly depressed by chlordecone treatment in both sexes in the pre- and postweaning periods. For Ss trained (Day 18) on 1-way active avoidance (OWA), chlordecone treatment increased the number of trials needed to attain the acquisition criterion; the effect was most pronounced in the males. A 72-hr retention test revealed a sex-dependent effect of chlordecone on response latency during the initial test trials. Acquisition of 2-way avoidance (TWA) (Days 28–30) was superior in females relative to males; chlordecone treatment significantly reduced this sex difference in Ss that had prior or no prior OWA training. However, following prior OWA training, vehicle-treated controls demonstrated a directional bias to make an avoidance response from a small to a large compartment, whereas chlordecone-treated Ss executed their avoidance responses in both directions at comparable rates. Similar evidence indicative of a selective retention deficit also characterized TWA performance when a "reversal" procedure was used. A final retention (extinction) session indicated that the chlordecone-treated Ss made fewer responses than vehicle-treated controls during the test trials. Plasma corticosterone levels of chlordecone-exposed Ss were significantly higher than control values when Ss were sacrificed 5 min after the final test. (32 ref).

303. Marban-Mendoza, Nahum. (1980). **Behavioral effects of selected non-fumigant nematicides, carbofuran and phenamiphos on *Pratylenchus vulnus* Allen and Jensen, 1951.** *Dissertation Abstracts International,* 40(10-B)), 4634.

304. Mattsson, Joel L.; Albee, Ralph R.; Eisenbrandt, David L. & Chang, Louis W. (1988). **Subchronic neurotoxicity in rats of the structural fumigant, sulfuryl fluoride.** 25th Annual Meeting of the Society of Toxicology (1986, New Orleans, Louisiana). *Neurotoxicology & Teratology,* 10(2), 127–133.
Exposed rats to sulfuryl fluoride for 13 wks. Treatment caused diminished weight gain; dental fluorosis; decreased grooming; decreased flicker fusion threshold; slowing of flash, auditory, and somatosensory evoked potentials; mild nasal and pulmonary inflammation; mild kidney effects; and mild vacuolation in the brain. Two months postexposure, evaluations of auditory brainstem responses and brain histology indicated that these effects were to a great extent reversible.

305. Mertens, H. W.; Lewis, M. F. & Steen, J. A. (1974). **Some behavioral effects of pesticides: Phosdrin and free-operant escape-avoidance behavior in gerbils.** *Aviation, Space, & Environmental Medicine,* 45, 1171–1176.
Studied effects of Phosdrin (mevinphos) on aversive behavior of gerbils in a free-operant escape-avoidance task with 2 levels of aversive shock. Dose-related decrements in avoidance behavior occurred at exposure levels which also caused overt somatic signs of poisoning; escape behavior was affected only by the highest dose. The findings of serious deficits in behavior which may occur before or with the 1st overt somatic signs of poisoning are applied as a caution to crop-duster pilots. (16 ref).

306. Mertens, H. W.; Steen, J. A. & Lewis, M. F. (1976). **Some behavioral effects of pesticides: The interaction of mevinphos and atropine in pigeons.** *Aviation, Space, & Environmental Medicine,* 47(2), 5 .
Examined the interaction of the organophosphate mevinphos and atropine in 2 pigeons performing in a VI schedule of reinforcement. When administered separately, both atropine and mevinphos produced a dose-related decrement in responding. The combined exposure to these drugs produced a performance decrement greater than that caused by exposure to each component drug alone. Findings suggest that prophylactic use of atropine may increase the detrimental behavioral effects of organophosphate exposure and that the atropine exposure alone may produce serious behavioral deficits.

307. Mertens, Henry W.; Steen, Jo A. & Lewis, Mark F. (1975). **The effects of mevinphos on appetitive operant behavior in the gerbil.** *Psychopharmacologia,* 41(1), 47-52.
Used a different pair of male gerbils in each of the following schedules of reinforcement: fixed response (FR) 25, FR 75, differential reinforcement of low rates (DRL) 12-sec, DRL 20-sec, and variable interval (VI) 1-min. Baseline performance in these tasks tended to be comparable to that of more common laboratory species but was more variable in the case of the VI 1-min task. The organophosphate pesticide, mevinphos, in intraperitoneal doses of .20 mg/kg and above produced observable somatic signs of poisoning and also dose-related decrements in performance in FR and VI tasks. Performance in the DRL schedule was affected only at a dose of .30 mg/kg. No performance deficits or overt somatic signs of poisoning were present at mevinphos doses of .10 mg/kg or lower. Results do not agree with those of an earlier study in which decrements in VI performance of pigeons and squirrel monkeys appeared at low mevinphos doses which did not produce overt somatic signs of poisoning. The possibility of variations in mevinphos effect as a function of species and task is discussed. (16 ref).

308. Mitchell, J. A.; Wilson, M. C. & Kallman, M. J. (1988). **Behavioral effects of Pydrin and Ambush in male mice.** *Neurotoxicology & Teratology,* 10(2), 113–119.
Assessed the effects of dermal and oral administration of the pyrethroid insecticide formulations Pydrin (30% fenvalerate) and Ambush (25.6% permethrin) in mice subjected to a conditioned taste aversion procedure. Fluid intake was not significantly altered. There were significant increases in nonambulatory, but not ambulatory activity.

309. Morison, Rufus. (1984). **The acute sublethal effects of the pesticides carbaryl and malathion on partial ethograms of the yellow bullhead (*Ictalurus natalis* (Lesueur)).** *Dissertation Abstracts International,* 45(5-B), 1368.

310. Moser, Virginia C. & MacPhail, Robert C. (1987). **Cholinergic involvement in the action of formetanate on operant behavior in rats.** *Pharmacology, Biochemistry & Behavior,* 26(1), 119–121.
Studied cholinergic involvement in the action of formetanate (FMT) on operant behavior in 7 adult male Long-Evans hooded rats. FMT is a formamidine acaricide-insecticide with a carbamate moiety in its molecular structure. Results suggest that FMT functions as an indirect agonist on central and peripheral muscarine receptors by inhibiting acetylcholinesterase to produce changes in schedule-controlled responding.

311. Nadzhimutdinov, K. N.; Kamilov, I. K. & Muzrabekov, Sh. M. (1974). **Influence of pesticides on the duration of hexobarbital-induced sleep.** *Farmakologiya i Toksikologiya,* 37(5), 533–537.
Concludes, after a series of experiments using 620 rats, that the hexobarbitol test is primarily an indicator of the functional state of the smooth endoplasmic reticulum of the hepacytes, and does not always reflect the degree of damage to the liver and disruption of its function. (English summary) (21 ref).

312. Olson, Kirsten L. (1978). **Effects of chronic pre- and postnatal exposure to pesticides on the behavior and learning ability in rats.** *Dissertation Abstracts International,* 38(7-B), 3108.

313. Paulsen, Karen; Adesso, Vincent J. & Porter, John J. (1973). **Report on pilot study of effects of DDT on maternal behavior.** *Bulletin of the Psychonomic Society,* 1(3), 205–206.
Examined the hypothesis that DDT would have an adverse effect on the behavior of 3 pregnant albino rats involved in the stressful and novel situation of giving birth for the 1st time. Ss were fed food containing DDT in concentrations of 0, 50, or 100 ppm. The maternal behavior of the DDT Ss, in the form of nest building, nursing (as measured by time spent nursing and weight of litters), retrieval, and activity level, as compared to control Ss, was as predicted by the hypothesis.

314. Paulsen, Karen; Adesso, Vincent J. & Porter, John J. (1975). **DDT: Effects on maternal behavior.** *Bulletin of the Psychonomic Society,* 5(2), 117–119.
Food containing concentrations of DDT was fed to 14 1-wk-pregnant primiparous albino rats to examine the hypothesis that DDT produces hyperexcitability, which in turn affects maternal behavior. Results show low DDT (50 ppm) Ss exhibited significantly less nursing and greater rejection than high DDT (100 ppm) and control (0 ppm) groups. It is concluded that poor maternal behavior, and not only DDT ingestion, caused harm to neonates. (15 ref).

315. Peele, David B. & Crofton, Kevin M. (1987). **Pyrethroid effects on schedule-controlled behavior: Time and dosage relationships.** *Neurotoxicology & Teratology,* 9(5), 387–394.
Investigated potential alterations in acquired (operant) behavior, by making acute dosage-effect and time-course determinations for permethrin (PMT, 100–400 mg/kg) and cypermethrin (CPM, 7.5–60 mg/kg), in 7 male rats. Findings show that while both compounds produced a decrease in rate of responding, the rate-decreasing effects of CPM (but not PMT) were dependent on underlying behavior.

316. Pfister, William R. et al. (1978). **Comparison of the behavioral effects of para-chloroamphetamine, chlordimeform, quipazine, and intraventricular serotonin in the rat.** *Communications in Psychopharmacology,* 2(4), 287–296.
Ss dosed with 5 mg/kg parachloroamphetamine exhibited the "serotonergic syndrome," which is purported to reflect increased central serotonergic transmission. Chlordimeform (80 mg/kg) also induced the syndrome. Intraventricular 5-hydroxytryptamine and the direct serotonin agonist, quipazine, failed to elicit the syndrome, even in doses that resulted in acute lethality.

317. Pfister, William R.; Hollingworth, Robert M. & Yim, George K. (1978). **Increased feeding in rats treated with chlordimeform and related formamidines: A new class of appetite stimulants.** *Psychopharmacology,* 60(1), 47–51.
Low doses of the formamidine pesticide chlordimeform (CDM) induced voracious daytime feeding in non-food-deprived Sprague-Dawley male rats. Anorexia accompanied by excessive CNS stimulation was noted with higher doses of CDM (above 40 mg/kg) and other formamidines. The formamidines constitute a new class of appetite stimulants, which should prove to be useful agents for the study of feeding behavior. (21 ref).

318. Pollack, Ellen H. (1985). **The effects of gypsy moth (*Lymantria dispar* L.) insecticides on the parasite,** *Cotesia melanoscelus.* *Dissertation Abstracts International,* 45(7-B), 2033.

319. Reischl, Peter. (1974). **Auditory detection behavior in parathion treated squirrel monkeys.** *Dissertation Abstracts International,* 34(10-B), 5046.

320. Roney, Paul L.; Costa, Lucio G. & Murphy, Sheldon D. (1986). **Conditioned taste aversion induced by organophosphate compounds in rats.** *Pharmacology, Biochemistry & Behavior,* 24(3), 737–742.
Three organophosphate compounds—dichlorvos, parathion, and diisopropylfluorophosphate—were tested as an unconditioned stimulus/stimuli (UCS) in the conditioned taste aversion (CTA) test. All organophosphates caused a dose-dependent CTA in male Sprague-Dawley rats at doses that did not induce any other signs of toxicity. Experiments with dichlorvos showed that the minimum dose that caused CTA did not alter the Ss' sensitivity to pain or their behavior in either an open field or an inclined plane. Cholinesterase activity was dose-dependently inhibited in brain and plasma after administration of the organophosphates, and CTA was correlated with the degree of plasma cholinesterase inhibition. Data indicate that CTA is a sensitive indicator of neurobehavioral effects of mild exposure to organophosphates that causes only 30–40% inhibition of plasma cholinesterase.

321. Rosecrans, John A.; Johnson, James H.; Tilson, Hugh A. & Hong, J. S. (1984). **Hypothalamic-pituitary adrenal (HPAA) axis function in adult Fischer-344 rats exposed during development to neurotoxic chemicals perinatally.** *Neurobehavioral Toxicology & Teratology,* 6(4), 281–288.
Administered chlordecone, an organochlorine insecticide, to rat mothers prenatally plus the 1st 12 days of the neonatal period (6 ppm in the diet) or neonatally via a single sc injection to rats at 4 days of age (1 mg/pup in 20 µg of dimethylsulfoxide [DMSO]). DMSO (20 µl/pup) and dexamethasone (100 µg/pup in 20 µl saline) were also injected on Day 4. HPAA function was evaluated at 70–80 days of age. Responsiveness of the HPAA to a repeated stressor was evaluated by exposing Ss of each treatment group to a 7-day stress-induced analgesia paradigm consisting of a daily 15-sec footshock (0.9mA) exposure preceded by a 15-sec white noise CS. The behavioral response to daily stress was evaluated by measuring tailflick latencies immediately before and/or after each stress exposure. The CR to stress was evaluated 24 hrs after the last of 7 daily footshock sessions in which Ss of each treatment and experimental group were exposed to the shock chamber only. Perinatal exposure to chlordecone did not significantly alter the behavioral and/or neuroendocrine responses to stress. Ambient hormone levels, however, were uniformly attenuated by chlordecone. Additional experiments suggest that chlordecone may alter HPAA function by releasing adrenal corticosterone and that inter- and intrastrain variables are important considerations in the study of HPAA function. (22 ref).

PESTICIDES

322. Ruppert, Patricia H.; Cook, Larry L.; Dean, Karen F. & Reiter, Lawrence W. (1983). **Acute behavioral toxicity of carbaryl and propoxur in adult rats.** *Pharmacology, Biochemistry & Behavior,* 18(4), 579–584.
Examined motor activity and neuromotor function in male CD rats exposed to either carbaryl or propoxur. Behavioral effects were compared with the time course of cholinesterase inhibition. Ss received an ip injection of either 0, 2, 4, 6, or 8 mg/kg propoxur or 0, 4, 8, 16, or 28 mg/kg carbaryl 20 min before testing. All doses of propoxur reduced 2-hr activity in a figure-8 maze, and crossovers and rears in an open field. For carbaryl, dosages of 8, 16, and 28 mg/kg decreased maze activity whereas 16 and 28 mg/kg reduced open field activity. To determine the time course of effects, Ss received a single injection of vehicle, 2 mg/kg propoxur, or 16 mg/kg carbaryl, and were tested for 5 min in a figure-8 maze. Immediately after testing, Ss were sacrificed and total cholinesterase was measured. Maximum effects of propoxur and carbaryl on blood and brain cholinesterase and motor activity were seen within 15 min. Maze activity had returned to control levels within 30 and 60 min, whereas cholinesterase levels remained depressed for 120 and 240 min for propoxur and carbaryl, respectively. Results indicate that both carbamates decrease motor activity, but behavioral recovery occurs prior to that of cholinesterase following acute exposure. (22 ref).

323. Schnorr, Janet K. (1973). **Effects of dieldrin on learning and retention of a visual discrimination task in sheep.** *Dissertation Abstracts International,* 33(8-B), 3995-3996.

324. Sharma, Raghubir P. (1973). **Brain biogenic amines: Depletion by chronic dieldrin exposure.** *Life Sciences,* 13(9), 1245-1251.
Conducted a chemical analysis of the brains of mallard ducks subjected to chronic dietary exposure to dieldrin. An appreciable depletion of brain serotonin, norepinephrine and dopamine, but not of gamma-aminobutyrate, was found. Such alterations may account for the toxic effects in animals following chronic pesticide exposure. It is suggested that changes in brain biogenic amines may be related to behavioral disorders (e.g., in mating behaviors) following exposure to such environmental contaminants. (15 ref).

325. Smith, Richard M. (1973). **Successive discrimination reversal and dieldrin toxicity in the squirrel monkey (Saimiri sciureus).** *Dissertation Abstracts International,* 33(8-B), 3997.

326. Stamper, Colleen R.; Balduini, Walter; Murphy, Sheldon D. & Costa, Lucio G. (1988). **Behavioral and biochemical effects of postnatal parathion exposure in the rat.** *Neurobehavioral Toxicology & Teratology,* 10(3), 261–266.
Preweanling rat pups were exposed daily to parathion (13 mg/kg or 1.9 mg/kg) or vehicle (corn oil) on Postnatal Days 5–20, a time period critical to development of behavioral and biochemical parameters of the cholinergic nervous system. This exposure resulted in dose-dependent reductions in acetylcholinesterase activity and muscarinic receptor binding in the cortex. Postweanling behavioral assessment revealed small deficits in tests of spatial memory in both the T-maze and the radial arm maze. Biochemical and behavioral deficits in cholinergic nervous system functioning occurred in the absence of severe signs of toxicity and in the absence of generalized nonspecific behavioral disturbances.

327. Stein, Elliot A.; Washburn, M.; Walczak, C. & Bloom, A. S. (1987). **Effects of pyrethroid insecticides on operant responding maintained by food.** *Neurotoxicology & Teratology,* 9(1), 27–31.
Male rats were trained on a VR25 schedule maintained by food pellets. Rats were injected intraperitoneally with 1 of 4 technical grade pyrethroids: permethrin, allethrin, deltamethrin, and fenvalerate. Results indicate that operant responding maintained by food is a sensitive measure of the behaviorally disruptive effects of subconvulsive doses of pyrethroids.

328. Uphouse, Lynda. (1986). **Single injection with chlordecone reduces behavioral receptivity and fertility of adult rats.** *Neurobehavioral Toxicology & Teratology,* 8(2), 121–126.
Studied the effects of intraperitoneal chlordecone (0, 25, 50, or 75 mg/kg) on fertility in 44 female Fischer-344 rats. The 2 highest doses significantly reduced fertility, and mating behavior was also decreased when exposure occurred on the morning of proestrus. Findings indicate that the failure of chlordecone-treated females to ovulate cannot totally account for the decreased fertility.

329. Vea, E. V.; Cutkomp, Laurence K. & Halberg, Franz. (1977). **Interrelationships of oxygen consumption and insecticide sensitivity.** *Chronobiologia,* 4(4), 313–323.
The circadian rhythms of oxygen consumption and insecticide sensitivity (i.e., to dichlorvos, a rapid-acting organophosphate) in adult confused flour beetles (*Tribolium confusum du Val*) were determined using a 12 hr–12 hr light–dark lighting regimen and other standardized conditions. The acrophase of oxygen consumption occurred on the average about 3 hrs after the middle of the daily dark span. Maximum insecticide sensitivity occurred about 2 hrs earlier. (36 ref).

330. Zaidi, Nikhat F.; Agrawal, Ashok K.; Anand, Mohini & Seth, Prahlad K. (1985). **Neonatal endosulfan neurotoxicity: Behavioral and biochemical changes in rat pups.** *Neurobehavioral Toxicology & Teratology,* 7(5), 439–442.
Repeated administration of 0.5 mg/kg endosulfan for 5 days/week to 3–5 wk old rat pups ($N=16$) produced no significant alteration either in the binding of ^{3}H-5-hydroxytryptamine (^{3}H-5-HT) to frontal cortical membranes or in footshock-induced fighting behavior. However, administration of 1 mg/kg endosulfan for 5 wks caused a significant increase in ^{3}H-5-HT binding as well as in footshock-induced aggressive behavior. The endosulfan-induced increase in aggressive behavior and increased binding of ^{3}H-5-HT were detectable 8 days after the cessation of endosulfan treatment. The endosulfan-induced fighting behavior was blocked by the pretreatment of Ss with methysergide, a 5-HT blocker. Results suggest an involvement of serotonergic systems in the neonatal neurotoxicity of endosulfan. (29 ref).

SOLVENTS

331. Field, Robert I. (1987). **Neuropsychological deficits in solvent encephalopathy and Alzheimer's Disease.** *Dissertation Abstracts International,* 48(4-B), 1150–1151.

332. Juntunen, Juhani. (1982). **Alcoholism in occupational neurology: Diagnostic difficulties with special reference to the neurological syndromes caused by exposure to organic solvents.** *Acta Neurologica Scandinavica,* 66(Suppl 92), 89–108.
Clinical syndromes caused by chronic exposure to organic solvents and by chronic abuse of alcohol share several common features. In practice, both develop insidiously, usually through repeated episodes of acute intoxication. It is difficult to diagnose them at their early stages. Careful history-taking that includes the occupational history and tests for possible nonneurologic signs of alcoholism are necessary for the correct diagnosis. Regular absenteeism, lack of efficiency at work, and changing jobs often are typical features of alcohol abuse. Difficulties in obtaining an adequate history of the patient's drinking habits are readily apparent, and considerable efforts are required. Alcohol abuse does not rule out the possible concomitant effects of chronic exposure to organic

solvents. The inadequacy of human data on exposure to various solvents and the consumption of alcohol makes it imperative that epidemiologic studies focus on these problems. Special emphasis should be placed on proper selection of sensitive techniques for the early detection of health impairments due to the consumption of alcohol and exposure to organic solvents. (49 ref).

333. Juntunen, Juhani. (1984). **Organic solvent intoxications in occupational neurology.** 25th Scandinavian Congress of Neurology: Occupational Neurology (1984, Bergen, Norway). *Acta Neurologica Scandinavica,* 69(98), 105–120.
Contends that there is a spectrum of clinical manifestations in chronic organic solvent poisoning ranging from mild cases to fatal ones. However, only a few clinically relevant applications can be extracted from the bulk of data accumulated from different studies on the nervous system effects of organic solvents. Rigorous clinical research is needed but is hampered by the inaccuracy of the data usually available on exposure and work conditions. The standardization of exposure estimation and the standardization of examination techniques are mandatory in order to improve the quality of neuroepidemiologic studies on organic solvent intoxication. (48 ref).

334. Ki Moon Bang. (1984). **Health effects of common organic solvents in the workplace.** *Family & Community Health,* 7(3), 15–29.
Notes that the most notable acute effects of occupational exposure to common organic solvents in the workplace are narcosis and other nerve dysfunctions. The most common symptoms of short-term exposure are fatigue, headache, nausea, sleep disturbances, and memory alterations. The following organic solvents are discussed: trichloroethylene, 1,1,1-trichloroethane, toluene, xylene, methyl ethyl ketone, acetone, isopropanol, and methylene chloride. (103 ref).

335. Lindström, Kari. (1982). **Behavioral effects of long-term exposure to organic solvents.** *Acta Neurologica Scandinavica,* 66(Suppl 92), 131–141.
A literature review indicates that epidemiological studies have detected an increased risk of neuropsychiatric diseases among groups occupationally exposed to organic solvents. Psychological studies of solvent-exposed workers have investigated both cognitive and sensorimotor functions. Most of these studies have dealt with trichloroethylene, toluene, styrene, and mixtures of organic solvents. A decline in sensorimotor functions has been observed in many studies. Of the cognitive functions, short-term memory in particular has proven to be sensitive to solvent exposure. Evidence of a decline in visuoconstructive abilities has also been found. It has been possible to analyze exposure–response and exposure–effect relationships between exposure and psychological findings only for some single studies, because reliable measures for long-term solvent exposure have usually not been available. The measurement of personality characteristics among solvent-exposure workers has been another neglected area. (30 ref).

336. Spencer, Peter S. & Schaumburg, Herbert H. (1985). **Organic solvent neurotoxicity: Facts and research needs.** International Conference on Organic Solvent Toxicity (1984, Stockholm, Sweden). *Scandinavian Journal of Work, Environment & Health,* 11(Suppl 1), 53–60.
Reviews the literature for evidence for the assertion that organic solvents are neurotoxic. While many organic solvents are capable of inducing an acute, reversible narcotic state in large doses, few unequivocally induce chronic, long-lasting, or irreversible changes in nervous system structure and/or function. For organic solvents with proven neurotoxic properties, the type of neurological damage is closely related to the structure of the chemical agent, while the degree of impairment and the extent of reversibility are related to the potency, dose, and duration of exposure. Examples include solvents containing n-hexane or methyl n-butyl ketone, which have caused occupational neuropathy. Chronic inhalation abuse of pure toluene produces irreversible cerebellar, brainstem, and pyramidal-tract dysfunction, but comparable changes have not been found in solvent workers occupationally exposed to toluene. Ototoxicity is found in experimental animals exposed to toluene, xylene, or styrene. Impure trichloroethylene can damage the trigeminal nerve; dichloroacetylene, a breakdown product of trichloroethylene, is probably responsible for this neurotoxic property. Prolonged occupational exposure to mixed solvents, notably white spirit, has been reported to induce a mild, nonprogressive dementing illness with or without peripheral nerve dysfunction, but supporting data from neuropathological and experimental animal studies are lacking. (59 ref).

Human Research

337. Arlien-Søborg, Peter. (1984). **Chronic toxic encephalopathy in house-painters.** *Acta Neurologica Scandinavica,* 69(Suppl 99), 105–113.
Evaluated behavioral and cognitive functioning in 70 24–63 yr old housepainters consecutively referred to a hospital neurological department for suspected chronic solvent intoxication or presenile dementia of an unknown origin. Ss' most common complaint was impaired learning and memory. Data from the administration of tests measuring immediate verbal memory span, verbal learning and memory, visual-spatial learning and memory, visual construction praxis, concept formation, and vigilance and psychomotor speed indicate that the symptoms were caused at least partly by the solvents' reduction of cerebral oxidative metabolism and blood flow. Symptoms may become permanent with continued solvent exposure. Alzheimer's disease and solvent-induced encephalopathy seem to have different etiologies. (27 ref).

338. Arlien-Søborg, P. et al. (1982). **Cerebral blood flow in chronic toxic encephalopathy in house painters exposed to organic solvents.** *Acta Neurologica Scandinavica,* 66(1), 34–41.
Studied cerebral blood flow (CBF) in 11 30–57 yr old controls and 9 24–59 yr old house painters occupationally exposed to organic solvents for a mean of 22 yrs. Ss completed neurological tests of memory, learning, and RTs. Results show that the painter group had mild to moderate intellectual impairment, no or only minor cerebral atrophy seen in a computerized tomography scan of the brain, and reduced CBF. Findings are discussed in relation to a chronic organic brain syndrome, the "chronic painters' syndrome." (30 ref).

339. Baker, Edward L.; White, Roberta F. & Murawski, Benjamin J. (1985). **Clinical evaluation of neurobehavioral effects of occupational exposure to organic solvents and lead.** *International Journal of Mental Health,* 14(3), 135–158.
Presents a conceptual and procedural framework for clinical evaluation of patients exposed to 2 types of environmental toxins (organic solvents and lead) and provides cases that demonstrate the application of this approach and identify characteristic neurobehavioral abnormalities seen following exposure to these substances. Methods for estimation of exposure intensity are given, and toxic disorders of the central nervous system (CNS) are described, including the acute organic mental disorders (acute intoxication and acute toxic encephalopathy) and the chronic organic mental disorders (organic affective syndrome, mild chronic toxic encephalopathy, and severe chronic toxic encephalopathy). The use of neuropsychological testing and the interpretation of data from this testing are also discussed. The cases of 5 males (aged 34–45 yrs) and a 29-yr-old female with exposure to lead or solvents are presented. It is concluded that information obtained from formal neuropsychological testing should be combined with an estimation of exposure based on detailed occupational

SOLVENTS

histories and appropriate biological monitoring; environmental monitoring may also be of value in some situations. (17 ref).

340. Beneš, V.; Frantík, E.; Horváth, M. & Kožená, L. (1985). **Adverse psychotropic effects and blood concentrations of toluene and trichloroethylene in model human exposures.** 26th Annual Psychopharmacological Meeting (1984, Jeseník, Czechoslovakia). *Activitas Nervosa Superior,* 27(1), 34–36.
Investigated the substances and conditions that impair the ability for humans to maintain alertness in a monotonous condition, using ethanol as a positive control. Substances were applied to healthy male volunteers (mean age 20 yrs), and blood concentrations of the applied substances were measured and related to doses and/or air concentrations and psychological effects. (6 ref).

341. Beneš, V.; Frantík, E.; Horváth, M. & Kožená, L. (1986). **Vigilance performance paralleled with blood levels of solvents: Acetone, styrene, tetrachloroethylene.** *Activitas Nervosa Superior,* 28(3), 234–236.
Examined the vigilance performance and blood concentrations of 20–21 yr old males who inhaled tetrachloroethylene (TE), styrene, and acetone vapors in increasing concentrations before, during, and after exposure. All 3 solvents improved performance compared with placebo; subjective ratings of sleepiness were rated by Ss higher in the exposed groups, especially in TE.

342. Bergholtz, L. M. & Ödkvist, L. M. (1984). **Audiological findings in solvent exposed workers.** Transactions of the XXIIth Congress of the Scandinavian Oto-Laryngological Society: Posters (1984, Copenhagen, Denmark). *Acta Oto-Laryngologica,* 412, 109–110.
Investigated the audiological effects of exposure to toxins in 14 painters, printers, and gasoline truck drivers (aged 32–63 yrs) with (Group A) and without (Group B) psycho-organic syndromes and in 9 persons (aged 41–64 yrs) exposed to jet fuel (Group C). Group A Ss showed decreased cerebellar functioning, positional nystagmus, pathological saccades, and vision suppression. Group C Ss experienced fatigue, unsteadiness, and memory and concentration problems. Group A Ss elicited pathological phase audiometry, and all Ss revealed pathological cortical response and interrupted speech audiometry.

343. Bælum, Jesper et al. (1985). **Response of solvent-exposed printers and unexposed controls to six-hour toluene exposure.** *Scandinavian Journal of Work, Environment & Health,* 11(4), 271–280.
43 male toluene-exposed printers (aged 29–50 yrs) and 43 age-, sex-, education-, and smoking-habit-matched controls were exposed once in a climate chamber to either 100 ppm of toluene or clean air for 6.5 hrs preceded by a 1-hr acclimatization period. The effects of toluene were measured from subjective votes with linear analog rating scales on 16 items and on the performance of 10 tests measuring psychomotor skills, perceptual skills, and vigilance. Results indicate that exposure to toluene compared with clean air caused discomfort with complaints of low air quality, strong odor, fatigue, sleepiness, a feeling of intoxication; and irritation of the eyes, nose, and throat. Ss exposed to toluene showed decreased manual dexterity, decreased color discrimination, and decreased accuracy in visual perception. (26 ref).

344. Cherry, Nicola et al. (1983). **The effects of toluene and alcohol on psychomotor performance.** *Ergonomics,* 26(11), 1081–1087.
Eight 22–50 yr old males took part in 4 experimental sessions in an exposure chamber to assess the effects of toluene (80 ppm) and alcohol (0.4 ml/kg), individually and in combination, on mood and 4 performance measures: simple RT, 4-choice RT, pursuit tracking, and visual search. Alcohol caused a significant deterioration over the exposure session in performance on pursuit-tracking and visual-search tasks and also in mood. Toluene had no significant effect on any of the behavioral measures, but examination of mean scores for each treatment suggested a tendency for performance and mood to deteriorate more when alcohol and toluene were administered together than when alcohol was taken alone. (French, German & Japanese abstracts) (10 ref).

345. Crossen, John R. & Wiens, Arthur N. (1988). **Wechsler Memory Scale—Revised: Deficits in performance associated with neurotoxic solvent exposure.** Special Issue: Initial validity studies of the new Wechsler Memory Scale—Revised. *Clinical Neuropsychologist,* 2(2), 181–187.
20 industrial painters with a history of solvent exposure and evidence of memory impairment on neuropsychological examination were administered the Wechsler Memory Scale—Revised (WMS—R). Although the more educated Ss had better WMS—R performance than the others, all educational groups performed at an impaired level relative to WMS—R education-adjusted norms. Employed Ss scored consistently higher on the WMS—R than unemployed Ss; these differences were not accounted for by age or education. Results support the construct and criterion validity of the WMS—R for assessment of chronic solvent encephalopathy.

346. Dager, Stephen R.; Holland, John P.; Cowley, Deborah S. & Dunner, David L. (1987). **Panic disorder precipitated by exposure to organic solvents in the work place.** *American Journal of Psychiatry,* 144(8), 1056–1058.
Describes 3 cases of idiosyncratic response to occupational solvent exposure, with symptoms characteristic of panic disorder (Diagnostic and Statistical Manual of Mental Disorders [DSM-III]). Ss were a 28-yr-old man and 2 females, aged 34 and 36 yrs. The specific treatment and prognostic implications of this panic-like reaction to solvents are discussed. Sodium lactate infusion is proposed as an objective test to aid in the diagnosis.

347. Dick, Robert B. (1988). **Short duration exposures to organic solvents: The relationship between neurobehavioral test results and other indicators.** *Neurotoxicology & Teratology,* 10(1), 39–50.
Discusses the use of behavioral tests in setting limits for exposure to industrial solvents with neurotoxic properties. It is noted that performance decrements have been found at exposure levels within currently acceptable levels, suggesting that ceiling levels for exposure need to be set more carefully. Neurobehavioral testing may offer promise for testing the potential of long-term development of solvent neurotoxicity from repeated exposure.

348. Dorndorf, W.; Kresse, M.; Christian, W. & Katritzki, G. (1975). **Dichloroethane poisoning with myoclonic syndrome, seizures and irreversible cerebral defects.** *Archiv fur Psychiatrie und Nervenkrankheiten,* 220(4), 373–379.
Describes the case of a 48-yr-old male who inadvertently took a sip of an ointment containing dichloroethane, survived, and showed a 2-phase course of toxic symptoms. After an initial narcosis and an interval with few pathological symptoms, seizures, myoclonia, and somnolence occurred. Irreversible final disturbances were lasting mental defects, cerebellar dysarthria, ataxia, and hydrocephalus. Concomitant diseases were acute liver dystrophy, nephropathy, and anemia. The clinical picture of dichloroethane poisoning is outlined, the pathogenesis of this particular cerebral lesion described, and the therapy discussed. (35 ref).

349. Eskelinen, Leena; Luisto, Marjaana; Tenkanen, Leena & Mattei, Osvaldo. (1986). **Neuropsychological methods in the differentiation of organic solvent intoxication from certain neurological conditions.** *Journal of Clinical & Experimental Neuropsychology,* 8(3), 239–256.

Compared the neuropsychological impairment and the subjective symptoms of 21 patients (mean age 44 yrs) with organic solvent intoxication with those of 47 patients with vertebrobasilar insufficiency, cerebral trauma, and headache. Measures included subtests from the Wechsler Adult Intelligence Scale (WAIS) and Wechsler Memory Scale; tests of motor speed and dexterity; drawing tasks; and scales assessing changes in mood, emotionality, and well-being. Although it was possible to differentiate between the 4 groups at group level, because of the variance in each group, no specific rule for individual diagnostics could be developed. At group level, a combination of 3 test variables (Block Design speed and failures and Digit Span forward) and 3 symptom scales (fatigue, sleep disturbances, and neurovegetative symptoms) yielded the most effective discrimination. Instead of the raw scores, subscores for the individual tests as well as detailed use of the symptom questionnaire were informative when the groups were compared. This approach may also be applicable to individual diagnostics. (26 ref).

350. Gamberale, Francesco. (1985). **Use of behavioral performance tests in the assessment of solvent toxicity.** International Conference on Organic Solvent Toxicity (1984, Stockholm, Sweden). *Scandinavian Journal of Work, Environment & Health,* 11(Suppl 1), 65–74.
Discusses the increasing use of behavioral performance tests in the assessment of solvent toxicity on the human nervous system. Since the use of psychometric techniques made it possible to link together deterioration of behavioral performance in humans and the inhalation of solvent vapor, psychometric tests or test batteries have been widely and successfully used to study solvent toxicity. Most of the evidence showing that low-dose exposure to industrial solvents can exert a depressant action on the nervous system has been obtained with psychometric tests. Results of experimental laboratory investigations, quasi-experimental field studies, and epidemiologic studies that used behavioral performance tests to investigate solvent toxicity are reviewed. The applicability of psychometric techniques to the different questions at issue in the study of the effects of solvent exposure on the nervous system is considered. Special attention is focused upon the interpretation of behavioral performance changes with regard to factors associated with the type of test used, the condition under which the tests are performed, the Ss' characteristics, and the study design. (58 ref).

351. Goldbloom, D. & Chouinard, Guy. (1985). **Schizophreniform psychosis associated with chronic industrial toluene exposure: Case report.** *Journal of Clinical Psychiatry,* 46(8), 350–351.
Presents the case history of a 29-yr-old male who developed irreversible schizophreniform psychosis following 5 yrs of continuous occupational exposure to toluene, a solvent commonly used in the workplace that has gained notoriety as a substance of abuse. Other effects that have been associated with chronic exposure to toluene include neurological abnormalities, personality changes, optic atrophy, pyramidal tract dysfunction, and cerebral and cerebellar atrophy. (8 ref).

352. Halonen, P.; Halonen, J.-P.; Lang, H. A. & Karskela, V. (1986). **Vibratory perception thresholds in shipyard workers exposed to solvents.** *Acta Neurologica Scandinavica,* 73(6), 561–565.
When vibratory perception thresholds (VPTs) were determined for 17 females and 73 males (aged 19–59 yrs), exposed in shipyard work to industrial solvents 1–44 yrs, 4 males but no females had bilaterally significantly increased VPTs in the lower limbs. Seven Ss had increased VPTs in the upper extremities only. Laboratory investigations of 15 Ss revealed abnormalities in Ss with increased VPTs in the lower limbs but not for Ss with increased VPTs in the upper limbs only.

353. Helmkamp, James C.; Forman, Samuel A.; McNally, Michael S. & Bone, Craig M. (1984). **Morbidity and mortality associated with exposure to Otto Fuel II in the U.S. Navy 1966–1979.** *US Naval Health Research Center Report,* 84-35, 22 p.
Otto Fuel II (OFII) is a liquid propellant used in preparing and maintaining US Navy torpedoes. The active component of medical concern is 1,2-propylene glycol dinitrate (PGDN). The present authors summarize studies that assessed whether excess morbidity and mortality, previously associated with compounds analogous to PGDN, would be found in Navy personnel, specifically torpedomen's mates (TPMs) exposed to OFII. Analyses were made of data collected for 14- and 10-yr periods. Findings show higher odds ratios for cardiovascular system (CVS) disorders in TPMs working with OFII than were found in 2 control groups. Results suggest that TPMs work in an environment that places them at increased risk for selected CVS, toxic, and neurological (e.g., tension and migraine headaches) disease outcomes. (29 ref).

354. Horváth, M.; Frantík, E. & Krekule, P. (1981). **Diazepam impairs alertness and potentiates the similar effect of toluene.** *Activitas Nervosa Superior,* 23(3), 177–179.
Assessed the single-dose effects of diazepam (5 or 10 mg/2 m^2 of body surface), toluene (a paint solvent; short-term inhalation of 240 ppm), or their combination in 63 male 20–21 yr old volunteers. Ethanol and pentobarbital were used as reference substances. The combination of the 2 substances resulted in the greatest impairment of alertness in monotonous conditions (an auditory click discrimination task), an effect that lasted 3–4 hrs. (10 ref).

355. Iregren, Anders. (1982). **Effects on psychological test performance of workers exposed to a single solvent (Toluene)—a comparison with effects of exposure to a mixture of organic solvents.** *Neurobehavioral Toxicology & Teratology,* 4(6), 695–701.
34 printers (mean age 38.4 yrs) occupationally exposed to toluene were examined with a psychological test battery that included measures of RT, dexterity, memory, and mental arithmetic. Their performance was compared to that of a matched group of spray painters exposed to a mixture of solvents and that of a control group of nonexposed industrial workers. While the performance of the painters was poorer than that of the controls on most tests, the performance of the printers was generally comparable to that of the nonexposed workers. However, in a simple RT test, the performance of the printers was clearly poorer than that of the other 2 groups. Results indicate that the risk for adverse effects on behavioral performance may be greater for workers exposed to solvent mixtures than for workers exposed to a single solvent. (27 ref).

356. Iregren, Anders. (1986). **Subjective and objective signs of organic solvent toxicity among occupationally exposed workers.** *Scandinavian Journal of Work, Environment & Health,* 12(5), 469–475.
A questionnaire consisting of 55 items concerning symptoms associated with exposure to organic solvents, as well as type and duration of exposure, was administered to 152 male spray painters (aged 19–64 yrs). 26 Ss with relatively high or low sensitivity to solvent exposure were matched with respect to age and number of years employed as a painter. Ss were experimentally exposed for 4 hrs to either 3.2 mmol/m^3 of toluene or a control condition in an exposure chamber. Effects on performance were assessed with a battery of 4 tests. Ratings of acute symptoms were also studied. The only difference found between the 2 groups was a higher frequency of symptoms of local irritation in the group that had reported high symptom frequencies on the questionnaire.

SOLVENTS

357. Iregren, Anders; Åkerstedt, Torbjörn; Anshelm Olson, Birgitta & Gamberale, Francesco. (1986). **Experimental exposure to toluene in combination with ethanol intake: Psychophysiological functions.** *Scandinavian Journal of Work, Environment & Health,* 12(2), 128–136.
Studied the effects of experimental exposure to toluene (300 mg/m^3) for 4.5 hrs and ethanol ingestion (15 mmol/kg) on the results of 4 performance tests, symptoms, mood, and physiological indices of wakefulness in 12 males (aged 22–44 yrs). Findings show that toluene exposure produced symptoms like headache and local irritation, as well as a weak depression of heart rate during rest but did not reduce performance capability. It was found that ethanol ingestion impaired performance on 2 of the tests and also increased heart rate. Mood was altered by ethanol, but no increase in subjective symptoms due to ethanol ingestion could be demonstrated. Physiological indices of wakefulness were not affected by toluene exposure or by ethanol intake. No interaction effects were found.

358. Jensen, Per B.; Mamsen, Pia & Pedersen, Grethe. (1985). **Hukommelsestræning af patienter med kronisk toksisk encefalopati. / Memory training of patients with chronic toxic encephalopathy.** *Nordisk Psykiatrisk Tidsskrift,* 39(6), 501–507.
Administered neuropsychological tests to 11 patients suffering from the aftereffects of exposure to organic solvents before, immediately after, and about 10 mo after memory training. Significant improvement in the learning and memory of verbal material was observed after training and was still present at follow-up. (English abstract).

359. Johansson, Barbro B. et al. (1984). **Vasoactive intestinal polypeptide (VIP) in cerebrospinal fluid from men after long-term exposure to organic solvents.** *Acta Neurologica Scandinavica,* 70(4), 317–318.
Measured VIP in (1) CSF from 14 men (mean age 48 yrs) with psycho-organic syndrome occupationally exposed to organic solvents for 7–38 yrs and (2) CSF from 8 neurologically healthy male volunteers (mean age 60 yrs). Findings reveal that the concentration of VIP in exposed Ss did not significantly differ from that of controls. Thus, determination of VIP in CSF appears to be of little value for detecting effects of long-term solvent exposure. (7 ref).

360. Juntunen, Juhani et al. (1985). **Nervous system effects of long-term occupational exposure to toluene.** *Acta Neurologica Scandinavica,* 72(5), 512–517.
43 male rotogravure printers (mean age 41.4 yrs) with long-term exposure to toluene (a neurotoxic organic solvent) and 31 male offset printers (mean age 41.4 yrs) without toluene exposure were interviewed and were administered neurological, autonomic nervous function, computerized axial tomography of the brain, and neurophysiological examinations and neuropsychological tests. Results show that toluene-exposed Ss had significantly more prevalent memory disturbance. Exposure to toluene also seemed to be associated with heavy drinking. (26 ref).

361. Juntunen, Juhani; Antti-Poika, Mari; Tola, Sakari & Partanen, Timo. (1982). **Clinical prognosis of patients with diagnosed chronic solvent intoxication.** *Acta Neurologica Scandinavica,* 65(5), 488–503.
80 patients (20–59 yrs old) with chronic organic solvent intoxication were evaluated in a 3–9 yr follow-up study. 31 Ss had slight neurological signs at diagnosis, while the remaining Ss had only neurophysiological or psychological disturbances. The most common subjective symptoms were headache, tiredness, and memory disturbances. Clinical disturbances occurred frequently in cerebellar functions, gait and station, and fine motor abilities. Psycho-organic alterations and neurasthenic signs were often found. Subjective symptoms decreased during follow-up, but objective clinical signs increased. (35 ref).

362. Juntunen, Juhani; Kaste, Markku & Härkönen, Hannu. (1984). **Cerebral convulsion after enfluran anaesthesia and occupational exposure to tetrahydrofuran.** *Journal of Neurology, Neurosurgery & Psychiatry,* 47(11), 1258.
Describes the case of a previously healthy 45-yr-old male, who after appendectomy surgery using enfluran anesthesia, had several generalized convulsions. Psychological tests given because of his occupational exposure to tetrahydrofuran, a solvent, revealed minor changes in visuomotor functions. Results suggest that the interactions of tetrahydrofuran and enfluran may provoke epileptic seizures; thus, it is important to consider the occupational history of recent exposure to some solvents as a risk factor for anesthesia. (4 ref).

363. Larsby, B.; Tham, R. & Ödkvist, L. M. (1982). **Influence on the vestibular system by industrial solvents.** *Acta Oto-Laryngologica,* 386, 246–248.
15 healthy volunteers (aged 19–30 yrs) were exposed to styrene or trichloroethylene (TCE) during light exercise and tested on 6 opto-vestibular tasks before, during, and after exposure. TCE produced no significant changes, whereas styrene altered response in the saccade and visual suppression tests. It is suggested that these results are due to the different chemical structures of the 2 solvents and resultant differences in action on the vestibulo-oculomotor pathways, and that these tests may be of value in recognizing early signs of intoxication from exposure to solvents. (12 ref).

364. Lindström, Kari; Antti-Poika, Mari; Tola, Sakari & Hyytiäinen, Asko. (1982). **Psychological prognosis of diagnosed chronic organic solvent intoxication.** *Neurobehavioral Toxicology & Teratology,* 4(5), 581–588.
Studied the psychological prognosis of 86 patients (aged 20–60 yrs at diagnosis) with previously diagnosed chronic solvent intoxication due to trichloroethylene, perchloroethylene, or solvent mixtures, after a follow-up period (mean 5.9 yrs). The mean duration of solvent exposure was 10.7 yrs. Tests for intelligence, short-term memory, and sensory and motor functions (e.g., WAIS, Wechsler Memory Scale) were applied. The group means of Ss' intellectual functions were increased after the follow-up period. At the group level, the scores on 1 sensorimotor task and tasks requiring manual dexterity were lower. Individual Ss performed better, worse, or equally when the results of the initial examination and the reexamination were compared. Overall prognosis of psychological test results was better with a longer follow-up period and younger age. Ss who used drugs with neurological effects had a poorer overall psychological prognosis. The characteristics of solvent exposure were related only to the prognosis of some single tests for sensory and motor functions. (17 ref).

365. Lindström, Kari & Wickström, G. (1983). **Psychological function changes among maintenance house painters exposed to low levels of organic solvent mixtures.** *Acta Psychiatrica Scandinavica,* 67(Suppl 303), 81–91.
219 maintenance house painters (mean age 42.4 yrs; mean exposure duration 22.5 yrs) and 229 nonexposed reinforcement workers (mean age 41.9 yrs) were administered a subjective symptom survey, an interview, and a psychological test battery that included subtests from the WAIS and the Wechsler Memory Scale and simple RT tasks. The groups were matched according to preexposure intellectual level. Painters' average exposure to white spirit was estimated to be 40 ppm. They were characterized by defects in short-term visual memory and prolonged simple RTs. Some slight relationships were found between low test performances and individual indices of long-term exposure to solvents. Results imply that adverse psychological effects existed even though the exposure level was much lower than the hygienic standard applied for white spirit in many countries. (14 ref).

366. Lindstrom, Kari. (1973). **Psychological performances of workers exposed to various solvents.** *Work-Environment-Health,* 10(3), 151-155.
Compared the performances of 168 male workers exposed to various common industrial solvents (e.g., tri- and tetrachloroethylene, toluene, xylene, and their mixtures), 50 unexposed controls, and 50 Ss with CS_2 poisoning on a battery of psychological tests. The performances of Ss exposed to the common solvents were inferior to those of the control group, but Ss suffering from CS_2 poisoning were even more disturbed. The parameters that varied most widely between the groups were sensorimotor speed performances and psychomotor performances. Visual accuracy was as poor in the group exposed to the common solvents as in the CS_2-poisoned group. In the group of solvent workers, those with verified or suspected poisoning had psychological performances, particularly in regard to sensorimotor speed, that were slightly inferior to those of the exposed Ss who displayed no symptoms of poisoning. The test battery seems to be a useful instrument for the registration of disturbances within groups of workers exposed to solvents.

367. Lorentzen, Per. (1987). **Kvalitative aspekter ved nevropsykologisk testing: Belyst ved to pasienter med sannsynlig løsemiddelskade. / Qualitative aspects of neuropsychological assessment.** *Tidsskrift for Norsk Psykologforening,* 24(1), 12–19.
Reports the use of qualitative analysis of neuropsychological test performance to distinguish between different deficits in 2 patients with probable central nervous system (CNS) damage caused by exposure to organic solvents. The Ss' symptoms are discussed in relation to their daily functioning. (English abstract).

368. Maizlish, Neil A. (1985). **A neurobehavioral evaluation of workers exposed to organic solvent mixtures.** *Dissertation Abstracts International,* 45(7-B), 2125.

369. Matikainen, E. & Juntunen, Juhani. (1984). **Autonomic dysfunction in toxic states: Alcohol and solvents.** 25th Scandinavian Congress of Neurology: Occupational Neurology (1984, Bergen, Norway). *Acta Neurologica Scandinavica,* 69(98), 130–133.
Examined 28 33–57 yr old male alcoholics and 34 27–61 yr old workers exposed to neurotoxic solvents (25 males, 9 females) to study the association between autonomic nervous system function and these conditions. Findings show that the autonomic nervous system is frequently involved in toxic states in association with disturbances of the peripheral nervous system. It is suggested that when peripheral neuropathy in toxic states is considered, detection of autonomic neuropathy should be included in the examinations. (2 ref).

370. Maximilian, V. Alexander et al. (1982). **Regional cerebral blood flow and verbal memory after chronic exposure to organic solvents.** *Brain & Cognition,* 1(2), 196–205.
Investigated regional cerebral blood flow (RCBF) in 32 right-handed male industrial workers (mean age 51 yrs) who had been exposed to organic solvents for an average of 24.5 yrs. The measurements were made at rest and during learning of associated word pairs. The resting flow level was 17% lower than expected for normal Ss of similar age and the activation-induced changes of RCBF during the test lacked the frontal activation normally seen. Significant correlations between age, length of exposure, and RCBF level were found. In order to control for the age factor, results were also calculated from 2 subgroups ($N=20$) of similar age but with different levels of exposure (13 and 31 yrs of average exposure). The 2 groups differed only slightly in resting RCBF. A marked difference was, however, seen during activation, with significant postcentral flow increases recorded in the lower-exposed group only. Results indicate the potential of the RCBF method for elucidating functional cortical changes related to neurotoxic effects of organic solvents. (31 ref).

371. Nielsen, Niels O. & Nielsen, Per. (1984). **Opløsningsmiddelforgiftning—kronisk toksisk encefalopati udvikling og prognose belyst ved litteraturstudium og efterundersøgelse. / Industrial solvent poisoning: Chronic toxic encephalopathy and a prognosis illustrated by literature and results of our own investigation.** *Psykologisk Skriftserie Aarhus,* 9(3), 128 p.
Presents results from a follow-up study of 26 patients diagnosed as suffering from chronic toxic encephalopathy after occupational exposure to organic industrial solvents. It was found that for most Ss, the condition had had considerable negative effects on their personal, social, and employment situations. Empirical studies on the CNS effects of solvent exposure are reviewed, focusing on studies that emphasized psychological test methods and on evidence pertaining to the emergence and development of associated subjective symptoms. (English abstract) (5 p ref).

372. Nishida, Hirobumi & Yamada, Hiroaki. (1984). **A case report of cerebellar ataxia due to the use of lacquer thinner.** *Kyushu Neuro-psychiatry,* 30(1), 55–61.
Reports the case study of a 28-yr-old female patient with neurologic symptoms caused by organic solvent intoxication. The patient had been inhaling the gas of organic solvents, including thinner, for more than 10 yrs and had recently started showing such symptoms as ataxic gait, dysarthria, and dysopsia after inhaling an unusually large quantity of the thinner. However, the symptoms, centering on the cerebellar ataxia, diminished after approximately 6 mo of treatment. The Durchgangs-Syndrome theory proposed by H. H. Wieck is evaluated in relation to the significance of the persistence of neurological symptoms. (34 ref).

373. Ödkvist, L. M. et al. (1982). **Vestibulo-oculomotor disturbances in humans exposed to styrene.** *Acta Oto-Laryngologica,* 94(5–6), 487–493.
Studied rotatory and optokinetic nystagmus, visual suppression, speed and accuracy of saccades, pulmonary uptake, and blood level of the solvent before, during, and 1 hr after 10 healthy Ss were exposed to styrene for 1 hr. The speed of the saccade was significantly enhanced, and visual suppression was disturbed. Results are consistent with the theory that some organic solvents block the cerebellar inhibition of the vestibulo-oculomotor system. (German abstract) (7 ref).

374. Ödkvist, L. M. et al. (1982). **Otoneurological and audiological findings in workers exposed to industrial solvents.** *Acta Oto-Laryngologica,* 386, 249–251.
11 men (aged 37–61 yrs) with a psycho-organic syndrome caused by exposure to industrial solvents were subjected to cerebellar tests, electronystagmography, and an audiological test battery. The presence of spontaneous or positional nystagmus in 7 Ss confirmed a CNS disturbance in these Ss. The positive cerebellar pathology in some Ss suggests that this might be the part of the brain most vulnerable to exposure to solvents. Some Ss had positive findings in oculomotor tests, but the most prominent pathology concerned the visual suppression test. In audiological testing, cortical response audiometry and interrupted speech discrimination were most frequently abnormal, reflecting the vulnerability of polysynaptic pathways. Normal brain-stem responses were found in 5 of the 6 Ss tested. Results suggest that the solvents block the inhibition of the vestibulo-ocular reflex presumably exerted by the cerebellum. (26 ref).

375. Olson, Birgitta A. (1982). **Effects of organic solvents on behavioral performance of workers in the paint industry.** *Neurobehavioral Toxicology & Teratology,* 4(6), 703–708.
47 industrial workers (aged 20–58 yrs) exposed daily to a mixture of organic solvents and 47 age-matched nonexposed

SOLVENTS

industrial workers were examined before and after a work day with a battery of tests including simple RT, perceptual speed, short-term memory, and critical flicker fusion. A questionnaire was used to assess subjective symptoms. The exposed group performed more poorly than the control group on all measures except critical flicker fusion at both times of testing. Significantly more exposed Ss reported tiredness, irritability, and impaired memory. The differences were most pronounced for Ss exposed to higher solvent concentrations and at the afternoon testing, which is interpreted as primarily due to an acute effect. (27 ref).

376. Ørbæk, Palle et al. (1985). **Effects of long-term exposure to solvents in the paint industry: A cross-sectional epidemiologic study with clinical and laboratory methods.** *Scandinavian Journal of Work, Environment & Health,* 11(Suppl 2), 1–28.
Examined the effects of organic solvents on 50 male workers (aged 27–64 yrs) who were exposed to such solvents over a period of 5–46 yrs. Ss were matched pairwise according to age and education with a group of 50 nonexposed Ss. An analysis of confounding factors confirmed good comparability between the 2 groups. Regional cerebral blood flow (RCBF) was measured, and the power spectrum of the Ss' EEGs was analyzed to determine degree of organic brain dysfunction in exposed Ss. Results indicate that RCBF was reduced 4% in exposed Ss and that EEGs demonstrated increased power in the delta and beta bands in the exposed group. Symptoms of brain dysfunction were significantly more frequent among the exposed Ss and showed an exposure-effect relationship. Neuropsychological tests revealed definite indication of brain dysfunction in 14% of the exposed Ss while no dysfunction was noted in the control Ss. Exposed Ss performed significantly worse than controls in tests measuring focused attention abilities. A neurophysiological examination of the peripheral nervous system showed no difference between the groups. Clinical chemistry demonstrated no differences that could be attributed to solvent exposure. (89 ref).

377. Petersen, Uwe. (1985). **Mentale følgevirkninger efter eksposition for organiske opløsningsmidler. / Mental effects due to exposure to organic solvents.** *Psykologisk Skriftserie Aarhus,* 10(5), 160 p.
Discusses the relationship between the neurological examination (computerized tomographic scanning) and the psychological examination of individuals with possible impairments of mental functions based on empirical research. Problems concerning diagnostic choice, definition of syndromes, and differential diagnosis are considered. (English abstract).

378. Putz-Anderson, Vernon; Setzer, James V. & Croxton, Jack S. (1981). **Effects of alcohol, caffeine and methyl chloride on man.** *Psychological Reports,* 48(3), 715–725.
Industrial workers are frequently exposed to organic solvents, such as methyl chloride, and also voluntarily ingest quantities of alcohol or caffeine, all of which affect the CNS. The present study assessed the behavioral effects of such substances alone and when combined. 84 18–32 yr olds were assigned to 1 of 6 treatment groups. Each S was then tested before and during both the treatment or control procedures on 3 performance tasks. Results indicate that an alcohol dose sufficient to register blood levels of 0.08% produced a significant impairment of 10% on all 3 tests, which included eye-hand coordination and alertness. A caffeine dose equivalent to 2 cups of coffee (200 mg) produced a small but significant impairment on only the eye-hand coordination test. However, Ss who were exposed to methyl chloride for 3.5 hrs at levels equivalent to the current legal standard did not experience any significant impairments on the tests. Moreover, when the solvent was combined with each drug individually, the effect was essentially equivalent to the sum of the separate effects; no behavioral interaction was found. (19 ref).

379. Risberg, Jarl & Hagstadius, Stefan. (1983). **Effects on the regional cerebral blood flow of long-term exposure to organic solvents.** *Acta Psychiatrica Scandinavica,* 67(Suppl 303), 92–99.
Regional cerebral blood flow (rCBF) was measured in 50 26–62 yr old male paint factory workers with a mean of 18 yrs of exposure to a mixture of organic solvents. 50 workers in a sugar refinery, matched for age and education, served as controls. Measurements were made during resting and during activation by mental tasks (word-pair learning). Results show slightly lower mean flow level in the exposed group. Largest differences were seen in frontotemporal areas. The difference between the exposed group and controls increased at higher dose levels. The largest rCBF increases during mental activation were seen in the exposed group, especially in the highest-exposed Ss. This finding might indicate mechanisms compensating for a somewhat defective brain function. Although the differences between groups were generally small with considerable overlap, results give some evidence of disturbances of brain blood flow and brain function likely related to the influence of organic solvents. (25 ref).

380. Rosengarten, Helene; Meller, Emanuel & Friedhoff, Arnold J. (1976). **Possible source of error in studies of enzymatic formation of dimethyltryptamine.** *Journal of Psychiatric Research,* 13(1), 23–30.
Describes an assay of an enzyme derived from red blood cells capable of catalyzing the formation of dimethyltryptamine (DMT) from C^{14}-S-adenosylmethionine (C^{14}-SAM) as a methyl donor and appropriate precursor. A hemoglobin free soluble fraction of the red cell was used as an enzyme source. Enzyme protein was incubated with C^{14}-SAM and N-methyltryptamine. Enzyme activity was low but reproducible, and over 80% of extractable radioactivity was authentic DMT product. The product of incubation was identified by chromatography and co-crystallization with authentic DMT carrier. In contrast, if hemoglobin rich undialysed supernate was used as the enzyme source, and C^{14}-SAM in ethanol as the methyl donor, only 11% of the recovered radioactivity migrated with authentic DMT carrier, and 89% was confined to 2-methyltetrahydrobetacarboline (THBC). In the hemoglobin rich fraction of the red cell supernate, formation of THBC predominates. Formation of C^{14}-formaldehyde from C^{14}-SAM via methanol in the red cell and nonenzymatic condensation with indoleamine substrates followed by formation of THBC is discussed. Proof of THBC formation is presented. (27 ref).

381. Ryan, Christopher M.; Morrow, Lisa A. & Hodgson, Michael. (1988). **Cacosmia and neurobehavioral dysfunction associated with occupational exposure to mixtures of organic solvents.** *American Journal of Psychiatry,* 145(11), 1442–1445.
Examined the interrelationships among occupational exposure to mixtures of organic solvents, neurobehavioral functioning, and complaints of cacosmia. The latter was defined as nausea, headaches, and subjective distress in individuals exposed to neutral environmental odors. The authors administered a battery of cognitive tests (including the Wechsler Memory Scale and subtests from the Wechsler Adult Intelligence Scale—Revised [WAIS–R]) to 17 men (mean age 41.5 yrs) with a history of solvent exposure, compared them with 17 age-matched men without such a history, and found exposed workers to be impaired across a wide range of cognitive domains. Multiple regression analyses of exposed workers demonstrated a highly significant relationship between a history of cacosmia and performance decrements on measures of learning and memory.

382. Schottenfeld, Richard S. & Cullen, Mark R. (1985). **Occupation-induced posttraumatic stress disorders.** *American Journal of Psychiatry,* 142(2), 198–202.
Describes a variant of posttraumatic stress disorder (PTSD) that presents as a somatoform disorder and its assessment in 21 patients (aged 23–58 yrs) who were severely disabled due

to multiple or vague recurrent or persistent symptoms (e.g., chest pain, nausea, fatigue) for which no organic etiology was discovered. By applying clearly specified diagnostic criteria, it was found that 7 Ss had atypical PTSD, while 3 Ss had typical PTSD, and the remainder suffered from somatoform disorders. All 3 Ss with typical PTSD had experienced acute, life-threatening occupational injury or exposure. Of the 7 Ss with atypical PTSD, 1 S had an acute exposure to a toxic substance at work, and the others had histories of chronic or repeated exposures to organic solvents or other volatile substances over extended periods. Analysis of these cases revealed specific exposure factors and personality characteristics that favor the development of atypical PTSD. Theoretical, clinical, and therapeutic advantages of this diagnosis are outlined. (16 ref).

383. Seppäläinen, Anna M. (1985). **Neurophysiological aspects of the toxicity of organic solvents.** International Conference on Organic Solvent Toxicity (1984, Stockholm, Sweden). *Scandinavian Journal of Work, Environment & Health,* 11(Suppl 1), 61–64.
Discusses the neurotoxic effects of exposure to organic solvents, which are the result of the systemic spread and metabolic transformation of the chemical. Among patients with solvent poisoning, abnormally slow nerve-conduction velocities are detected. Electromyography (EMG) reveals denervation activity in early axonopathy; loss of motor units is detectable at a later stage. Hexacarbons (e.g., n-hexane) have caused changes in visual evoked potentials (i.e., prolonged latencies and decreased amplitudes), probably due to axonal lesions within the central nervous system (CNS). Among patients, actual EEG abnormalities, mainly diffuse or local slow-wave abnormalities, are frequent. (25 ref).

384. Singh, Jaya; Dwivedi, Kamal & Saxena, V. B. (1987). **Memory and subjective symptoms in automobile painters.** *Indian Psychological Review,* 32(2), 5–12.
Investigated the effect of long-term exposure to a mixture of organic solvents in paint thinner on the scores of 24 automobile painters who were administered a memory questionnaire and a questionnaire of subjective symptoms. Scores were compared with those from 24 unexposed workers in the upholstery department of the same automobile workshop. Unexposed Ss performed significantly better in 4 areas of memory, with memory attention and concentration the most affected. Although only 3 of 40 symptoms showed significant differences between the groups, results indicate some degree of deterioration in psychological functioning in Ss exposed to organic solvents.

385. Stollery, Brian T. & Flindt, Michael L. (1988). **Memory sequelae of solvent intoxication.** *Scandinavian Journal of Work, Environment & Health,* 14(1), 45–48.
Conducted a retrospective study on 9 female workers accidentally intoxicated by organic solvents (toluene and aliphatic hydrocarbons) to evaluate residual memory impairment. 10 unexposed female workers served as control Ss. Assessments of memory included paired-associate, serial-position, and word-recall tasks. Testing was performed 2 mo after the intoxication with a follow-up 6 mo later to assess recovery. Ss showed normal patterns of performance on tests of learning and short- and long-term memory, but difficulties were observed when attention had to be allocated between 2 resource-competing tasks. There was no evidence of recovery by the follow-up session. Results indicate that solvent intoxication can cause neuropsychological sequelae lasting for over 8 mo.

386. Struwe, Göran & Wennberg, Arne. (1983). **Psychiatric and neurological symptoms in workers occupationally exposed to organic solvents: Results of a differential epidemiological study.** *Acta Psychiatrica Scandinavica,* 67(Suppl 303), 68–80.
80 laquerers exposed to a mixture of industrial solvents (average hygienic effect 0.3) and 37 printers exposed almost only to toluene (average hygienic effect 1.0) were compared with a control group of 80 age-matched nonexposed Ss. In psychiatric interviews, the painters showed more mental symptoms. Fatigue, nervousness, and lack of manual dexterity were most important and formed a typical neurasthenic syndrome. A general decrease in conduction velocity and action potential amplitude was observed for the peripheral nerves. Printers showed a large decrease of the nerve action potential amplitude only for the sural nerve. No EEG abnormalities were found, nor could any increase in mental symptoms be detected through psychiatric interviews compared to the controls. Results are interpreted as evidence for a CNS affect with consequent neuropsychiatric signs and symptoms after long-term occupational exposure to mixtures of industrial solvents below the current threshold limit values (TLV) but not after exposure to a single substance like toluene at about the TLV. The differential effects may be explained by synergistic amplification of the toxicity of solvent mixtures. (16 ref).

387. Swanson, Joan R. (1985). **The psychological and educational implications of formaldehyde toxicology.** *Dissertation Abstracts International,* 45(11-A), 3325.

388. Tariot, Pierre N. (1983). **Delirium resulting from methylene chloride exposure: Case report.** *Journal of Clinical Psychiatry,* 44(9), 340–342.
Reports a case of a 52-yr-old male suffering from delirium resulting from work-related exposure to methylene chloride, a widely used organic solvent. Inhalation of its vapors caused toxic effects via endogenous carbon monoxide production, which, it is concluded, caused S's symptoms. Follow-up evaluation and EEG 6 wks after discharge were normal. (15 ref).

389. Turbiaux, Marcel. (1980). **Contribution à l'étude des effets psychologiques de l'exposition chronique au trichlorethylène en milieu industriel. / Study of the psychological effects of chronic exposure to trichloroethylene in the workplace.** *Bulletin de Psychologie,* 33(347), 997–1007.
Investigated the effects of trichloroethylene on intelligence (WAIS), attention span (BG 10 Test), and apperception of general physical and psychological health (Cornell Index, Form N2) of chronically exposed workers. Deterioration on WAIS performances was found among Ss having relatively low levels of trichloroethylene per liter of blood. Chronically exposed Ss reported more psychological disturbances on the Cornell Index. However, the absence of signs of organicity on the Rorschach protocols of Ss presenting psychometric deterioration reinforced the hypothesis that such effects are transitory and reversible. While the effects of trichloroethylene on susceptible individuals are uncontestable, the study was not designed to establish levels of susceptibility. Suggestions are made, though, for prevention and control of trichloroethylene exposure. (32 ref).

390. Vinař, O.; Frantík, E. & Horváth, M. (1981). **Subjectively perceived effects of diazepam, toluene and their combination.** *Activitas Nervosa Superior,* 23(3), 179–182.
With reference to the authors' (1981) previous study, which showed that diazepam and toluene (a paint solvent) impaired performance and alertness in an auditory discrimination task, the present study reports on the subjective effects of the single-dose diazepam and toluene treatments (both alone and combined) perceived by 49 healthy male volunteers. While hypnotic effects, impaired performance on another auditory discrimination task and a visuomotor feedback task, fatigue, and tension reduction were reported by the Ss, there were no statistically significant correlations between subjective effects and performance. (7 ref).

SOLVENTS

391. White, Roberta F. (1987). **Differential diagnosis of probable Alzheimer's disease and solvent encephalopathy in older workers.** *Clinical Neuropsychologist,* 1(2), 153–160.
Presents 4 case histories to illustrate the differential diagnosis of the effects of exposure to industrial solvents vs Alzheimer's disease and discusses research findings with regard to assessing cognitive problems in older workers. Issues discussed include the prevalence of such problems, patterns of neuropsychological dysfunction, and proposed principles of diagnosis. These principles concern the assessment of IQ, language, retrograde memory, attention and visuospatial skills, and progression of cognitive decline.

392. Winneke, Gerhard. (1982). **Acute behavioral effects of exposure to some organic solvents: Psychophysiological aspects.** *Acta Neurologica Scandinavica,* 66(Suppl 92), 117–129.
Previous findings indicate that acute low-level exposure to organic solvent vapors may result in prenarcotic states of CNS depression, often characterized by behavioral dysfunction. The author reviews behavioral findings from experimental acute human exposures to toluene, trichloroethylene (TCE), and methylene chloride (MC). Perceptual (e.g., CFF), sustained attention (vigilance), psychomotor performance (e.g., RT, motor speed, and coordination), and EEG measures illustrate the main effects from such studies. A progressive increase of RT was observed at toluene exposures of only 300 ppm (30 min). No consistent behavioral deficit has been reported for TCE below 300 ppm; instead, visual and auditory EPs were affected at TCE vapor concentrations between 50 and 100 ppm (3½–7½ hrs of exposure). CFF depression, vigilance decrements, and disruptions of psychomotor performance have previously been observed during MC exposure (200–800 ppm; 2–4 hrs). Although such behavioral effects are usually considered reversible and of no demonstrated pathological impact, they may nevertheless contribute to accident-prone behavior in occupational settings. (28 ref).

Animal Research

393. Bushnell, Philip J. & Peele, David B. (1988). **Conditioned flavor aversion induced by inhaled *p*-xylene in rats.** *Neurobehavioral Toxicology & Teratology,* 10(3), 273–277.
Male Long-Evans rats were placed on a restricted water schedule (30 min/day). 10 days later, all Ss received 0.1% saccharin in place of water and were exposed immediately either to filtered air or to 50, 100, 200, 400, 800, or 1,600 ppm *p*-xylene for 4 hr or to air or 400 ppm *p*-xylene for 0.5, 1, 2, 4, or 8 hr. Results show that inhalation of all concentrations of *p*-xylene reduced relative saccharin intake, with maximal aversion at 800 and 1,600 ppm.

394. Colotla, Victor A.; Bautista, Samuel & Torres Cházaro, Octavio. (1980). **Behavioral recovery after toluene exposure in rats.** *Revista Mexicana de Análisis de la Conducta,* 6(1), 103–111.
Reports results of the behavioral recovery after toluene exposure in laboratory rats. The data on toluene exposure have been previously reported (V. A. Colotla et al, 1979): A differential effect of toluene was found in the 2 components of the multiple schedule employed: an increase in response rate in the differential reinforcement of low rate (DRL) component and a decrease in the FR component. During the recovery sessions DRL performance decreased to baseline levels, but FR performance remained at low levels. During the timeout periods there was an increase in responses during exposure to the solvent, which decreased to baseline in the postdosage session. An analysis of local rates indicated that, whereas DRL performance did not vary throughout the session, the ratio performance changed progressively: Response rate decreased as the session advanced and increased progressively in the postdosage session. (9 ref).

395. Dyer, Robert S. et al. (1984). **Neurophysiological effects of 30 day chronic exposure to toluene in rats.** *Neurobehavioral Toxicology & Teratology,* 6(5), 363–368.
Male Long-Evans hooded rats were exposed to 1,000 ppm toluene ($n = 51$) or 0 ppm toluene ($n = 51$) for 6 hrs/day, 5 days/week for 30 days. Following removal from the exposure conditions (18–26 hrs) flash-EPs were recorded to paired light flashes, and pentylenetetrazol (PTZ) seizure properties were examined. No alterations were found in the response to the 1st flash, but alterations in the recoverability of the nervous system were demonstrated by significant latency shifts in the response to the 2nd of the paired flashes, using 1st-flash latencies as covariates. No significant alterations were found in PTZ seizures. Data indicate that at these exposure levels, toluene produced a small but significant alteration in brain function, even after toluene had been completely metabolized. The negative PTZ test findings contrast with a study by Y. Takeuchi and H. Suzuki (1975). (20 ref).

396. Dyer, Robert S.; Bercegeay, Mark S. & Mayo, Lieser M. (1988). **Acute exposures to p-xylene and toluene alter visual information processing.** *Neurotoxicology & Teratology,* 10(2), 147–153.
Evaluated the functional integrity of the visual system in hooded rats exposed to single doses of toluene at 0, 250, 500, and 1,000 mg/kg and to p-xylene at 0, 125, 250, 500, 1,000, and 2,000 mg/kg and to inhalation of p-xylene for 4 hrs at 0, 800, or 1,600 ppm using flash-evoked potentials (FEPs). Data indicate a significant depression in amplitude of FEP peak N3 at 250 mg/kg and higher dosages of toluene and p-xylene. A similar depression in peak N3 amplitude was observed following inhalation exposure to 1,600 ppm p-xylene. The effects produced by oral administration of 500 mg/kg p-xylene or toluene lasted at least 8 hrs, while the effect of inhaled p-xylene dissipated within 75 min of removal from the exposure. It is suggested that the effects of p-xylene and toluene on FEPs, while indicative of altered processing of visual information, may be secondary to changes in arousal or excitability.

397. Dyer, Robert S.; Boyes, William K. & Hetzler, Bruce E. (1986). **Acute sulfolane exposure produces temperature-independent and dependent changes in visual evoked potentials.** *Neurobehavioral Toxicology & Teratology,* 8(6), 687–693.
Studied the effects of acute injections of sulfolane on the visual system of male Long-Evans hooded rats, measuring flash evoked potentials (EPs) and pattern reversal EPs. Sulfolane produces a variety of acute neurobehavioral effects in the rat. This study showed that sulfolane caused a clear increase in visual EP latencies and more complex changes in response amplitudes, as it caused hypothermia. No single mechanism explains these results.

398. Evans, H. L.; Bushnell, P. J.; Pontecorvo, Michael J. & Taylor, J. D. (1985). **Animal models of environmentally induced memory impairment.** *Annals of the New York Academy of Sciences,* 444, 513–514.
Examined the effects of toxicants and drugs on memory in macaques and pigeons using a 3-choice, variable-delay matching-to-sample (DMS) procedure. Delayed matching of previously trained pigeons was evaluated following daily inhalation of toluene or n-hexane. Inhalation of 3,000 ppm toluene reduced matching accuracy after 1–2 wks of daily exposure; recovery occurred within 2 wks after the exposure stopped. Acute inhalation of toluene by monkeys during performance of the DMS task produced immediate decrements in accuracy and reaction time (RT). A decrement in DMS also occurred in monkeys and pigeons after acute exposure to trimethyltin. (10 ref).

399. Gade, Anders & Jensen, Hans H. (1985). **State-dependent learning during chronic trichloroethylene exposure.** *Scandinavian Journal of Work, Environment & Health,* 11(6), 495–497.
Discusses the behavioral phenomenon of state-dependent learning, in which reproduction of behavior learned under the influence of a drug may be facilitated by a similar drug state during the test of retention. It is posited that state-dependent learning during solvent exposure may be erroneously interpreted as behavioral impairment indicative of brain lesions. To illustrate the phenomenon and how readily it can be misinterpreted, the authors reanalyze data from an experiment by P. Kjellstrand et al (1980).

400. Geist, Charles R.; Drew, Kelly L.; Schoenheit, Carolyn M. & Praed, Jeffrey E. (1983). **Learning impairments following postnatal exposure to benzene.** *Perceptual & Motor Skills,* 57(3, Pt 2), 1083–1086.
16 male hooded Sprague-Dawley rats were administered 550 mg/kg, ip of benzene in corn oil or pure corn oil on Days 9, 11, and 13 postpartum. When tested on problems of the Hebb-Williams closed-field maze-learning task, Ss previously exposed to benzene manifested significantly impaired learning ability when compared to controls in the total number of error zones entered over the 12 test problems. No significant differences were found in food consumption, water consumption, or weight gain. None of the overt manifestations characteristic of acute or chronic benzene exposure were observed. Learning deficits were exhibited at levels of exposure previously considered subtoxic. Findings extend those reported by H. A. Tilson et al (1980). (12 ref).

401. Geller, I.; Hartmann, R. J. & Gause, E. M. (1983). **Effect of exposure to high concentrations of toluene on ethanol preference of laboratory rats.** *Pharmacology, Biochemistry & Behavior,* 19(6), 933–937.
15 Holtzman Sprague-Dawley rats were given 10-min exposures to high concentrations of toluene (TL) twice a week at 10–30 days of age. Another 15 Ss served as sham-exposed littermate controls. The rate of acquisition of ethanol preference did not differ for the 2 groups. Once ethanol preference curves were established, Ss were exposed to high concentrations of TL over a 5-day period; an increase in ethanol intake occurred irrespective of early TL exposures at 10–30 days of age. (11 ref).

402. Geller, I.; Hartmann, R. J.; Mendez, V. & Gause, E. M. (1983). **Toluene inhalation and anxiolytic activity: Possible synergism with diazepam.** *Pharmacology, Biochemistry & Behavior,* 19(5), 899–903.
Toluene exposure (10,000, 20,000, or 30,000 ppm) or injections of diazepam (0.75–8.0 mg/kg) reinstated leverpress that had been suppressed by punishment in male albino Sprague Dawley rats. When concentrations of toluene or diazepam that were ineffective or minimally effective in this paradigm were administered in combination, they produced a qualitatively similar effect that was much greater than the total of effects produced by the same amount of either substance alone. Observations suggest an anxiolytic action for toluene and a possible synergism between the 2 substances. (10 ref).

403. Geller, Irving; Hartmann, Roy J.; Mendez, Victor & Gause, Emily M. (1985). **Toluene and ethanol effects on baboon match-to-sample performance: Possible synergistic action.** *Pharmacology, Biochemistry & Behavior,* 22(4), 583–588.
Examined whether exposure to toluene and ethanol vapors would produce qualitatively similar effects on 4 male juvenile baboons' (*Papio cynocephalus*) performance of a match-to-sample (MTS) task, and the possible effects of exposure to combinations of ineffective concentrations of toluene and ethanol. Ss were trained to respond for banana pellet rewards on an MTS discrimination task. Exposure of the Ss to a range of concentrations of either toluene or ethanol vapor resulted in a slowing of response times and a reduction in the percent trials attempted for some concentrations of either vapor. When behaviorally ineffective (subthreshold) concentrations of each vapor were combined, effects upon response times and trials attempted were similar to the effects produced by the higher concentrations of the individual vapors. However, while high concentrations of ethanol vapor produced errors in half of the Ss, combinations of ethanol and toluene did not increase this effect. Data suggest an ethanol potentiation of toluene effects, rather than the reverse. (15 ref).

404. Ghilardi, M. Felice; Chung, Eunyong; Bodis-Wollner, Ivan; Dvorzniak, Mark et al. (1988). **Systemic 1-methyl,4-phenyl,1-2-3-6-tetrahydropyridine (MPTP) administration decreases retinal dopamine content in primates.** *Life Sciences,* 43(3), 255–262.
MPTP produced bradykinesia, tremor, and postural abnormality (parkinsonian syndrome); altered visual evoked potential and electroretinogram measurements; and reduced retinal dopamine and dihydroxyphenylacetic acid levels in 4 monkeys. Dopamine may have a function in the visual system of primates.

405. Ghosh, T. K. & Pradhan, S. N. (1987). **Comparison of effects of xylene and toluene inhalation on fixed-ratio liquid-reinforced behavior in rats.** *Research Communications in Psychology, Psychiatry & Behavior,* 12(4), 205–214.
Studied the effects of xylene (XYL) or toluene (TOL) inhalation on an operant behavior maintained by an FR liquid-reinforced schedule in 4 male rats. Ss were exposed to each of the 3 graded concentrations of either XYL (116, 214, or 442 ppm) or TOL (121, 211, or 496 ppm) for 2 hrs in a dynamic inhalational behavioral chamber. The reinforcement rate was decreased significantly at 1 hr during exposure to XYL at all concentrations. TOL also showed a similar effect during exposure only to 211 and 496 ppm. A comparison of decreases of the reinforcement rates following XYL or TOL inhalation showed that the effects of these solvents were not significantly different.

406. Gibbons, Barbara H. & Gibbons, I. R. (1981). **Organic solvents modify the calcium control of flagellar movement in sea urchin sperm.** *Nature,* 292(5818), 85–86.
Results of a study of sea urchin sperm indicate that low concentrations of various organic solvents interacted with the mechanism by which Ca ions induce waveform asymmetry. The solvents studied fell into 2 groups of which the first, consisting of methanol, 2-propanol, and ethylene glycol, mimicked the effect of Ca ions and increased the asymmetry; whereas the 2nd group, N,N-dimethylformamide, formamide, and paradioxane, blocked the increase in asymmetry induced by Ca ions. However, all solvents in both groups acted similarly in decreasing the flagellar beat frequency. (23 ref).

407. Himnan, Donald J. (1984). **Tolerance and reverse tolerance to toluene inhalation: Effects on open-field behavior.** *Pharmacology, Biochemistry & Behavior,* 21(4), 625–631.
Exposed 20 male Long-Evans rats by inhalation to extremely high concentrations of toluene vapors twice daily for 6 wks, as an animal model of organic solvent abuse. Six Ss were in a sham-exposure group. At preset intervals during repeated exposure, Ss were exposed to test concentrations of toluene and effects on behavior in an open field were measured. Concentration–effect curves were determined during Weeks 4–6 of repeated exposure. Tolerance to toluene was measured as a decreased response to the test exposure and a shift of the concentration–effect curve to the right. Reverse tolerance was measured as an increased response to the test exposure and a shift of the concentration–effect curve to the left. Results demonstrate that the effects of repeated exposure to toluene showed behavioral selectivity: Tolerance developed to ataxia, hindlimb myoclonus, and inhibition of rearing; reverse toler-

SOLVENTS

ance developed to headshakes and increased locomotor activity. (35 ref).

408. Hinman, Donald J. (1987). **Biphasic dose-response relationship for effects of toluene inhalation on locomotor activity.** *Pharmacology, Biochemistry & Behavior,* 26(1), 65–69.
Studied the effects of toluene inhalation on the spontaneous locomotor activity of adult male Long-Evans hooded rats during a randomized, crossover, graded-dose experiment. Ss were exposed to graded concentrations of toluene, and locomotor activity was measured continuously before, during, and after administration. Results indicate that behavioral responses to extremely high concentrations of toluene are characterized by biphasic actions as demonstrated both by analysis of concentration–response and time–action factors. The biphasic effects produced by toluene inhalation are dependent on both the concentration of toluene and the duration of exposure. Exposure to concentrations of toluene similar to those used in this study occurs during organic solvent abuse and glue-sniffing in humans.

409. Howd, Robert A.; Rebert, Charles S.; Dickinson, Julie & Pryor, Gordon T. (1983). **A comparison of the rates of development of functional hexane neuropathy in weanling and young adult rats.** *Neurobehavioral Toxicology & Teratology,* 5(1), 63–68.
Chronic inhalation exposure of adult rats to hexane causes neural toxicities to develop over several weeks. Because the developing organism is more vulnerable to toxic insult than the adult, and children make up a substantial proportion of the population of solvent abusers, the effects of exposing weanling (21 days old) and young adult (80 days old) male Fischer-344 rats to 1,000 ppm of hexane for 24 hrs/day, 6 days/wk for 11 wks were studied. Within 2 wks of exposure, significant decreases in body weight and grip strength were observed in Ss of both ages. However, the subsequent effects of the treatment on these indices of toxicity were greater in the young adults than in the Ss exposed as weanlings. The older Ss also exhibited earlier and more severe signs of hindlimb flaccid paralysis. In contrast, the effects of hexane on tail nerve-conduction time and on the brain-stem auditory evoked response were about the same at both ages, with latencies increasing compared to controls over the exposure period. The relative resistance of the weanling rats to hexane neuropathy may be due to shorter, smaller-diameter axons or to a greater rate of growth and repair in their peripheral nerves compared to those of adults. (22 ref).

410. Ishikawa, Terry T. & Schmidt, Hans. (1973). **Forced turning induced by toluene.** *Pharmacology, Biochemistry & Behavior,* 1(5), 593-595.
Conducted an experiment with 30 male Sprague-Dawley albino rats, in which repeated daily toluene inhalation produced circling. It is suggested that this effect may be specific to toluene since xylene failed to elicit turning. The turning followed toluene inhalation and was not associated with histological lesions of the brain. Forced circling was reestablished more rapidly 15 days after the last toluene inhalation than 21 or 30 days thereafter. These conditions required as many exposures to toluene as were required to institute turning originally.

411. Kjellstrand, Per. (1986). **Comment on the interpretation of effects caused by chronic trichloroethylene exposure.** *Scandinavian Journal of Work, Environment & Health,* 12(2), 154–155.
Replies to comments made by A. Gade and H. H. Jensen (1985) who referred to a previous article by the present author and colleagues (1980) as an example of how readily state-dependent learning can cause misinterpretation in experiments using behavior to explore the central nervous system (CNS). The present authors note that the original experiments were not purported to be the correct explanation of the phenomenon of state dependent learning.

412. Lockard, Joan S.; Levy, René H.; Congdon, William C. & DuCharme, Larry L. (1979). **Efficacy and toxicity of the solvent polyethylene glycol 400 in monkey model.** *Epilepsia,* 20(1), 77–84.
Evaluated the possibility that polyethylene glycol 400 (PEG 400) might be efficacious, toxic, or both. 11 rhesus monkeys rendered epileptic by aluminum hydroxide were administered PEG 400 by constant rate (1 ml/hr) iv infusion for 3–4 wks, preceded and followed by several weeks of baseline. At a concentration of 60%, PEG 400 significantly reduced seizure frequency, but also exhibited severe side effects (i.e., toxicity). Findings suggest that experimental testing of anticonvulsants may be compromised when this or similar solvents are used chronically. (12 ref).

413. Lorenzana-Jimenez, Marte & Salas, Manuel. (1983). **Neonatal effects of toluene on the locomotor behavioral development in the rat.** *Neurobehavioral Toxicology & Teratology,* 5(3), 295–299.
128 male Wistar rats were exposed to toluene twice a day for 15 min on Days 2–32 of postnatal life. The subsequent effects on swimming ability, escape latency from water, locomotor activity, and physical development were evaluated. Maturation of swimming behavior and physical development were delayed about 3–4 days in experimental Ss. Moreover, escape from water showed prolonged mean latencies until 24 postnatal days, and the locomotor activity was increased during the 60 min following toluene exposure compared with nonexposed littermate controls. Data suggest that neonatal toluene exposure appears to be primarily interfering with the development of those cortical and brain-stem structures underlying swimming and locomotor activities. (27 ref).

414. Miyake, Hirotsugu. (1983). **Slow learning in rats due to long-term inhalation of toluene.** *Neurobehavioral Toxicology & Teratology,* 5(5), 541–548.
Male Wistar rats were exposed to toluene (1,000, 4,000 and 7,000 ppm) for 1 hr/day, 6 days/wk for 154 days. Behavioral tests on a test battery were carried out after the termination of 154 days' exposure. The performance level of FR-1, extinction of the FR-30 schedule, wheel running activity, scores of open-field test, and body weight were not influenced. Slow acquisition of the timing behavior of a DRL-12 sec schedule in toluene-exposed Ss was revealed: higher responses from the 1st session onward, lower percent of reinforced responses from the 1st session onward, and higher relative frequency of shorter interresponse times (IRT) from the 9th to 12th sessions, respectively, than those of the controls. At the 33rd session onward, the highest relative frequency of IRT of the DRL-12 sec schedule was at around 12 sec in all groups except the group exposed to 7,000 ppm. (24 ref).

415. Moser, Virginia C. (1983). **A comparative behavioral pharmacology of inhaled solvents; toluene, 1,1,1-trichloroethane, halothane, and ethanol.** *Dissertation Abstracts International,* 44(3-B), 766.

416. Moser, Virginia C. & Balster, Robert L. (1986). **The effects of inhaled toluene, halothane, 1,1,1-trichloroethane, and ethanol on fixed-interval responding in mice.** *Neurobehavioral Toxicology & Teratology,* 8(5), 525–531.
Adult male CD-1 mice were trained to leverpress under an FI-60-sec schedule for milk presentation during 15-min sessions. Concentration–effect curves were determined at termination of 30-min inhalation exposures to various volatile agents—halothane, toluene, trichloroethane (TCE), and ethanol. Ss were also tested after ethanol administered orally. Each compound produced both response-rate increases and

decreases, initially or during the recovery phase. Recovery from the response-rate-decreasing effects generally occurred during the 15-min sessions. The highest concentration of toluene and the high dose of oral ethanol produced the longest duration of effects. Findings indicate that the effects of toluene and TCE are qualitatively similar to those of 2 volatile central nervous system (CNS) depressants, halothane and ethanol.

417. Moser, Virginia C. & Balster, Robert L. (1985). **Effects of toluene, halothane and ethanol vapor on fixed-ratio performance in mice.** *Pharmacology, Biochemistry & Behavior,* 22(5), 797–802.
Studied the behavioral effects of inhalation of the vapors of volatile compounds representative of different chemical groups in male CD-1 mice under conditions where behavior and exposure concentrations could be concurrently monitored. The magnitude and time course of the effects of toluene, halothane, and ethanol inhalation on fixed-ratio (FR) responding were compared. Ss were trained to leverpress under a FR-100 schedule of water reinforcement. Daily operant sessions took place in the exposure chambers, and solvent exposures were conducted once a week. The test exposures lasted for 20 min, and the sessions continued until the Ss resumed baseline rates of responding to give a measure of recovery. All solvents produced concentration-dependent response rate decreases, and only halothane showed any evidence of response rate increases at low concentrations. Halothane quickly produced maximal response rate-decreasing effects and recovery was rapid, while the effects of toluene became progressively greater during the exposure and recovery was prolonged. Ethanol displayed the most rapid onset and recovery of effects. Thus, these solvents produced somewhat similar effects on FR responding but displayed potency and time course differences. (29 ref).

418. Nelson, B. K.; Brightwell, W. S.; Burg, J. R. & Massari, V. John. (1984). **Behavioral and neurochemical alterations in the offspring of rats after maternal or paternal inhalation exposure to the industrial solvent 2-methoxyethanol.** *Pharmacology, Biochemistry & Behavior,* 20(2), 269–279.
18 male Sprague-Dawley rats were exposed to 25 ppm of the industrial solvent 2-methoxyethanol (2ME) for 7 hrs/day, 7 days a week for 6 wks. Ss were then mated with untreated females who were allowed to deliver and rear their young. In addition, groups of 15 pregnant rats were exposed 7 hrs/day on Gestation Days 7–13 or 14–20 to the same amounts of the solvent and allowed to deliver and rear their young. Results of this exposure to the current US permissible occupational exposure limit show no effect on paternal or maternal Ss or on the weight of live offspring. Behavioral testing of pups revealed significant differences from controls only in avoidance conditioning of offspring of female Ss exposed on Days 7–13. Neurochemical deviations were observed in brains from 21-day-old offspring from both groups of exposed parents; changes were numerous in the brain stem and cerebrum but fewer in the cerebellum and midbrain. (45 ref).

419. Nelson, B. K.; Brightwell, W. S. & Setzer, J. V. (1982). **Prenatal interactions between ethanol and the industrial solvent 2-ethoxyethanol in rats: Maternal and behavioral teratogenic effects.** *Neurobehavioral Toxicology & Teratology,* 4(3), 387–394.
60 pregnant Sprague-Dawley rats were given 10% ethanol in the drinking water with or without concomitant inhalation exposure to 100 ppm ethoxyethanol during Gestation Days 7–13 or 14–20. 16 Ss were exposed to 200 ppm ethoxyethanol on Days 7–13. 43 sham-exposed controls were included for both gestation periods. Ethanol alone on Days 14–20 and 200 ppm ethoxyethanol reduced overall weight gain during pregnancy. As in previous research, pregnancy duration was extended in the groups given ethoxyethanol but not in groups given ethanol alone. Neuromotor ability was reduced by 200 ppm ethoxyethanol and by ethanol alone on Days 7–13. The group given ethanol plus ethoxyethanol on Days 14–20 spent more time in the start area of an open field, and this group as well as that given 200 ppm ethoxyethanol were less active than controls in the open field and shuttle box. Findings indicate that ethanol administration early in gestation may reduce the effects, but later in gestation may enhance the effects, of prenatal ethoxyethanol. (20 ref).

420. Nelson, Benjamin K. (1988). **Effects of 2-methoxyethanol on fetal development, postnatal behavior, and embryonic intracellular pH of rats.** *Dissertation Abstracts International,* 48(10-B), 2943–2944.

421. Nelson, Jeffrey L. (1988). **Trichloroethylene: Possible opioid involvement.** *Dissertation Abstracts International,* 48(10-B), 3144.

422. Nelson, Jeffrey L. & Zenick, Harold. (1986). **The effect of trichloroethylene on male sexual behavior: Possible opioid role.** *Neurobehavioral Toxicology & Teratology,* 8(5), 441–445.
Trichloroethylene (TCE) is a solvent used as an industrial degreasing agent. Workers exposed to TCE often exhibit symptoms similar to those produced by narcotics. The present 3 studies evaluated the effects of TCE exposure on measures of male sexual behavior in male Long-Evans rats. Data indicate that TCE (1,000 mg/kg orally) 4 hrs before testing produced an increased ejaculation latency effect on copulatory behavior. Naltrexone (2.0 mg/kg), given intraperitoneally 15 min before testing, blocked this TCE-induced effect. Ss given chronic TCE administration showed tolerance to TCE's effect by the end of 2 wks. Cross-tolerance to morphine was also demonstrated. Quaternary naloxone failed to block any of the TCE-induced effects. Data suggest that many of TCE's effects may be mediated by the endogenous opioid system at the central nervous system (CNS) level.

423. Pryor, Gordon T.; Dickinson, Julie; Feeney, Ellen M. & Rebert, Charles S. (1984). **Hearing loss in rats first exposed to toluene as weanlings or as young adults.** *Neurobehavioral Toxicology & Teratology,* 6(2), 111–119.
48 male Fischer-344 rats were exposed by inhalation to 1,200 ppm toluene for 14 hrs/day, 7 days/week for 5 wks beginning just after weaning or as young adults. During the 5th week of exposure, they were trained to perform a multisensory conditioned pole-climb avoidance response (CAR) task using a 4-kHz tone, a change in the intensity of the test chamber light, or a nonaversive current on the grill floor as the stimuli. When tested the week after the exposures ended, both groups of toluene-exposed Ss were deficient in their performance of the CAR to a 20-kHz tone. This effect was significantly greater for the Ss exposed beginning just after weaning than it was for the young adult Ss. Subsequent behavioral and electrophysiologic audiometry confirmed the presence of a toluene-induced high-frequency hearing loss in both groups with the more severe deficits occurring in the younger Ss. Preliminary morphologic examinations revealed loss of, and/or damage to, hair cells in the basal turn of the cochlea of the younger toluene-exposed Ss. Findings are considered in relation to the potential effects of solvent abuse in humans. (17 ref).

424. Pryor, Gordon T.; Dickinson, Julie; Howd, Robert A. & Rebert, Charles S. (1983). **Neurobehavioral effects of subchronic exposure to weanling rats to toluene or hexane.** *Neurobehavioral Toxicology & Teratology,* 5(1), 47–52.
Several behavioral and neurophysiologic tests were used to examine the effects of subchronic inhalation exposure of male Fischer-344 rats to toluene and to compare them with the effects of the known neurotoxicant hexane. Ss were exposed to toluene (900 or 1,400 ppm) or hexane (2,000 ppm) 14 hrs/

SOLVENTS

day, 7 days/wk for 14 wks. Both solvents inhibited weight gain. Hexane caused a neurotoxic syndrome characterized by reductions of grip strength (especially hindlimb), motor activity, and startle responses and increased latencies of several EP components. Initial acquisition of a conditioned avoidance response (CAR) was also impaired, but subsequent performance was intact. Toluene did not cause the peripheral motor symptoms associated with exposure to hexane. However, a component of the brain-stem auditory evoked response was depressed and CAR acquisition was impaired along with the acquisition of a tone-intensity discrimination task when tested within hours after the daily exposure ended. (22 ref).

425. Pryor, Gordon T.; Dickinson, Julie; Howd, Robert A. & Rebert, Charles S. (1983). **Transient cognitive deficits and high-frequency hearing loss in weanling rats exposed to toluene.** *Neurobehavioral Toxicology & Teratology,* 5(1), 53–57.
In the authors' (1983) previous experiment, weanling rats subchronically exposed to toluene by inhalation were deficient in learning a multisensory conditioned avoidance response (CAR) and a tone-intensity discrimination task when trained several hours after each daily 14-hr exposure ended. The present experiment determined whether this deficit represented a residual pharmacologic effect or more persisting nervous system damage. Independent groups of male Fischer-344 rats were trained on the CAR task either during the last week of a 5-wk exposure to 1,400 or 1,200 ppm toluene (14 hrs/day, 7 days/wk) or during the 1st or 3rd wks after the exposures ended. None of the 3 groups of toluene-exposed Ss acquired the auditory CAR, whereas they learned the visual and somesthetic CARs. (The frequency of the tone was 20 kHz in the present experiment, whereas it had been 4 kHz in the previous experiment). When the frequency and intensity of the tone were varied, hearing in these Ss was unimpaired at 4 kHz, slightly impaired at 8 kHz, and markedly impaired at 12 kHz and above. Thus, although toluene is relatively innocuous as a toxicant, this solvent should be examined further, especially with regard to its frequent abuse by humans. (18 ref).

426. Pryor, Gordon T.; Howd, Robert A.; Uyeno, Edward T. & Thurber, Andrea B. (1985). **Interactions between toluene and alcohol.** *Pharmacology, Biochemistry & Behavior,* 23(3), 401–410.
Examined interactions between toluene and alcohol in male Fischer-344 rats exposed by inhalation to air or 2,000 ppm toluene for 8 hrs each day for 2 wks. Subgroups had access to water or 6% alcohol as their only fluid sources, respectively. Ss exposed to both toluene and alcohol subsequently showed a marked preference for 6% alcohol in 2-bottle choice tests that persisted for up to 20 days for some Ss. Ss exposed to toluene without access to alcohol and control Ss (exposed to air and water) showed a marked aversion to the alcohol solution, and only 2 of 12 Ss forced to drink alcohol without exposure to toluene preferred alcohol in the preference tests. Exposure to both toluene and alcohol also caused greater inhibition of weight gain than exposure to either substance alone, accompanied by greater signs of organ toxicity as indicated by clinical blood chemistries. Exposure to toluene caused marked hearing loss as assessed by a behavioral technique (conditioned avoidance), and there was a trend toward enhancement of this ototoxic effect by forced consumption of alcohol. (41 ref).

427. Pryor, Gordon T. & Howd, Robert A. (1986). **Toluene-induced ototoxicity by subcutaneous administration.** *Neurobehavioral Toxicology & Teratology,* 8(1), 103–104.
Male weanling Fischer-344 rats were injected subcutaneously twice daily with a control liquid or with 1.5 or 1.7 gm/kg toluene for 7 days and measured for behavioral auditory response thresholds. Results indicate that noise was not a major factor in toluene-induced hearing loss and that direct penetration of the toluene vapors through the external ear structure, as might occur during inhalation exposure, was not a necessary condition for inducing the hearing loss.

428. Pryor, Gordon T.; Rebert, Charles S.; Dickinson, Julie & Feeney, Ellen M. (1984). **Factors affecting toluene-induced ototoxicity in rats.** *Neurobehavioral Toxicology & Teratology,* 6(3), 223–238.
Conducted 7 experiments with 308 young male Fischer rats to examine concentration and exposure parameters sufficient to cause toluene-induced ototoxicity. Hearing loss, measured by behavioral and electrophysiologic methods, was repeatedly observed after as few as 2 wks of exposure to 1,000 ppm toluene for 14 hrs/day, but lower concentrations (400 and 700 ppm) were without effect, even after 16 wks of exposure. Three-day exposures to 1,500 ppm for 14 hrs/day or 2,000 ppm for 8 hrs/day were ototoxic, whereas single exposures to 4,000 ppm for 4 hrs or 2,000 ppm for 8 hrs were without effect. Intermittent exposure to 3,000 ppm for 30 min every hour for 8 hrs/day caused hearing loss within 2 wks, but a similar exposure schedule for 4 hrs/day was ineffective even after 9 wks. Results confirm that toluene causes hearing loss in rats and are discussed in terms of their relevance to industrial exposure, industrial accidents, and voluntary, high-level exposure by solvent abusers. (18 ref).

429. Rank, Jette. (1985). **Xylene induced feeding and drinking behavior and central adrenergic receptor binding.** *Neurobehavioral Toxicology & Teratology,* 7(5), 421–426.
Eight NMRI-BOM mice were exposed to 1,600 parts per million of metaxylene (MX) 4 hrs/day, 5 days/week for 7 wks. At the end of exposure, binding of ^{3}H-clonidine to 4 brain regions was measured, and it was found that the binding was significantly decreased in the hypothalamus region but not altered in the diencephalon, cortex, and cerebellum. During MX exposure, Ss ate and drank more than the control group ($n = 8$), which resulted in a loss of weight for the controls compared to the exposed Ss, when weighed before and after the 4 hrs of exposure. Results show that MX can induce eating and drinking responses in mice, suggesting that there is a connection between this phenomenon and the decrease in alpha-receptor binding in the hypothalamus region. (22 ref).

430. Rea, Thomas M. (1983). **Neurobehavioral and neurochemical investigation of toluene, monochlorobenzene, and styrene inhalation in the rat.** *Dissertation Abstracts International,* 43(12-B), 3932.

431. Rebert, Charles S. & Sorenson, Sally S. (1983). **Concentration-related effects of hexane on evoked responses from brain and peripheral nerve of the rat.** *Neurobehavioral Toxicology & Teratology,* 5(1), 69–76.
Sensory evoked responses (SERs) were studied in 32 chronically implanted male Fischer-344 rats to characterize the electrophysiologic concomitants of hexacarbon polyneuropathy. The action potential (AP) of the ventral caudal (tail) nerve, the brain-stem auditory evoked response (BAER), and cortical somatosensory (SER), auditory, and visual evoked responses were recorded from Ss exposed to air or 500, 1,000, or 1,500 ppm hexane for 24 hrs/day, 5 days/wk, for 11 wks. Concentration-related latency increases occurred within each sensory modality. The most pronounced effects were on the AP and SER. Latency of the 5th, but not the 1st, component of the BAER was prolonged, indicating an effect on central auditory tract conduction time. Amplitudes of response components were variable and rarely affected significantly by exposure to hexane. (30 ref).

432. Rebert, Charles S.; Sorenson, Sally S.; Howd, Robert A. & Pryor, Gordon T. (1983). **Toluene-induced hearing loss in rats evidenced by the brainstem auditory-evoked response.** *Neurobehavioral Toxicology & Teratology,* 5(1), 59–62.

In the authors' (1983) previous study, toluene caused hearing loss in rats. This finding precipitated the present electrophysiologic study of the auditory thresholds of these rats using the brain-stem auditory evoked response (BAER). 23-day-old male Fischer-344 rats had been exposed to 1,400 or 1,200 ppm toluene 14 hrs/day for 4 or 5 wks, while a control group was exposed only to air. Ss were tested 2.5 mo after termination of the exposures. BAERs, recorded with 25-gauge needle electrodes placed over the nose and posterior skull, were evoked by 100-μsec-duration clicks and 1-msec-duration tone pips at 8 intensities. Thresholds for the appearance of BAERs in the toluene-exposed Ss were elevated by 13 to 27 db, and latency–intensity functions were consistent with the occurrence of sensorineural hearing loss. The amplitudes of the 3rd and 5th components of the BAER were attenuated at high stimulus intensities in the toluene-exposed Ss. These behavioral and electrophysiologic results are apparently the first to indicate the ototoxicity of toluene in experimental animals. (8 ref).

433. Rees, David C. (1985). **Behavioral determinants of tolerance to toluene or *d*-amphetamine.** *Dissertation Abstracts International,* 45(12-B, Pt 1), 3761.

434. Rees, David C.; Coggeshall, Ellen & Balster, Robert L. (1985). **Inhaled toluene produces pentobarbital-like discriminative stimulus effects in mice.** *Life Sciences,* 37(14), 1319–1325.
Investigated the hypothesis that the abuse of volatile solvents may be due to their ability to produce an intoxication similar to that produced by classical central nervous system depressants such as the barbiturates and ethanol. 10 CD-1 male mice were trained to discriminate pentobarbital from saline injections in a 2-lever operant task. Stimulus generalization was examined following 20-min inhalation exposures to toluene (300–5,400 ppm). Findings show that in 8 of 10 Ss, pentobarbital-lever responding occurred following toluene exposure, indicating an overlap in the discriminative stimulus properties of toluene and pentobarbital. (38 ref).

435. Rees, David C.; Coggeshall, Ellen M.; Dragan, Yvonne; Breen, Timothy J. et al. (1986). **Acute effects of some volatile nitrites on motor performance and lethality in mice.** *Neurobehavioral Toxicology & Teratology,* 8(2), 139–142.
Male CD-1 mice were examined for effects on lethality and motor performance on an inverted screen test following inhalation exposure to isoamyl, n-butyl, and isobutyl nitrite. Isoamyl and isobutyl nitrite were equally potent on both lethality and motor performance measures, whereas n-butyl nitrite was significantly more potent than isoamyl and isobutyl for lethality. Slope estimates of the concentration-effect curves for lethality were significantly greater than those of the motor performance measure. Data suggest that behaviorally active concentrations of volatile nitrites may put solvent abusers at risk to other health consequences.

436. Sherman, A. D. & Gál, E. M. (1977). **Cerebral metabolism of intraventricular [³H]-fenfluramine.** *Neuropharmacology,* 16(5), 309–315.
The time course of the cerebral metabolism of intraventricularly injected [³H]-fenfluramine (FE) was followed in 109 Sprague-Dawley rats. Four hours after injection, 99% of cerebral FE was dealkylated to norfenfluramine (NFE). NFE had reached all areas of brain and was still detectable at 3 days. Two toluene-extractable metabolites (FE_2 and FE_3) could be isolated from the brain. Experiments in vitro confirmed the cerebral synthesis of FE_2. Distributional studies indicated that the level of FE_3 in neocortex was twice as high as that in brain stem. In Ss injected with Lilly 110140, the cerebral conversion of intraventricular FE to FE_3 and FE_2 did not take place. Iprindole given alone or in combination with Lilly 110140 increased cerebral levels of FE_2 and FE_3. FE_2 and FE_3 were recoverable from urine but not from liver of Ss given ip or intraventricular FE. Ip injection of FE did not lead to the appearance of FE_2 and FE_3 in brain. Administration of iprindole increased the urinary output of FE_2 and FE_3 but not of FE and NFE. 20% of all FE_3 and 10% of all NFE appeared in the synaptosomal fraction. The marked differences in the metabolism of FE and para-chloroamphetamine, both neurotoxic agents, are discussed. (20 ref).

437. Wada, Hiromi; Hosokawa, Toshiyuki & Saito, Kazuo. (1986). **Effects of single exposure to toluene on shock avoidance and time estimation in rats.** *Neurobehavioral Toxicology & Teratology,* 8(6), 727–730.
Studied the effects of a single exposure to toluene on time estimation and shock avoidance behavior in 12 male Wistar rats. After acquisition training in time estimation and shock avoidance in a shuttle box, Ss were exposed through inhalation to toluene vapor at 8,000, 4,000, or 2,000 parts per million (ppm). Maintenance of shock avoidance and time estimation were examined for up to 6 hrs after the 4-hr exposure. Avoidance response, eliminated initially after 8,000 ppm, was recovered by 3 hrs. Other concentrations increased the percentage of avoidance response and shortened response latencies. In addition to the excitatory effects of toluene, the Ss may have estimated the time interval to be longer than the real time.

438. Wimolwattanapun, S.; Ghosh, T. K.; Mookherjee, S.; Copeland, R. L. et al. (1987). **Effect of inhalation of xylene on intracranial self-stimulation behavior in rat.** *Neuropharmacology,* 26(11), 1629–1632.
Studied the effect of the inhalation of 4 successively graded concentrations of xylene on intracranial self-stimulation behavior in male rats in a flow-through (dynamic) inhalational behavioral chamber. The rate of leverpressing showed a dose-dependent decrease during exposure to 192, 419, and 623 ppm of xylene. After 4 days the depressant effect was attenuated, showing the development of tolerance.

METALLIC ELEMENTS

439. Barlow, Charles F. (1984). **Mental Retardation Research Center, Children's Hospital—Boston.** *American Journal of Mental Deficiency,* 88(5), 559–560.
The program of the Mental Retardation Research Center at Boston Children's Hospital consists of research in 2 major areas: neuroscience and genetics, with related laboratories in behavioral science, epidemiology, and clinical neurophysiology. The major efforts in the behavioral epidemiologic laboratories have centered on the long-term effects of postnatal low-level lead exposure on the cognitive and classroom behavior of children, a study that has been extended to consider the effect of lead on the prenatal brain.

440. Bland, Jeffrey. (1980). **Through the looking glass darkly: A story of trace mineral-induced behavioral disturbance and hair mineral analysis.** *Journal of Orthomolecular Psychiatry,* 9(1), 24–32.
Discusses the characters in Lewis Carroll's books as examples of behavioral dysfunction caused by various imbalances of essential minerals or by toxic mineral excesses. Two clinical cases illustrate how hair trace mineral analysis (HTMA) can identify causes of misbehavior and suggest nutritional treatment. Criticisms of HTMA have charged that the technique is unreliable because the results do not take sufficiently into account variations due to hair color, the part of the scalp from which a sample is taken, the effect of various beauty treatments, environmental influences, methods of washing the hair, and unstandardized procedures among commerical laboratories making the analyses. Some of these objections are examined in detail and challenged by experimental evidence. Recent research on the levels of lead, cadmium, cobalt, chro-

METALLIC ELEMENTS

mium, and lithium in children's hair differentiated learning-disabled Ss from normals with 98% accuracy. It is concluded that although HTMA is not a panacea and cannot diagnose all metabolic problems, it does offer another valuable tool, similar to blood and urine analyses, for use by the diagnostician. (10 ref).

441. Evans, Hugh L.; Laties, Victor G. & Weiss, Bernard. (1975). **Behavioral effects of mercury and methylmercury.** *Federation Proceedings,* 34(9), 1858-1867.
Notes that intoxication by elemental mercury or by methylmercury is revealed primarily by changes in behavior and by neurological signs. Disorders of movement and posture have been most widely reported, both in animals and humans. Specific sensory symptoms are also prominent in human methylmercury poisoning. Recent data indicate similar symptoms in monkeys during long-term exposure to methylmercury. Variations in the profile of behavioral and neurological effects are discussed in terms of differences in species and differences between acute and long-term exposure. The latter condition poses the most difficult questions for human health, yet has been less frequently studied. Procedures are suggested that may help to resolve these problems (e.g., tests of learned behavior). (55 ref).

442. Feldman, Robert G. (1982). **Neurological manifestations of mercury intoxication.** *Acta Neurologica Scandinavica,* 66(Suppl 92), 201–209.
Previous research suggests that the pathological changes resulting from chemical toxicity of mercury may be the reduction of amino acid incorporation into brain tissue and reduced production of neuronal RNA. The present author discusses acute and chronic intoxication and low-level chronic exposure to mercury. Findings indicate that the extent and possible degree of reversibility depends on the severity and duration of exposure and the particular form of mercury. (27 ref).

443. Feldman, Robert G. (1982). **Neurological picture of lead poisoning.** *Acta Neurologica Scandinavica,* 66(Suppl 92), 185–199.
A literature review suggests that impairment caused by exposure to lead can be found at lower exposure levels than previously considered safe. Some type of neural damage does exist in "asymptomatic" children. It is therefore important to consider the various clinical presentations of lead toxicity in adults and children so that potential victims of exposure to the many sources of lead may be identified. Case histories are presented, illustrating lead poisoning and neuropsychological deficits attributable to lead intoxication. (30 ref).

444. Feldman, Robert G. (1982). **Central and peripheral nervous system effects of metals: A survey.** *Acta Neurologica Scandinavica,* 66(Suppl 92), 143–166.
Discusses several neurological syndromes that have been associated with metal accumulation. Specifically, disorders of the cerebral hemisphere (e.g., headache), memory and behavior, extrapyramidal system, and the peripheral nervous system are reviewed. (114 ref).

445. Hänninen, Helena. (1982). **Behavioral effects of occupational exposure to mercury and lead.** *Acta Neurologica Scandinavica,* 66(Suppl 92), 167–175.
Discusses the neurotoxic effects of long-term exposure to lead and mercury in terms of psychomotor disturbances, deterioration of intellectual capacities, and emotional alterations. Research suggests that the early behavioral effects of lead and mercury have much in common. Results have been consistent in regard to tasks calling for some cognitive manipulation of visual stimulus material. (21 ref).

446. Hanson, Mats. (1983). **Amalgam—hazards in your teeth.** *Journal of Orthomolecular Psychiatry,* 12(3), 194–201.
Contends that amalgam, an alloy commonly used in dental fillings, gives off mercury in the form of gas, ions, and abraded particles that can lead to chronic mercurialism. Early symptoms of chronic mercurialism are largely subjective and mental: tiredness, reduced energy, irritability, loss of short-term memory, and shyness or depression. Diagnosis is difficult because no way has been found to measure the body burden of mercury. Composite plastics, although far from ideal, are the best alternatives to amalgam at the present time. (63 ref).

447. Heilbronn, E.; Eriksson, H. & Häggblad, J. (1982). **Neurotoxic effects of manganese: Studies on cell cultures, tissue homogenates and intact animals.** *Neurobehavioral Toxicology & Teratology,* 4(6), 655–658.
Summarizes some of the neurotoxic effects of manganese, discusses a model of its toxicological action, and presents data indicating that chronic administration of manganese in the rat leads to increased motor activity. The literature indicates that the central catecholaminergic system is attacked by manganese compounds, and in humans 3 effects of chronic exposure have been described: (1) early symptoms of tiredness, sleep disturbances, aggressivity, and behavioral disturbances; (2) neurological disturbances and a syndrome resembling Parkinson's disease, and (3) peripheral nerve lesions. (20 ref).

448. Hellberg, Jan. (1978). **A method of measurement of critical flicker fusion intensity (cffi) in scotopic vision.** *Psychological Research Bulletin, Lund U.,* 18(1), 13 p.
Measured (a) critical flicker fusion intensity (CFFI) in scotopic vision and (b) level of dark adaptation, using a modified automatic adaptometer. Flicker was held constant at 10 cps. Light of 2 different wavelengths was used. The 22 male and 27 female Ss were mainly university student volunteers. CFFI for the 2 wavelengths was compared to results of an earlier investigation. Results show that time of the day did not influence CFFI. A significant increase of CFFI occurred when the wavelength was changed. An extrapolation was made that pointed to a 72% gain in sensitivity of the apparatus if a light source emitting a wavelength of 5,000 angstroms was used. This is considered important since the apparatus is meant to be used as a diagnostic instrument in epidemiological investigations of populations exposed to methyl mercury.

449. Hellberg, Jan. (1978). **The influence of fatigue and different light wavelengths on critical flicker fusion intensity in scotopic vision.** *Psychological Research Bulletin, Lund U.,* 18(2), 10 p.
Investigated an apparatus for semiautomatic testing of the level of dark adaptation and critical flicker fusion intensity in 2 slightly different ways when flicker was held constant at 10 cycles/sec. The aim was to establish a standardized test procedure and normative values that would allow the apparatus to be used as a diagnostic instrument in epidemiological investigations of populations exposed to methyl mercury. 50 non-exposed Ss, mean age 25.5 yrs, were randomly divided into 3 different subgroups and were tested on 3 occasions by 3 testers. Results suggest a standardized procedure simpler than the one used in the investigation. Reliability was found to be sufficient. Further investigations should concern the effects of fatigue and what can be gained by changing the wavelength of the stimulus light toward the optimum for rod sensitivity.

450. Laties, Victor G. & Evans, Hugh L. (1980). **Research strategies for assessing the effects of methylmercury on behavior.** *Revista Mexicana de Análisis de la Conducta,* 6(1), 27–37.
Outlines a strategy for dealing with the problem of assessing the toxic effects of methylmercury on behavior, which is complicated by the ways in which the substance affects many organ systems simultaneously. The strategy consists of producing in other ways some of the signs that characterize methylmercury poisoning and contrasting the behavioral ef-

fects of these procedures with those of the methylmercury. Examples are drawn from work with pigeons engaged in schedule-controlled behavior. (Spanish abstract) (18 ref).

451. Lowenstein, L. F. (1982). **Effects of lead poisoning.** *British Journal of Clinical & Social Psychiatry,* 1(1), 13–15.
Discusses the long- and short-term effects of ingestion of minimal dosages of lead. Results from studies with animals and humans indicate that perceptual and especially discriminatory powers are affected by lead intoxication. Poisoning may cause hyperactivity, night blindness, and loss of appetite, and it may also affect motivation, concentration, attention, and verbal ability. Lead-chelating agents may play a role in the treatment of hyperactivity in children. (14 ref).

452. Marlowe, Mike. (1986). **Metal pollutant exposure and behavior disorders: Implications for school practices.** *Journal of Special Education,* 20(2), 251–264.
Suggests that metal pollutants at low levels, far below those associated with clinical metal poisoning, are associated with a spectrum of behavior disorders. A literature review addresses a set of environmental and diet variables to reduce metal exposure that are within the realm of control of child, parent, and health or educational professional working with the family.

453. Marlowe, Mike. (1985). **Low lead exposure and learning disabilities.** *Research Communications in Psychology, Psychiatry & Behavior,* 10(1–2), 153–169.
Argues that childhood exposure to lead routinely encountered in the environment is an issue of importance to the field of learning disabilities. Lead at low levels, far below those associated with clinical lead poisoning, is associated with a spectrum of behavioral alterations involving psychometric intelligence; auditory, visual, and language processing; fine motor performance; attention; quantitative EEGs; and classroom behavior. It is concluded that the question of whether lead at low doses is associated with central nervous system (CNS) dysfunctions and learning disabilities no longer needs or deserves prolonged debate. Protective social action on lead would benefit the future of all children. (41 ref).

454. Needleman, Herbert L. (1982). **Lead and impaired abilities.** *Developmental Medicine & Child Neurology,* 24(2), 196–197.
Contends that the editorial accompanying the report of Yule et al (1982), finding a relationship between blood lead levels and intelligence, serves only to confuse the issue. It is concluded that the editorial creates a false dilemma, implying that the concern about the physical and chemical environment of children can obscure other social factors important to the healthy development of the child. (4 ref).

455. Pleva, Jaro. (1983). **Mercury poisoning from dental amalgam.** *Journal of Orthomolecular Psychiatry,* 12(3), 184–193.
Contends, on the basis of the author's experience, that silver amalgam as a dental filling is not a stable alloy and that symptoms of mercury poisoning may result when it corrodes. Symptoms may include amnesia, reduced capacity for intellectual work, and increased need for sleep, in addition to physical ills. Case reports and data in the literature, as well as studies of corroded amalgam fillings, are presented to support this contention. It is concluded that the use of gold and other metals with amalgam should be stopped and that studies of amalgam corrosion should be started. (38 ref).

456. Silbergeld, Ellen K. (1983). **Indirectly acting neurotoxins.** *Acta Psychiatrica Scandinavica,* 67(Suppl 303), 16–25.
The role of toxic substances in causing CNS dysfunction is discussed with a focus on effects that are mediated indirectly through other organ systems that affect the brain. Neurochemical measurements of brain function and the use of neuropharmacological probes of behavior are illustrated using examples of lead poisoning (as a case of chemical porphyria) and estrogenization (as a case of hormonal dysfunction). (30 ref).

457. Silbergeld, Ellen K. & Chisolm, J. Julian. (1976). **Lead poisoning: Altered urinary catecholamine metabolites as indicators of intoxication in mice and children.** *Science,* 192(4235), 153–155.
Whether neuropsychological impairment occurs in children with increased lead absorption who are without clinical symptoms is of current concern. This issue, which involves potentially large numbers of children, remains unresolved, in part because of the lack of sensitive biochemical indicators of the effects of lead on the nervous system. In the present study, experimental subclinical lead poisoning in CD-1 mice led to significant increases in homovanillic acid and vanillylmandelic acid in brain and urine. In 6 asymptomatic and mildly symptomatic 16–42 mo olds with increased lead absorption, these acids were measured in urine collected quantitatively under controlled dietary conditions; preliminary results show fivefold increases in the daily output of these compounds compared to findings in 6 3–10 yr old controls. Data suggest that the altered catecholamine metabolism also occurs in children. (21 ref).

458. Spyker, Joan M. (1975). **Assessing the impact of low level chemicals on development: Behavioral and latent effects.** *Federation Proceedings,* 34(9), 1835-1844.
There is growing evidence that nervous tissue, especially the brain, is more sensitive to many foreign chemical substances than has previously been suspected, and that toxic effects may be manifested as subtle disturbances of behavior long before any classical symptoms of poisoning become apparent. Early detection of an insidious toxic process (behavioral toxicology) may enable the prevention or attenuation of harm to humans and other organisms. There is also increasing evidence that individuals are more vulnerable to adverse factors during the period of development (conception to puberty) than at any other time in life. Subtle functional disturbances in organisms exposed while immature (behavioral teratology) may be one of the most sensitive indicators of chemical toxicity. Examples of the effects of pre- and postnatal exposure to methylmercury are presented for a thorough assessment of the impact of certain low level chemicals on human health. (38 ref).

459. Winder, Christopher; Carmichael, Neil G. & Lewis, Paul D. (1982). **Effects of chronic low level lead exposure on brain development and function.** *Trends in Neurosciences,* 5(6), 207–209.
Previous evidence from Ss with lead levels beneath those at which encephalopathy occurs suggests that the nervous system may be very sensitive to this metal. These findings have given rise to the rather confusing but widely used term "subclinical" lead poisoning. The present study reviews evidence that such low-level exposure may indeed perturb brain development and function. Attempts to investigate the effects of low doses of lead on animal behavior however have produced no clear-cut conclusions. (39 ref).

Human Research

460. ———. (1986). **Workers' compensation: Mental and physical disabilities.** *Mental & Physical Disability Law Reporter,* 10(1), 37–38.
Describes 2 decisions dealing with the nature of compensation for employees who were severely disabled on the job. In *Sanchez v. Molycorp, Inc.,* 703 P.2d 925 (N.M. Ct. App. 1985), the court held that a brain injury—accompanied by chronic, severe headaches; dizziness; difficulty in functioning; and depression—was compensable as a work-related accident.

METALLIC ELEMENTS

In *Perez v. Pennsuco Cement & Aggregates,* 474 So. 2d 293 (Fla. Dist. Ct. App. 1985), the court reversed a decision that denied attendant care services to a claimant who was a victim of manganese intoxication poisoning sustained while he was employed as a welder.

461. ———. (1986). **Lead linked to hearing loss in children.** *International Journal of Biosocial Research,* 8(2), 113–114.
Proposes lowering the definition of excessive absorption of lead by children due to its relationship with diminished height, intelligence, and hearing and associated impairment in neurological functioning.

462. Accardo, Pasquale; Whitman, Barbara; Caul, Jefferies & Rolfe, Ursula. (1988). **Autism and plumbism: A possible association.** *Clinical Pediatrics,* 27(1), 41–44.
Presents 6 cases of inner-city Black 3–5 yr olds with both infantile autism and lead poisoning. In 3 cases, developmental deviance seemed to have been present before the possible impact of lead toxicity. In 2 cases the lead poisoning may have contributed to the onset or acceleration of developmental symptomatology, while in the remaining case the temporal sequence remained unclear. The potential contribution of pica to the development of lead poisoning among autistic children and the possibility that lead poisoning can result in mental retardation, severe communication disorder, and autistic features is discussed.

463. Agnew, Jacqueline. (1985). **Neurobehavioral performance of workers exposed to lead for less than one year.** *Dissertation Abstracts International,* 46(6-B), 1859.

464. Almirall Hernández, Pedro & Ibarra Fernández de la Vega, Enrique. (1981). **La prueba de Bender y su relación con algunas alteraciones bioquímicas en la intoxicación por plomo. / The Bender test and its relation to some biochemical changes in lead poisoning.** *Boletín de Psicología (Cuba),* 4(3), 59–68.
Administered the Bender Visual Motor Gestalt Test to 21 workers (mean age 36.6 yrs) who had been exposed to lead fumes for an average of 8.9 yrs. Blood lead levels were analyzed, and delta-aminolevulinic acid and coproporphyrin were measured in urine. Bender test results revealed psychological problems in more than 70% of the sample. A significant relationship was found between Bender test results and biochemical results, but not between Bender results, age, and length of lead exposure. The findings corroborate the usefulness of the Bender test in the diagnosis of lead poisoning. (English abstract) (15 ref).

465. Bailey, Kent G.; Lazar, Joel M. & Edinger, Jack. (1977). **Intelligence test potential: Analysis of breadth, depth, and differential prediction.** *Journal of Consulting & Clinical Psychology,* 45(3), 492–493.
In a study with 40 undergraduates, 2 measures of "breadth" and 3 measures of "depth" were derived, based on special administration and scoring of the WAIS Similarities subscale. Factor analyses performed on the Similarities indices, the Concept Mastery Test, and Guilford's Tin Can item, indicated that breadth and depth can be distinguished statistically, and multiple regression analyses revealed that the derived measures contributed to improved predictive efficiency.

466. Baker, Edward L.; Feldman, Robert G.; White, Roberta G. & Harley, J. Preston. (1983). **The role of occupational lead exposure in the genesis of psychiatric and behavioral disturbances.** *Acta Psychiatrica Scandinavica,* 67(Suppl 303), 38–48.
In a prospective study of lead neurotoxicity, 107 exposed foundry workers and 65 non-lead-exposed referents were evaluated using a comprehensive neurobehavioral battery that included the WAIS, Wechsler Memory Scale, and Profile of Mood States. Other performance indexes were obtained by questionnaire, physical examination, and nerve-conduction testing. Results show increased rates of depression, confusion, anger, fatigue, and tension among Ss with blood levels over 40 mcg/dl. Other aspects of neurobehavioral function, including verbal-concept formation, memory, and visual/motor performance were also impaired. In view of the large number of individuals exposed to lead in their work, attention should be given by practitioners to correctly diagnosing lead-induced disorders manifesting themselves as neuropsychiatric illness. Specific inquiries should be made of individuals with affectual complaints to clarify the nature of their work and workplace exposure to lead. (31 ref).

467. Baloh, Robert; Sturm, Randall; Green, Bonnie & Gleser, Goldine. (1975). **Neuropsychological effects of chronic asymptomatic increased lead absorption: A controlled study.** *Archives of Neurology,* 32(5), 326–330.
27 asymptomatic children (mean age 67.23 mo) with confirmed chronic increased lead absorption were compared with 27 matched control children (mean age 68.27 mo) for evidence of neuropsychological impairment. Evaluation of each child included a complete history, physical examination, quantitative neurological tests, and comprehensive psychological tests (e.g., WISC or Wechsler Preschool and Primary Scale of Intelligence, McCarthy Scales of Children's Abilities, and the Early Childhood Matching Familiar Figures Test). There was significantly increased incidence of hyperactive behavior in Ss with increased lead levels, but there was no significant difference in any of the quantitative test results. Uncontrolled variables, especially lead absorption in infancy and adverse environmental pressures other than lead, still leave questions about the relationship between chronic lead exposure and behavior or intelligence. (27 ref).

468. Barrett, Rowland P. (1978). **Auditory-visual integration, intelligence, and reading achievement in normal and subclinically lead poisoned children.** *Dissertation Abstracts International,* 39(3-B), 1451–1452.

469. Bellinger, David C. et al. (1984). **Early sensory-motor development and prenatal exposure to lead.** *Neurobehavioral Toxicology & Teratology,* 6(5), 387–402.
As part of a longitudinal study of the early developmental effects of exposure to lead, the authors administered the Bayley Scales of Infant Development to 249 infants when they were 6 mo old and classified them into 3 groups based on their umbilical cord blood lead levels: low (mean 1.8 μg/dl), mid (mean 6.5 μg/dl), and high (mean 14.6 μg/dl). No S had a cord blood lead level greater than 30 μg/dl, the level currently regarded as the upper limit of normal for young children. Multiple regression analyses indicated that high cord blood lead levels at birth were associated with lower covariance-adjusted scores on the Mental Development Index at 6 mo. Scores on the Psychomotor Development Index were not significantly related to cord blood lead level. The level of lead in blood at 6 mo of age was not associated with scores on either the Mental or Psychomotor Development Index. These data are compatible with the hypothesis that low levels of lead delivered transplacentally are toxic to infants. (69 ref).

470. Bellinger, David; Leviton, Alan; Waternaux, Christine; Needleman, Herbert et al. (1987). **Longitudinal analyses of prenatal and postnatal lead exposure and early cognitive development.** *New England Journal of Medicine,* 316(17), 1037–1043.
On the basis of lead levels in umbilical-cord blood, 249 infants were assigned to low, medium, or high prenatal-exposure groups. Development was assessed semiannually from 6 mo to 2 yrs, using the Mental Development Index (MDI) of the Bayley Scales of Infant Development. Regression analyses indicated that, at all ages, infants in the high-exposure group had lower MDI scores than infants in the low and medium groups. MDI scores were not related to postnatal exposure. Results indicate that the fetus may be adversely affected at

blood lead concentrations well below the 25 μg/dl level currently defined by the Centers for Disease Control as the highest acceptable level for young children.

471. Bellinger, David C.; Leviton, Alan; Needleman, Herbert L.; Rabinowitz, Michael et al. (1986). **Low-level lead exposure and infant development in the first year.** *Neurobehavioral Toxicology & Teratology,* 8(2), 151–161.
Assessed the developmental impact of prenatal and early postnatal low-level lead exposure in a prospective study of 249 middle and upper-middle class infants with umbilical cord blood-lead levels in the range currently considered normal. Ss were tested with the Bayley Scales of Infant Development at 6 and 12 mo of age. Results show that prenatal exposure to lead levels relatively common among urban populations appears to be associated with less favorable development through the 1st yr of life.

472. Bellinger, David C. & Needleman, Herbert L. (1985). **Prenatal and early postnatal exposure to lead: Developmental effects, correlates, and implications.** *International Journal of Mental Health,* 14(3), 78–111.
Discusses the developmental sequelae of high- and low-level lead exposure and describes efforts to identify factors that predict children's blood lead levels within the range 0–20 μg/dl. The clinical significance of the observed developmental sequelae of low-level lead exposure and their implications for developmental models and public health policy are discussed. (6 p ref).

473. Besser, R.; Krämer, G.; Thümler, R.; Bohl, J. et al. (1987). **Acute trimethyltin limbic-cerebellar syndrome.** *Neurology,* 37(6), 945–950.
An acute limbic-cerebellar syndrome was seen in 6 industrial workers (aged 34–51 yrs) who inhaled trimethyltin. Clinical features included hearing loss, disorientation, confabulation, amnesia, aggressiveness, hyperphagia, disturbed sexual behavior, complex partial and tonic-clonic seizures, nystagmus, ataxia, and mild sensory neuropathy. Severity paralleled maximal urinary organotin levels. One patient died and 2 remained seriously disabled.

474. Blouin, Arthur G.; Blouin, Jane H. & Kelly, Teresa C. (1983). **Lead, trace mineral intake, and behavior of children.** *Topics in Early Childhood Special Education,* 3(2), 63–71.
Exposure to lead and nutritional inadequacy have been found to be related to learning and behavioral disorders in children. The bulk of the research on this relation is correlational, however, rendering the existence (and direction) of causality unknown. The treatment studies in this area generally have not included appropriate placebo controls or double-blind conditions. In addition, studies of lead exposure tend to exclude consideration of dietary factors in spite of the fact that competition between lead and trace minerals has been demonstrated. The cumulative effects of mineral insufficiency and exposure to lead are examined, and it is suggested that sound nutrition not only may affect psychological development but may also reduce susceptibility to the effects of environmental neurotoxins. (59 ref).

475. Bonithon-Kopp, C.; Huel, G. & Moreau, T. (1986). **Plomb et développement psychomoteur de l'enfant. Analyse critique des arguments d'origine épidémiologique. / Lead and psychomotor development in children: Critical analysis of arguments of epidemiologic origin.** *Neuropsychiatrie de l'Enfance et de l'Adolescence,* 34(8–9), 383–394.
Discusses the main epidemiologic studies conducted since the 1970s on the effect of moderate exposure to lead on children's psychomotor development (cognitive and verbal faculties, perceptuo-motor and fine motor capacities, global motor skills, scholastic achievement, and behavior). Weaknesses, interpretation problems, and the validity of the causal hypothesis are considered. (English, German & Spanish abstracts).

476. Buiatti, Eva et al. (1985). **A case control study of lung cancer in Florence, Italy: I. Occupational risk factors.** *Journal of Epidemiology & Community Health,* 39(3), 244–250.
Conducted a case control study of lung cancer in Florence to investigate occupational risk factors for 36 female and 340 male patients with primary lung cancer and 75 female and 817 male control patients with discharge diagnoses other than lung cancer or attempted suicide. Ss were similar in age and smoking status. Logistic regression models were used to calculate odds ratios for specific occupations (e.g., retail, administrative, metal work, agriculture, electrical) compared to all others. Among men, the lung cancer risk for bricklayers using firebrick and other refractory materials was elevated. Female hatmakers, probably exposed to arsenic while making felt hats, had an elevated risk of lung cancer. (11 ref).

477. Chaiklin, Harris. (1979). **The treadmill of lead.** *American Journal of Orthopsychiatry,* 49(4), 571–573.
Argues that while lead poisoning may be the most widespread and destructive children's disease in the US, it is not one of the most popular environmental causes. Large numbers of children appear particularly sensitive to even slightly elevated levels of lead; they not only have difficulty in learning but are often misdiagnosed as minimally brain damaged. (13 ref).

478. Chaiklin, Harris; Cook, Jeanne J.; Hayes, Margaret E. & Scanland, Vera B. (1974). **Recurrence of lead poisoning in children.** *Social Work,* 19(2), 196-200.
To study the importance of family dynamics and social environment on lead poisoning in children, hospital records of 10 single-ingestor cases and 10 recidivist lead poisoning cases were compared. No significant differences were found in demographic data; both groups had socioeconomic characteristics associated with poverty. In terms of family diagnoses, single-ingestor families tended to be inadequate whereas recidivist families were unsocial and exhibited more severe pathology. Most families were below normal on all areas of family functioning (e.g., marital relationships and child-rearing practices). In all of the unsocial families and in 4 of the inadequate families the child continued to ingest foreign substances. Inadequate families followed directions for their child's treatment more than recidivist families, who exhibited aggressive resistance to treatment. It is concluded that family type is a significant variable in both the onset and recidivism of lead poisoning, and that family and social therapy is as important as medical procedures in treating the disease.

479. Chaiklin, Harris; Mosher, Barbara S. & O'Hara. David M. (1985). **The social and the emotional in the etiology of childhood lead poisoning.** *Journal of Sociology & Social Welfare,* 12(1), 62–78.
The extensiveness of lead poisoning in the US and its relationship to hyperactivity and learning disabilities are described. Social, emotional, cultural, and economic factors that play a role in its etiology are discussed. To examine the role of maternal anxiety in childhood lead poisoning, 15 mothers of normal children and 15 mothers of children diagnosed as having toxic lead blood levels were administered the Taylor Manifest Anxiety Scale. Children were aged 2–5 yrs. An association was found between maternal anxiety and children's lead levels. It is suggested that the high anxiety scores of mothers with children with elevated lead levels may come from the fact that their child had received a diagnosis. Public policy recommendations include providing social and material services to families with lead poisoning that need this help, and treating/working with the whole family when an individual is diagnosed as lead poisoned.

METALLIC ELEMENTS

480. Conrad, Mary K. (1980). **An examination of the environmental and psychological correlates of lead poisoning in young children.** *Dissertation Abstracts International,* 41(5-A), 2012-2013.

481. David, Oliver J. (1984). **The relationship of lead to learning and behavioral disabilities.** *Advances in Learning & Behavioral Disabilities,* 3, 41-56.
Reviews studies that examined the hypothesis that lower levels of lead than those previously used as a definition for lead poisoning (60 μg Pb/dl Hb) can also be toxic. This toxicity, however, will be less acutely florid and less severe than that associated with higher lead levels. It is argued that at levels between 25 and 55 μg Pb/dl Hb, heretofore regarded as elevated but nontoxic, a number of CNS disorders develop. Mechanisms through which the body absorbs lead are outlined. Studies that researched a population identified as having increased lead levels for CNS symptomatology have indicated a significant decrease in CNS functions in association with increases in blood lead levels. Such studies, however, have made little or no provision for the effects of biological variability, an important aspect of lead-related CNS dysfunction. Host resistance factors must be taken into account. It is noted that some lead-related conditions may cause CNS dysfunctions that are not as well-known or destructive as the classic encephalopathic or preencephalopathic states. Studies that have implicitly acknowledged host susceptibility as an important variable have also demonstrated a relation between lead and various types of CNS dysfunction. The examination of children who present with hyperactivity, learning disabilities, mental retardation, conduct disturbances, and various CNS dysfunctions for elevated blood lead levels is advocated. (45 ref).

482. David, Oliver J. et al. (1976). **Lead and hyperactivity. Behavioral response to chelation: A pilot study.** *American Journal of Psychiatry,* 133(10), 1155-1158.
Used lead-chelating medication to treat 13 6-10 yr old hyperkinetic school children whose blood and urine lead levels were in an elevated but "nontoxic" range. Six Ss with histories of etiologically relevant perinatal or developmental complications showed relatively little improvement. Seven others with unremarkable histories, and for whom a lead etiology could thus be entertained, showed marked improvement. It is concluded that (a) lead may play an important role in the etiology of some cases of hyperactivity; (b) lead-chelating agents may have a major place in the treatment of hyperactivity; and (c) the medical workup of hyperactivity should include lead level measurements and careful consideration of other possible etiological factors.

483. David, Oliver J.; Grad, Gary; McGann, Barbara & Koltun, Arnold. (1982). **Mental retardation and "nontoxic" lead levels.** *American Journal of Psychiatry,* 139(6), 806-809.
Studied the blood level concentrations of 83 4-12 yr olds with WISC or Stanford-Binet Intelligence Scale scores of 58-84 who were divided according to the presence or absence of a probable etiology for their retardation. 40 age-matched controls were employed for comparison. There was a significant negative correlation between IQ and lead levels in the retarded children with unknown etiologies; that is, as IQ scores decreased, the lead levels increased. The correlation among the retarded Ss with probable etiologies was not significant. (23 ref).

484. Davis, J. Michael & Svendsgaard, David J. (1987). **Lead and child development.** *Nature,* 329(6137), 297-300.
Discusses prospective studies conducted to measure the effects of prenatal low-level lead exposure on later child development. Particular attention is devoted to a group of longitudinal studies conducted in 3 US cities and 1 Australian city. Results show a correlation between prenatal lead exposure and lower performance on the Mental Development Index of the Bayley Scales of Infant Development at 6, 12, 18, and 24 mo of age. The Australian study suggested a possibly greater influence of postnatal lead exposure; several technical and environmental explanations for this outcome are offered. It is concluded that prenatal lead exposure impairs neurobehavioral development, reduces gestational age, and lowers birth weight.

485. de Mol, J.; Loseke, N. & Leleux, C. (1979). **Mental disturbances in bismuth encephalopathy: A case report.** *Acta Psychiatrica Belgica,* 79(2), 185-197.
Presents the case of a 63-yr-old male with bismuth encephalopathy, with emphasis on the S's neuropsychological and neurolinguistic disturbances. An analysis is made of the related literature in reference to the clinical picture in its prodromic phase, state phase, differential diagnosis, course, and potential neuropsychological complications. (English, Flemish, German, Italian, & Spanish summaries) (17 ref).

486. Dietrich, Kim N.; Krafft, Kathleen M.; Bier, Mariana; Succop, Paul A. et al. (1986). **Early effects of fetal lead exposure: Neurobehavioral findings at 6 months.** *International Journal of Biosocial Research,* 8(2), 151-168.
Tested the hypothesis that prenatal exposure to lead (Pb) would be related to sensorimotor developmental deficits at 6 mo, using 305 lower socioeconomic status (SES) mothers (mean age 22.7 yrs) residing in Pb-hazardous areas. A set of potentially confounding covariables was assessed (e.g., home stimulation, perinatal health) and included in multiple regression and structural equation analyses. Results show an independent inverse relationship between both prenatal and neonatal blood Pb levels and performance of Ss' infants at 6 mo. Male infants and those from the poorest families appeared to be especially sensitive to psychoteratogenic influences. It is reported that early Pb-related neurobehavioral deficits were partly mediated through lowered birth weight and shortened gestational age.

487. Duva, Nicholas A. (1977). **Effects of asymptomatic lead poisoning of psychoneurological functioning of school-age urban children: A follow-up study.** *Dissertation Abstracts International,* 38(1-A), 168.

488. Ernhart, Claire B. (1986). **"Lead levels: Comment": Reply.** *Journal of Learning Disabilities,* 19(6), 322-323.
Responds to criticism by H. L. Needleman (1985) regarding the present author and colleagues' (1985) reanalysis of the data they obtained in a 1981 study of subclinical lead level and development deficit and contends that the errors receiving criticism belong instead to Needleman. (5 ref).

489. Ernhart, Claire B. (1987). **Lead levels and child development: Statement by Claire B. Ernhart.** *Journal of Learning Disabilities,* 20(5), 262-264.
Argues that H. L. Needleman (1986) published misrepresentations of both an earlier study on the relation of subclinical lead levels and child development by the present author and colleagues (1981) and a reanalysis of the data by the present author et al (1985). The present author contends that findings from the study are not sufficient to accept the hypothesis that low level lead exposure is detrimental to child development.

490. Ernhart, Claire B.; Landa, Beth & Wolf, Abraham W. (1985). **Subclinical lead level and developmental deficit: Re-analyses of data.** *Journal of Learning Disabilities,* 18(8), 475-479.
The authors reanalyzed data from the following 2 studies: (1) the report by J. Perino and the 1st author (1974) that moderate levels of lead exposure in 80 preschool urban Black children were related to cognitive impairment (the McCarthy Scales of Children's Abilities); and (2) the reexamination by the 1st author and colleagues (1981) of 63 of these children 5 yrs later, which found no significant association between preschool lead level and outcome measures, including cognitive

measures, reading tests, and teacher behavior ratings. The positive findings of the preschool study were not substantiated in reanalysis, and the school-age lead data required technical adjustment. Additional variables were generated, including change scores, combinations, and interactions. Of 66 analyses, 2 tests of the lead effect were significant. The first depended on a deviant case; the second was an uninterpretable interaction. It is concluded that if these results are due to a lead effect, the effect is minimal. There was no evidence of an effect of moderate blood lead levels in the preschool period and any school-age outcome measure. (18 ref).

491. Ernhart, Claire B.; Morrow-Tlucak, Mary; Marler, Matthew R. & Wolf, Abraham W. (1987). **Low level lead exposure in the prenatal and early preschool periods: Early preschool development.** *Neurotoxicology & Teratology,* 9(3), 259–270.
Fetal lead exposure was measured in maternal and cord blood while preschool lead level was measured in venous blood samples at ages 6 mo, 2 yrs, and 3 yrs in 285 Ss. These blood lead measures (PbB) were related to concurrent and ensuing scores on developmental measures at 6 mo, 1 yr, 2 yrs, and 3 yrs. Results show that, with statistical control of covariate measures (age, sex, race, birth weight, birth order, gestational exposure to other toxic substances, maternal intelligence, and several indicators of the quality of the caretaking environment) as well as potentially confounding risk factors (gestational exposure to alcohol and other toxic substances), most significant associations of PbB with concurrent and later development were completely attenuated. It is concluded that the relationship between lead level and measures of development was primarily a function of the dependence of each on the quality of the caretaking environment.

492. Ewert, T.; Beginn, U.; Winneke, G.; Hofferberth, B. et al. (1986). **Sensible Neurographie, visuell und somatosensorisch evozierte Potentiale (VEP und SEP) an bleiexponierten Kindern. / Sensory nerve conduction and visual and somatosensory evoked potentials in children exposed to lead.** *Nervenarzt,* 57(8), 465–471.
Examined neurophysiological, neuropsychological, and biochemical effects of lead exposure in 114 6–7 yr olds who lived near a lead-zinc smelter. Ss were administered anamnestic, clinical, neurophysiological, psychological, and biochemical laboratory tests. Lead levels in Ss' blood were consistently below the critical threshold. Increasing lead levels in blood resulted in a significant increase in sensory nerve and radial nerve conduction velocity, a lesser increase in the nervus medianus, and a significant decrease in P_2 latency of visual evoked potentials. The causes of these symptoms may have been due to activation of the enzymes of the central and peripheral nervous system in the presence of lighter lead absorption. Psychological tests revealed significant reactive behavior disorders in Ss with actual increasing lead levels in blood, although no correlations could be proven between intelligence impairment and lead exposure.

493. Fergusson, D. M.; Fergusson, J. E.; Horwood, L. J. & Kinzett, N. G. (1988). **A longitudinal study of dentine lead levels, intelligence, school performance and behaviour: II. Dentine lead and cognitive ability.** *Journal of Child Psychology & Psychiatry & Allied Disciplines,* 29(6), 793–809.
Examined the relationship between dentine lead levels and measures of cognitive ability for a birth cohort of New Zealand children studied from birth to 9 yrs. There were small, consistent, and stable correlations between dentine lead measures and all measures of cognitive ability including intelligence, word recognition, and teacher ratings of school performance. After adjustment for the effects of confounding covariates, sample selection factors and possible reverse causal effects, the correlations between intelligence and dentine lead levels became nonsignificant. However, small but significant correlations persisted between dentine lead values and all measures of school performance after adjustment for sources of confounding. It is concluded that the weight of the evidence from this analysis favors the hypothesis that low level lead exposure may have deleterious effects on levels of achievement in children.

494. Fergusson, D. M.; Fergusson, J. E.; Horwood, L. J. & Kinzett, N. G. (1988). **A longitudinal study of dentine lead levels, intelligence, school performance and behaviour: I. Dentine lead levels and exposure to environmental risk factors.** *Journal of Child Psychology & Psychiatry & Allied Disciplines,* 29(6), 781–792.
Obtained dentine lead levels for 996 children (aged 6+ yrs) who were participants in a longitudinal study of child development. Mean dentine lead levels were just over 6 µg g^{-1} and had a log normal distribution. The relationship between dentine lead values and a number of variables (social background, residence in old weatherboard housing, residence on busy roads, pica) describing exposure to sources of lead was analyzed. Findings show that all factors made small but significant contributions to variations in dentine lead values and that collectively these factors explained 10% of the variance in lead values.

495. Fergusson, D. M.; Fergusson, J. E.; Horwood, L. J. & Kinzett, N. G. (1988). **A longitudinal study of dentine lead levels, intelligence, school performance and behaviour: III. Dentine lead levels and attention/activity.** *Journal of Child Psychology & Psychiatry & Allied Disciplines,* 29(6), 811–824.
Examined the relationship between dentine lead levels and maternal/teacher ratings of inattentive/restless behavior in 888 children for a birth cohort of New Zealand children. Ss were studied at birth, 4 mo, and annual intervals to age 9 yrs. There were small but relatively consistent and stable correlations between dentine lead values and behavior ratings. After correction for errors of measurement in dentine lead values and behavior ratings, it was estimated that the correlation between lead levels and inattentive/restless behavior was in the region of +0.18. However, after control for various sources of confounding, there was only a small but significant correlation of +0.08 between lead levels and inattention/restlessness in children. It is concluded that the weight of the evidence favors the view that there is a very weak causal association between lead levels and attention and activity levels in children.

496. Finney, Jack W.; Russo, Dennis C. & Cataldo, Michael F. (1982). **Reduction of pica in young children with lead poisoning.** *Journal of Pediatric Psychology,* 7(2), 197–207.
Investigated the use of behavioral procedures to reduce pica (the ingestion of inedible materials) in young children with lead poisoning. Four children (aged 2 yrs 3 mo to 5 yrs 8 mo) hospitalized for high blood lead levels received a sequential training program of discrimination training and DRO. In 2 cases, a 3rd phase involving DRO and overcorrection was also used. Results show a reduction of pica during hospitalization. Contact with materials remained similar across conditions in all Ss, indicating continued environmental exploration. Results are considered in light of developmental, ethical, and educational concerns involved in behavioral treatment for young children. (27 ref).

497. Fitzgerald, Michael; O'Rourke, Michael & Murphy, Michael. (1987). **Blood lead level of children attending an Urban Child Guidance Clinic.** *Irish Journal of Psychiatry,* 8(2), 4–13.
Evaluated blood lead and erythrocyte protoporphrin of 40 primary school children attending a child guidance clinic in a disadvantaged suburban area of Dublin, Ireland and 37 primary school controls. Results are discussed in terms of the association between blood lead levels, classroom behavior problems, and cognitive impairment.

METALLIC ELEMENTS

498. Garruto, Ralph M.; Swyt, Carol; Yanagihara, Richard; Fiori, Charles E. et al. (1986). **Intraneuronal co-localization of silicon with calcium and aluminum in amyotrophic lateral sclerosis and parkinsonism with dementia of Guam.** *New England Journal of Medicine,* 315(11), 711–712.
Reports the correlation of silicon with calcium and aluminum in hippocampal neurons bearing neurofibrillary tangles in 2 Guamanian patients with amyotrophic lateral sclerosis and 5 with parkinsonism with dementia. It is suggested that the epidemiology of these disorders among 3 genetically and geographically distinct populations in the western Pacific region implicates environmental factors in their causation.

499. Ghafour, Siham Y.; Khuffash, Faisal A.; Ibrahim, Hanem S. & Reavey, Philip C. (1984). **Congenital lead intoxication with seizures due to prenatal exposure.** *Clinical Pediatrics,* 23(5), 282–283.
Reports the case of a newborn female presenting with frequent tonic spasms. A diagnosis of congenital plumbism was supported by the finding of a high maternal blood lead level. When chelation therapy was initiated, S's blood level dropped to normal and looked clinically normal at 16 mo of age. However, a basic developmental screening at S's 2 yrs of age showed poor language development. (8 ref).

500. Gilewski, Michael J. (1985). **Probable behavioral side effects of a mercury preparation.** *Clinical Gerontologist,* 3(4), 69–71.
Discusses the case of a 69-yr-old man who presented at a counseling center for older adults complaining of memory problems possibly related to long-term use of an over-the-counter psoriasis ointment containing mercury. Although a definite diagnosis was not established, the S's pattern of psychological deficits paralleled those observed in patients suffering from a chronic exposure to low levels of mercury (motor tremors, intellectual deterioration, and alterations in emotional state). (2 ref).

501. Gillberg, Christopher; Norén, J. G.; Wahlström, J. & Rasmussen, Peder. (1982). **Heavy metals and neuropsychiatric disorders in six-year-old children: Aspects of dental lead and cadmium.** *Acta Paedopsychiatrica,* 48(5), 253–263.
Analyzed dental lead and cadmium with a potentiometric stripping technique in exfoliated deciduous teeth of 98 5–6 yr olds. Ss were also assessed for any neurological dysfunctions, RT, language disorders, and attention deficits. Ss' mothers completed questionnaires on Ss' health, development, and behavior. The 10 Ss with the highest lead levels showed significant prolongation of mean RT when compared with Ss with the lowest lead levels. All 10 Ss in the high-lead group lived in heavy traffic areas compared with only half of the Ss in the low-lead group. It is concluded that RTs may be prolonged by high brain levels of lead, and this might increase vulnerability for psychiatric disturbance. (French, German & Spanish abstracts) (26 ref).

502. Glickman, Linda A. (1982). **Oculomotor indicators of inorganic lead neurotoxicity.** *Dissertation Abstracts International,* 42(10-B), 4236.

503. Gordon, Cynthia M. (1984). **Blood pressure in college students as related to dietary influences, certain hair and saliva element concentrations, psychological profile, and taste acuity.** *Dissertation Abstracts International,* 45(1-B), 131.

504. Gowdy, John M. & Demers, Francois X. (1978). **Whole blood mercury levels in mental hospital patients.** *American Journal of Psychiatry,* 135(1), 115–117.
Investigated the possibility that chronic mercury accumulation might be a factor in some mental diseases. Measurements of whole blood mercury levels in 81 male and 10 female (mean ages 45.5 and 69.8 yrs, respectively) hospitalized psychiatric patients in a VA hospital show no statistically significant differences in mercury levels among Ss with various diagnoses; race, duration of hospitalization, or clinical severity also had no relation to mercury levels.

505. Greenless, Robert M. (1987). **The relationship between airborne lead and performance on standardized tests.** *Dissertation Abstracts International,* 48(4-A), 875.

506. Gregory, Robert J. & Mohan, Philip J. (1977). **Effect of asymptomatic lead exposure on childhood intelligence: A critical review.** *Intelligence,* 1(4), 381–400.
Outlines criteria for evaluating studies of asymptomatic lead exposure and childhood intelligence. When these criteria were applied to 9 recent studies on the intellectual consequences of asymptomatic lead exposure, all of the studies were found to have significant deficiencies. It is concluded that the intellectual consequences of asymptomatic lead exposure are simply unknown. Suggestions for improving future research by assessing information processing capacities are offered. (42 ref).

507. Harvey, P. G. (1984). **Lead and children's health: Recent research and future questions.** *Journal of Child Psychology & Psychiatry & Allied Disciplines,* 25(4), 517–522.
From measurements of lead in children's teeth, researchers have found that low levels are associated with higher IQ, while high levels of lead are associated with lower IQ and with behavioral problems. However, some of these results are confounded by SES variables. After accounting for SES variables, the data support the position that at the levels shown there is no significant relationship between body burden of lead and various indicators of children's behavior and cognitive performance. (37 ref).

508. Harvey, P. G.; Hamlin, M. W.; Kumar, R.; Morgan, G. et al. (1988). **Relationships between blood lead, behaviour, psychometric and neuropsychological test performance in young children.** *British Journal of Developmental Psychology,* 6(2), 145–156.
Assessed 201 inner-city dwelling children (aged 5.5 yrs) on cognitive, performance, neuropsychological, and behavioral measures. Extensive sociodemographic and family indices were also examined. Body burden of lead was derived from a venous sample of blood. Results show that the initial correlations between blood lead and the outcome measures were generally few and low. No significant relationship was found between overall IQ and blood lead, and the marginally significant association found when the sample was split by father's occupation proved nonsignificant. The only outcome measures that showed significant association with blood lead were tests requiring motor skills (where performance generally speeded up with increasing blood lead) and a reaction time (RT) measure where the converse was obtained.

509. Hawk, B. A. et al. (1986). **Relation of lead and social factors to IQ of low-SES children: A partial replication.** *American Journal of Mental Deficiency,* 91(2), 178–183.
Attempted to replicate S. R. Schroeder's (1985) study and clarify the relationships of blood lead (PbB) levels, social factors, and IQ in a more homogeneous group (75 3–7 yr old Blacks) of low socioeconomic status (SES) at risk for Pb exposure. Ss' families were evaluated in a single-blind protocol that included an extensive demographic history related to Pb exposure; the Stanford-Binet Intelligence Scale; maternal IQ, using the Peabody Picture Vocabulary Test—Revised; neurological and electrophysiological testing; and blood samples. Ss' mean PbB level was 20.8 μg/dl. Analyses showed no significant interactions between PbB and age, sex, maternal IQ, home environment, or SES. There was a highly significant negative relationship between both mean and maximum PbB levels and IQ: IQ decreased linearly as PbB increased. The most accurate and precise regression model included Pb, maternal IQ, home environment, and gender, which differs from Schroeder and colleagues' finding that only PbB and SES were significant variables.

510. Hawk, Barbara A. (1987). **Interactive effects of lead burden and social factors on IQ in children.** *Dissertation Abstracts International,* 47(8-B), 3523–3524.

511. Hebel, J. R.; Kinch, Denise & Armstrong, Eileen. (1976). **Mental capability of children exposed to lead pollution.** *British Journal of Preventative & Social Medicine,* 30(3), 170-174.
"Eleven-plus" school examination scores were obtained for 851 Birmingham (England) 11-yr-olds residing since birth in a lead-polluted area and for 1,642 residing in 2 similar but unpolluted areas. It was found that the children in the lead-polluted area actually scored higher on the average than children in the control areas. Within the area of lead contamination, children living closest to the source of pollution did not have significantly lower scores than children living further away. Results indicate that lead pollution of the magnitude reported in this investigation did not have a demonstrable effect on the mental capabilities of children in the affected community.

512. Huggins, Hal A. (1982). **Mercury: A factor in mental disease?** *Journal of Orthomolecular Psychiatry,* 11(1), 3–16.
Reviews studies that suggest that mercury leaching out of dental amalgam filling can affect the peripheral nervous system, immune system, and cardiovascular system, and that mercury in a biological system appears to create or mimic many disorders in these 3 areas. The case of a 17-yr-old girl, who, at the suggestion of various professionals, was to be placed in a mental institution for her physical and emotional problems, but who in fact was suffering from mercury toxicity, is also presented. (30 ref).

513. Hunt, Thomas J. (1978). **Caretaker attitude as related to pica and lead poisoning.** *Dissertation Abstracts International,* 38(10-B), 4988.

514. Iștoc-Bobiș, Mariana & Gabor, Silvia. (1987). **Psychological disfunctions in lead- and mercury-occupational exposure.** *Revue Roumaine des Sciences Sociales - Série de Psychologie,* 31(2), 183–191.
Evaluated neuropsychological changes in 206 workers exposed to lead and in 106 workers exposed to mercury. Ss were administered a battery of cognitive, personality, and motor tests, including the Wechsler Adult Intelligence Scale (WAIS), the Eysenck Personality Inventory, and the Raven Progressive Matrices. Exposure to lead exerted marked dysthymic trends, manifested by loneliness, and depressive and obsessive phenomena associated with general impairment in intellectual performance. Exposure to mercury induced dominating tendencies, impulsiveness, aggressiveness, and seizures accompanied by alteration of some intellectual structural factors.

515. Jonderko, G. et al. (1979). **Psychological and neurological disturbances and an increased accident rate among workers exposed to high manganese concentration.** *International Review of Applied Psychology,* 28(1), 33–36.
Statistical investigations were made for a 6-yr employment period for 199 persons working in ferromanganese and silicomanganese alloys and 199 matched controls. Psychological examinations were conducted using 17 Ss with increased blood manganese concentrations. Results indicate that deficiency of intellectual capacity, emotional disturbances, and a decreased sense of criticism should be classified as the early symptoms of manganese poisoning. For antitrauma prophylaxis, the continued use of psychological examinations is suggested, especially among workers employed in contact with manganese on dangerous jobs requiring a great deal of concentration. (5 ref).

516. Kelkar, S. A. (1975). **Psychomotor skill changes in workers exposed to mercury.** *Indian Journal of Psychology,* 50(1), 17-24.
Studied hand–eye coordination and force-loaded forearm tremor in 36 control male worker volunteers and in 75 other volunteers who were exposed to mercury vapor in their work in chemical plants but exhibited no classical clinical symptoms of mercurialism. Significant differences appeared between experimental and control Ss in 11 of the 16 performance parameters measured. It is suggested that this lack of consistency in performance may indicate that damage due to exposure to mercury may be occurring at the CNS level. The use of psychomotor skill tests is recommended to protect workers against adverse effects of toxic substances and other environmental hazards. (15 ref).

517. Kirkconnell, Shirley C. & Hicks, Lou E. (1980). **Residual effects of lead poisoning on Denver Developmental Screening Test scores.** *Journal of Abnormal Child Psychology,* 8(2), 257–267.
Administered the Denver Developmental Screening Test to 22 low-income preschoolers who had been lead-poisoned, then medically deleaded. Pretest (i.e., before blood lead elevations occurred) scores were comparable to those of a matched control group, but posttest scores (i.e., after deleading) on the Fine Motor-Adaptive subtest declined, indicating significant residual effects of lead poisoning. (21 ref).

518. Knafle, June D. (1976). **Children's learning of words as a function of minimum contrasts in variable letter positions.** *Journal of Reading Behavior,* 8(2), 205–220.
Presents results of an experimental task which measured children's learning of consonant-vowel-consonant (CVC) words when employed with minimum contrasts in 1st, middle, and last letter positions (e.g., tin, win, vs pan, pen vs pit, pig). Ss were 41 male and 43 female kindergarten and 1st-grade pupils who knew the alphabet but who had not yet learned to read. The visual and oral tasks provided measures of transfer, recognition, recall, delayed recognition, and delayed recall. For the sexes separately and combined, 1st letter position contrasts (rhyming words) were superior to letter contrasts in the middle or last letter positions; middle letter position contrasts were least effective. Last letter position contrasts were more effective for females than males. Results suggest that the teaching of rhyming words is the most efficient initial presentation of CVC words for beginning readers. (27 ref).

519. Kracke, Kevin R. (1982). **Biochemical bases for behavior disorders in children.** *Journal of Orthomolecular Psychiatry,* 11(4), 289–296.
Investigated to what extent, if any, biochemical differences occur among groups of psychotic, neurotic, and control children using hair analysis (atomic absorption spectroscopy). The total sample was comprised of 37 boys and 20 girls (aged 7 yrs 5 mo to 12 yrs 6 mo). 20 Ss were assigned to psychotic or neurotic groups on the basis of responses to the Child Behavior Checklist. Results indicate that molybdenum, chromium, cobalt, vanadium, and lead were significantly different across diagnostic groups. Copper, sodium, and manganese all demonstrated trends towards differing signficantly across groups. Controls had significantly elevated cobalt and vanadium levels and depressed molybdenum and chromium levels as compared to the psychotic and neurotic groups. The neurotic group had significantly more lead than the psychotic and control groups. The biochemical influences of these substances are discussed. (49 ref).

520. Krall, Vita et al. (1980). **Effects of lead poisoning on cognitive test performance.** *Perceptual & Motor Skills,* 50(2), 483–486.
47 lead-poisoned children (mean age 8 yrs), treated and without encephalopathy, were compared with 45 sibling controls on perceptual-verbal pattern comparisons of subtests of the WISC to determine whether there had been brain damage. The groups did not differ significantly on comparisons of

these patterns, and they appeared to be similar to each other in WISC functioning. The conclusion is that lead-poisoning, treated and without encephalopathy, does not result in detectable brain damage by means of these pattern analyses. (11 ref).

521. Landis, Theodor; Graves, Roger; Benson, D. Frank & Hebben, Nancy. (1982). **Visual recognition through kinaesthetic mediation.** *Psychological Medicine,* 12(3), 515–531.
Reports the case of a 30-yr-old male in whom mercury intoxication produced visual symptoms with an unusual compensation. The similarity of this patient to Schn. (K. Goldstein and A. Gelb, 1918), a much reported neuropsychiatric case, was striking and prompted correlation of the 2 cases. A battery of tests indicated that in both cases, rather than hysterical or learned exaggerations, Ss' behavior was the product of a partially successful attempt to compensate for a serious disruption of cerebral function. (52 ref).

522. Lester, Michael L.; Horst, Richard L. & Thatcher, Robert W. (1986). **Protective effects of zinc and calcium against heavy metal impairment of children's cognitive function.** *Nutrition & Behavior,* 3(2), 145–161.
Investigated the effects of heavy metal pollutants on cognitive function, using spectrometer analysis of hair samples obtained from 149 children (aged 5–16 yrs). Analyses in which the environmental heavy metal pollutants and essential elements were evaluated as predictors of cognitive function (IQ) indicated a significant interaction between the essential and nonessential elements with reference to cognition. It is concluded that the study provides evidence for an interaction between cadmium and zinc and between lead and calcium in relation to cognitive function in children.

523. Lin-Fu, Jane S. (1973). **Vulnerability of children to lead exposure and toxicity: I.** *New England Journal of Medicine,* 289(23), 1229-1233.

524. Mac Isaac, David S. (1976). **Learning and behavioral functioning of low income, Black preschoolers with asymptomatic lead poisoning.** *Dissertation Abstracts International,* 37(5-A), 2747.

525. Madden, Nancy A.; Russo, Dennis C. & Cataldo, Michael F. (1980). **Behavioral treatment of pica in children with lead poisoning.** *Child Behavior Therapy,* 2(4), 67–81.
Employed behavior modification procedures to eliminate pica (the ingestion of nonedible substances) in 3 2-yr-old Black females with lead poisoning. Three kinds of procedures were used: (1) discrimination training, in which the S was taught to recognize that paint and several objects were not edible; (2) reinforcement for the absence of pica; and (3) overcorrection for the occurrence of pica. Pica was eliminated in all 3 Ss. (28 ref).

526. Madden, Nancy A.; Russo, Dennis C. & Cataldo, Michael F. (1980). **Environmental influences on mouthing in children with lead intoxication.** *Journal of Pediatric Psychology,* 5(2), 207–216.
The relationship of mouthing behavior to different environmental conditions was evaluated for 3 Black children with asymptomatic lead poisoning: 2 males aged 2 yrs 8 mo and 2 yrs 9 mo, and 1 female, age 1 yr 11 mo. The amount of mouthing; involvement with materials, adults, and other children; and noninvolvement were measured across daily sessions in group play, individual impoverished play, and individual enriched play, using an interval-recording system. For each S, results indicate that mouthing was exhibited significantly more frequently in the impoverished setting as compared to either group play or individual enriched environments. Results suggest that simple environmental enrichment may hold promise in the reduction of mouthing and pica. Further research evaluating procedures for reduction of mouthing and pica is suggested. (9 ref).

527. Maghazaji, H. I. (1974). **Psychiatric aspects of methylmercury poisoning.** *Journal of Neurology, Neurosurgery & Psychiatry,* 37(8), 954-958.
Studied 43 patients with methylmercury poisoning. Results indicate that 74.4% of the patients showed some degree of depression; their blood levels of mercury were higher than the average values for the whole group and considerably higher than the blood levels of the nondepressed patients. Irritability was observed in 44.2% of the patients, all except one of the 19 being under 30 yrs old. There was general improvement in the mental states of the patients who were hospitalized. Mercury binding compounds did not seem to have a significant effect in enhancing recovery from the depressive state. The possibility of there being 2 distinct syndromes, due to organic and inorganic mercury poisoning, is discussed.

528. Mantere, P.; Hänninen, Helena & Hernberg, S. (1982). **Subclinical neurotoxic lead effects: Two-year follow-up studies with psychological test methods.** *Neurobehavioral Toxicology & Teratology,* 4(6), 725–727.
16 lead workers were examined at the beginning of their employment and after 2 yrs; 31 workers not exposed to lead served as controls. Whereas the control group displayed pronounced performance improvement due to training for most of the tests, a sizeable portion of the exposed group exhibited performance deterioration. The most sensitive indicators of psychological impairment among the lead workers were Block Design and Digit Span subtests of the WAIS and the Santa Ana Coordination Test. It is concluded that the impairment of CNS function was caused by lead exposure. No exact threshold for impaired performances could be estimated. (4 ref).

529. Marlowe, Mike et al. (1985). **Main and interaction effects of metallic toxins on classroom behavior.** *Journal of Abnormal Child Psychology,* 13(2), 185–198.
Investigated the relationships of metal levels and metal combinations to 80 1st–6th grade children's classroom behavior. Hair-metal concentrations of lead, arsenic, mercury, cadmium, and aluminum were determined in Ss, who were also rated by their classroom teacher on the Walker Problem Behavior Identification Checklist (WPBIC). Parents were interviewed to control for confounding variables that may have affected behavioral development. Regression analysis indicated that the set of metals was significantly related to increased scores on 4 of 5 WPBIC subscales and on the total scale, with lead being a major contributor to 4 of 6 dependent measures. Metal combinations were significantly related to increased WPBIC scores on subscales measuring acting-out, disturbed peer relations, and immaturity as well as on the total scale. It is concluded that a continuing reexamination of metal-poisoning concentrations is needed because metal levels and combinations previously thought harmless may be associated with nonadaptive classroom behavior. (32 ref).

530. Marlowe, Mike; Cossairt, Ace; Welch, Ken & Errera, John. (1984). **Hair mineral content as a predictor of learning disabilities.** *Journal of Learning Disabilities,* 17(7), 418–421.
Investigated the relationships between hair mineral elements and childhood learning disabilities and determined which minerals, if any, separated 26 learning disabled (LD) from 24 normal 5–12 yr olds. The LD group had significantly raised hair-lead concentrations. There were also differences in the mean levels of 10 other minerals. Discriminant function analysis revealed that by using lead, calcium, silicon, aluminum, vanadium, mercury, and zinc, Ss could be correctly classified as normal controls or LD with 91.7% and 76.1% accuracy, respectively. The relationships between hair mineral element patterns and childhood learning disabilities are discussed. It is suggested that lead poisoning concentrations need to be reex-

amined because concentrations previously thought harmless may have to be considered as an etiological factor in neurobehavioral dysfunctions. (16 ref).

531. Marlowe, Mike; Errera, John; Stellern, John & Beck, Dave. (1983). **Lead and mercury levels in emotionally disturbed children.** *Journal of Orthomolecular Psychiatry,* 12(4), 260–267.
Investigated possible relationships of metal levels to emotional disturbance in children without demonstrable cause for their emotional deficit by comparing 37 emotionally disturbed (ED) children (mean age 9.5 yrs) with 107 non-ED (NED) children (mean age 8.7 yrs). Hair metal concentrations of lead, arsenic, mercury, cadmium, and aluminum were examined; each S was also rated on the Walker Problem Behavior Identification Checklist (WPBIC). Results indicate that ED Ss had significantly higher hair lead and mercury levels. Discriminant function analysis revealed that by using levels of lead, mercury, arsenic, and aluminum as indicators, Ss could be correctly classified as ED or NED with 77.8% accuracy. Significant positive correlations emerged between lead and the WPBIC scales measuring acting-out, withdrawal, distractibility, disturbed peer relations, and immaturity, and between mercury and acting-out, disturbed peer relations, and immaturity. It is concluded that levels of metal previously thought harmless may be associated with emotional disturbances in children. (30 ref).

532. Marlowe, Mike; Errera, John & Jacobs, Jim. (1983). **Increased lead and cadmium burdens among mentally retarded children and children with borderline intelligence.** *American Journal of Mental Deficiency,* 87(5), 477–483.
Investigated the relationship between subtoxic metal levels and mild mental retardation and borderline intelligence. Hair metal concentrations in 135 4–16 yr olds with mild retardation or borderline intelligence (IQ 55–84) and 71 4–15 yr old nonretarded controls were compared. Ss in the retarded/borderline group had significantly higher lead and cadmium concentrations. Sources of lead and cadmium exposure are discussed. Although not establishing an etiological relationship, findings suggest the need for a continuing reexamination of lead and cadmium poisoning concentrations because levels of these metals previously thought harmless may be associated with mental retardation and impaired intelligence. (20 ref).

533. Marlowe, Mike; Errera, John; Ballowe, Tom & Jacobs, Jim. (1983). **Low metal levels in emotionally disturbed children.** *Journal of Abnormal Psychology,* 92(3), 386–389.
Investigated possible relationships of metal levels to childhood behavioral disorders. Hair-metal concentrations in 22 emotionally disturbed children (mean age 8.72 yrs) were compared to hair-metal levels in 25 control Ss (mean age 8.4 yrs) drawn from the general school population. Each S was also rated on the Walker Problem Behavior Identification Checklist (WPBIC). Disturbed Ss had significantly higher hair-lead levels. Correlations were run between hair-metal levels and WPBIC ratings for the 2 groups. Arsenic, cadmium, and aluminum levels correlated positively and significantly with the WPBIC total scale score for the disturbed group. A continuing reexamination of metal-poisoning concentrations is needed because metals levels previously thought harmless may be associated with behavioral impairments in children. (12 ref).

534. Marlowe, Mike & Errera, John. (1982). **Low lead levels and behavior problems in children.** *Behavioral Disorders,* 7(3), 163–172.
Compared lead levels in hair samples taken from 26 children (aged 6–14 yrs) identified by their teachers as having behavior problems and 29 control children not exhibiting behavior problems. Ss were also rated by their teachers on the Walker Problem Behavior Identification Checklist (WPBIC). Behavior-problem Ss had significantly higher hair lead levels than did controls. Significant positive correlations were found between lead levels and WPBIC scales measuring distractibility, aggression, disturbed peer relations, and immaturity. It is concluded that a reexamination of lead poisoning levels is needed because lead levels previously thought harmless may be associated with neurobehavioral impairments. (38 ref).

535. Marlowe, Mike; Errera, John & Case, James C. (1986). **Hair selenium levels and children's classroom behavior.** *Journal of Orthomolecular Medicine,* 1(2), 91–96.
Investigated the relationship between children's hair-selenium (HS) levels and their behavioral performance, using 120 1st to 6th graders. Ss' HS levels were correlated with teachers' ratings of the Ss on the Walker Problem Behavior Identification Checklist (WPBIC). Parents were also interviewed. Results show that increasing HS values correlated significantly with increased scores on the WPBIC scales measuring acting out, withdrawal, and total scale score. It is concluded that a continuing examination of selenium exposure in the young is needed to determine the margin of safety between potentially toxic and nutritionally required levels and to control adverse behavioral effects (e.g., hyperirritability).

536. Marlowe, Mike; Folio, Rhonda; Hall, Debra & Errera, John. (1982). **Increased lead burdens and trace-mineral status in mentally retarded children.** *Journal of Special Education,* 16(1), 87–99.
Investigated the relationship between low-level lead absorption and mild and borderline mental retardation and evaluated the relationships among nutrient minerals, heavy metals, and increased lead burdens. Hair trace-mineral concentrations were compared in 40 retarded children (mean age 11 yrs; IQs 55–84) and in 27 nonretarded Ss (mean age 11.07 yrs). Findings indicate that (1) the retarded group had significantly raised hair-lead concentrations and (2) there were indications that lead and other toxic metals occurred together in the retarded. It is concluded that continuing research is needed to study the relationship between retardation and lead burdens. (33 ref).

537. Marlowe, Mike; Moon, Charles; Errera, John & Stellern, John. (1983). **Hair mineral content as a predictor of mental retardation.** *Journal of Orthomolecular Psychiatry,* 12(1), 26–33.
Investigated the relationship between mineral elements and mild and borderline mental retardation in 64 4–16 yr old mentally retarded Ss (IQ 55–84) and 71 4–15 yr old controls. Results of comparisons of hair element concentrations show that mentally retarded Ss had significantly raised hair-lead and hair-cadmium concentrations. Differences in the mean levels of Mg, Ni, Se, Co, Mo, Na, and Zn were also found. Ss could be correctly classified as nonretarded or retarded with 83.1 and 75% accuracy, respectively. (21 ref).

538. Marlowe, Mike; Moon, Charles E.; Errera, John; Jacobs, Jim et al. (1986). **Low mercury levels and childhood intelligence.** *Journal of Orthomolecular Medicine,* 1(1), 43–49.
Studied 59 children in Grades 1–4 to determine the relationship between mercury levels and performance of the Ss on the Wechsler Intelligence Scale for Children—Revised (WISC—R). Ss were asked to submit a small sample of hair (about 400 mg) for trace mineral analysis. Samples were collected from as close to the scalp as possible. Mercury levels were determined using the atomic absorption spectrophotometer, the graphite furnace, and the induction coupled plasma torch. Results indicate that with increased mercury levels, decreases were found in full-scale, performance, and verbal IQ, as well as in scores on 6 of the 10 WISC—R subtests. It is suggested that the developing central nervous system (CNS) is especially vulnerable to mercury toxicity and that future studies should examine possible adverse developmental effects.

METALLIC ELEMENTS

539. Marlowe, Mike; Stellern, John; Moon, Charles & Errera, John. (1985). **Main and interaction effects of metallic toxins on aggressive classroom behavior.** *Aggressive Behavior,* 11(1), 41–48.
Hair-metal concentrations of lead, arsenic, mercury, cadmium, and aluminum were determined in 80 randomly selected elementary-age children. Each child was also rated by his/her classroom teacher on the Acting-out subscale of the Walker Problem Behavior Identification Checklist. Ss' parents were interviewed to control for confounding variables that may affect behavioral development. Regression data indicated that the set of metals was significantly related to increased scores on the Acting-out subscale with lead being the major contributor; the metal combinations were also significantly related to increased Acting-out scores with the interaction of lead-cadmium being the major contributor. It is concluded that a continuing reexamination of metal-poisoning concentrations is needed, because metal levels and metal combinations previously thought harmless may be associated with aggressive classroom behavior. (30 ref).

540. Mayfield, Sandra A. (1983). **Language and speech behaviors of children with undue lead absorption: A review of the literature.** *Journal of Speech & Hearing Research,* 26(3), 362–368.
A review of the literature on the effects of chronic undue or low-lead absorption (LLA) on the speech and language behavior of children indicates that, while the effects of high-level lead poisoning have been documented, the effects of chronic LLA remain controversial. It is concluded that the evidence supports the presence of speech and language problems in some children with LLA. The severity, duration, and specific nature of the problems, however, are not clear. (72 ref).

541. McCracken, James T. (1987). **Lead intoxication psychosis in an adolescent.** *Journal of the American Academy of Child & Adolescent Psychiatry,* 26(2), 274–276.
Presents a case of a schizophreniformlike psychosis in a 14-yr-old adolescent with secondary to moderate lead intoxication. S showed severe and persistent anxiety, distracted and lost concentration, speech and language problems, and paranoid ideation. Four days of chelation therapy proved effective. This represents a possible manifestation of lower levels of lead not previously discussed in the literature. Psychobiological vulnerability to the effects of lead and implications for screening and treatment are discussed.

542. Milar, Christopher R. (1980). **Behavioral correlates of increased lead burden in children.** *Dissertation Abstracts International,* 41(1-B), 360.

543. Milar, Christopher R. et al. (1980). **Contributions of the caregiving environment to increased lead burden of children.** *American Journal of Mental Deficiency,* 84(4), 339–344.
14 12–30 mo old and 12 31–78 mo old children showing increased lead burden were compared to a sample of children matched for age, sex, and socioeconomic status but showing no evidence of increased lead burden. All Ss were screened at a local county health department because of suspected lead exposure or as part of the Early and Periodic Screening, Diagnosis, and Treatment Program. The quality of the caregiving environment was assessed using the Home Observation for Measurement of the Environment (HOME) Inventory. A measure of maternal intelligence was also obtained. For the younger Ss, significant deficits in maternal IQ and quality of the caregiving environment were associated with increased lead burden. In particular, the subscales of the HOME inventory dealing with emotional and verbal responsivity of the mother and maternal involvement with the child were significantly lower for Ss with increased lead burden. For the older Ss there was no significant association between lead burden and home environment or maternal IQ. Results suggest that intellectual deficits previously attributed to lead toxicity may be related to compromised home environment. (19 ref).

544. Milar, Christopher R.; Schroeder, Stephen R.; Mushak, Paul & Boone, Lois. (1981). **Failure to find hyperactivity in preschool children with moderately elevated lead burden.** *Journal of Pediatric Psychology,* 6(1), 85–95.
40 10 mo–6.5 yr old children evidencing moderately increased lead burden were compared to 48 same-age Ss not evidencing increased lead burden on 3 measures of hyperactivity. All Ss were screened at a local county health department because of suspected lead exposure or as part of an early and periodic screening, diagnosis, and treatment program. The 3 measures of activity were the D. K. Routh et al (1974) free-field measure of gross motor activity, the C. K. Conners (1970) Parent Rating Scale, and the Werry-Weiss-Peters Activity Rating Scale; both of the latter were completed by the parents. As in previous research, a consistent age effect in gross motor activity was found. No difference was found between the groups in gross motor activity or in parental report of activity level. Results suggest that using the aforementioned measures of hyperactivity, moderate lead exposure does not result in overactivity in preschoolers. (18 ref).

545. Miller, Terry P.; Davies, Helen D.; Yesavage, Jerome A. & Tinklenberg, Jared R. (1984). **Presenile dementia associated with elevated aluminum and zinc levels: A case report.** *Clinical Gerontologist,* 2(3), 55–59.
Reports a failure of an attempted treatment of a 43-yr-old male patient with progressive dementia associated with markedly elevated serum, urine, and CSF levels of aluminum with the aluminum chelating agent tetracycline (1,000 mg) for 3 mo. Implications are discussed in terms of the role of aluminum in Alzheimer's disease. (2 ref).

546. Moon, Charles; Marlowe, Mike; Stellern, John & Errera, John. (1985). **Main and interaction effects of metallic pollutants on cognitive functioning.** *Journal of Learning Disabilities,* 18(4), 217–221.
Investigated possible relationships of metal levels and metal combinations with 69 elementary school aged children's cognitive functioning. Hair-metal concentrations of lead, arsenic, mercury, cadmium, and aluminum were determined. Ss were administered the Wide Range Achievement Test, Reading and Spelling tests and the Bender Visual-Motor Gestalt Test. Parents of Ss were interviewed to control for confounding variables that may have affected cognitive development. Regression data indicate that increases in arsenic and the interaction of arsenic with lead were significantly related to decreased reading and spelling achievement, and increases in aluminum and the interaction of aluminum with lead were significantly related to decreased visual-motor performance. It is concluded that metal levels and metal combinations previously thought harmless may be associated with cognitive deficits. (26 ref).

547. Moore, M. R. (1980). **Exposure to lead in childhood: The persisting effects.** *Nature,* 283(5745), 334–335.
Discusses the effects of environmental lead exposure on children. In the earliest studies of childhood overexposure to lead, it was found that classroom performance was poorer than in children who had not been exposed. Thereafter, studies showed that mental retardation could be linked with overexposure to lead in drinking water and with high concentrations of blood lead at about the time of birth. In the most recent studies (e.g., H. L. Needleman et al, 1979), a diminished learning ability (IQ drop of 4–7 points) and behavioral changes (e.g., diminished attention span) have been associated with increased concentrations of lead in teeth. (11 ref).

548. Moore, Michael R. et al. (1982). **A prospective study of the neurological effects of lead in children.** *Neurobehavioral Toxicology & Teratology,* 4(6), 739–743.

Describes an ongoing study of the cognitive and behavioral development of 151 children subdivided into 3 groups according to the level of lead exposure during early in utero development. Current data include measurement of psychometric function and postnatal development at the ages of 1 and 2 yrs, information about attitudes and relationships within the home setting, and biochemical measures of lead exposure. Assessment will continue through to early scholastic performance and will include measurement of deciduous tooth lead concentration as an integrated measure of long-term exposure. (31 ref).

549. Needleman, Herbert L. (1983). **Lead at low dose and the behavior of children.** *Acta Psychiatrica Scandinavica,* 67(Suppl 303), 26–37.
Over 3,000 1st and 2nd graders attending public schools were classified as to past lead exposure according to the concentrations of lead in their teeth. Ss in the highest and lowest deciles for lead were evaluated by a broad battery of neuropsychologic outcome measures. 39 additional variables that could affect outcome were controlled either by matching or ANCOVA. High-lead Ss were significantly impaired on IQ, auditory processing, and RT under varying intervals of delay. Teacher's rating scales showed a dose-related increase in nonadaptive classroom behavior with no evidence of a threshold. EEG scores and observations of Ss in class demonstrated differences in high- and low-lead Ss. Three-year follow-up indicated that high-lead Ss spent more time in distracted, off-task activity, looking at peers, the observer, or away from their work. (13 ref).

550. Needleman, Herbert L. (1973). **Lead poisoning in children: Neurologic implications of widespread subclinical intoxication.** *Seminars in Psychiatry,* 5(1), 47–54.
Discusses exogenous toxins, and lead in particular, that have been implicated in causing impaired brain function. Those children in whom the elevated body lead content is unrecognized due to asymptomatic behavior still endure neurological and psychological impairment. The onset and symptomatology of lead poisoning are discussed. Concentration of lead in the blood is the generally accepted standard of toxicity. It is suggested, however, that other signs of lead poisoning and vulnerability (e.g., tooth lead levels and age) have been noted. Minor degrees of perceptual and cognitive impairment, motor incoordination, and disturbances in attention can easily escape detection. The health threat is especially great among the urban poor, where exposure to lead is likely and detection is unlikely. The need for social and medical action is emphasized. (38 ref).

551. Needleman, Herbert L. (1982). **The neurobehavioral consequences of low lead exposure in childhood.** *Neurobehavioral Toxicology & Teratology,* 4(6), 729–732.
2,335 1st and 2nd graders were classified according to the concentration of lead in their shed deciduous teeth. Ss in the lowest and highest tenth percentile were studied with a detailed neuropsychological battery under blind conditions. 39 nonlead covariates were controlled either by matching or in the biostatistical analysis. High-lead Ss tended to have significantly lower WISC-R Verbal IQs, impaired auditory and language processing, increased RTs at longer intervals of delay, and an increased incidence of disordered classroom behavior. EEG analysis demonstrated decreased midline alpha and increased midline delta in high-lead Ss. Observations of a subsample of high-lead Ss during classroom activities at a 4-yr follow-up showed them to spend less time on task and to be more distractible than their classmates. (10 ref).

552. Needleman, Herbert L. (1982). **The neuropsychiatric implications of low level exposure to lead.** *Psychological Medicine,* 12(3), 461–463.
Previous research suggests that exposure to lower doses of lead in children may result in CNS alterations that manifest themselves as learning disorders, attentional deficits, or behavioral problems. The symptoms of lead poisoning (e.g., behavioral change and clumsiness) are nonspecific and easily misdiagnosed. Mental retardation, learning disorders, and behavioral problems occur more frequently in areas with higher environmental levels of lead. (21 ref).

553. Needleman, Herbert L. et al. (1979). **Deficits in psychologic and classroom performance of children with elevated dentine lead levels.** *New England Journal of Medicine,* 300(13), 689–695.
To measure the neuropsychologic effects of unidentified childhood exposure to lead, the performance of 58 1st and 2nd graders with high and 100 with low dentine lead levels was compared. Ss with high lead levels scored significantly less well on the WISC-R than those with low lead levels. This difference was also apparent on verbal subtests, 3 other measures of auditory or speech processing, and a measure of attention. An ANOVA showed that none of these differences could be explained by any of the 39 other variables studied. Also evaluated by a teachers' questionnaire was the classroom behavior of all children (2,146 in number) whose teeth were analyzed. The frequency of nonadaptive classroom behavior increased in a dose-related fashion to dentine lead level. Lead exposure, at doses below those producing symptoms severe enough to be diagnosed clinically, appears to be associated with neuropsychologic deficits that may interfere with classroom performance. (36 ref).

554. Needleman, Herbert L. (1987). **Lead levels and child development: Statement by Herbert L. Needleman.** *Journal of Learning Disabilities,* 20(5), 264–265.
Refers to the study by J. Perino and C. B. Ernhart (1974) in which it was reported that lead was significantly related to lesser IQ scores in asymptomatic children and also discusses 2 follow-up reanalyses by Ernhart et al (1981; 1985) in which these findings were negated. The present author disagrees with the findings of the reanalyses and suggests that 2 methodological questions are to be considered.

555. Needleman, Herbert L. (1986). **Lead levels: Comment.** *Journal of Learning Disabilities,* 19(6), 322.
Discusses 3 "errors of fact and inference" that are contended to exist in a paper by C. B. Ernhart et al (1985) in which they reanalyzed data from their 1981 study of subclinical lead levels and development deficit. (3 ref).

556. Needleman, Herbert L. (1985). **The neurobehavioral effects of low-level exposure to lead in childhood.** *International Journal of Mental Health,* 14(3), 64–77.
Discusses the effects of low-level exposure to lead, noting problems in the design or execution of studies in this area, such as (1) use of an inadequate marker of lead exposure, (2) use of insensitive or inappropriate measures of outcome, (3) neglect of variates that can confound, (4) neglect of the possibility of ascertainment bias, and (5) lack of statistical power. Studies that confront these design problems are also reviewed; the data converge on the finding that IQ scores, behavioral measurements, and reaction time (RT) are impaired at levels of lead too small to bring the Ss to medical attention. It is noted that some investigators have evaluated the same group of studies and have concluded that no lead effect has been demonstrated or that if it has, it is of little magnitude. Epistemic issues on which this argument relies are examined, including (1) building nonveridical causal models, (2) ignoring prior information, and (3) assigning shared variance exclusively to the control variable. The question of why progress toward control of environmental sources of lead at low doses has been less than aggressive is addressed. (21 ref).

METALLIC ELEMENTS

557. Needleman, Herbert L.; Geiger, Susan K. & Frank, Richard. (1985). **Lead and IQ scores: A reanalysis.** *Science,* 227(4688), 701–704.
The authors respond to criticism by the Environmental Protection Agency (see L. Grant et al, 1983) concerning their (1979) finding that asymptomatic children exposed to high lead concentrations had significantly lower WISC IQ scores than low-exposure children, after controlling for 39 socioeconomic covariates. To the criticism that fathers' education rather than SES should have been controlled for and that multiple regression analysis with backwards elimination should have been used to examine the data, the authors reply that such a reanalysis of Performance and Full-Scale IQ showed effects similar to those shown in the original study. (3 ref).

558. Nolan, Kevin R. (1983). **Copper toxicity syndrome.** *Journal of Orthomolecular Psychiatry,* 12(4), 270–282.
Discusses the finding in a general medical practice (Vancouver, British Columbia) that a significant number of patients showed increased copper levels as measured by hair mineral analysis. It was noted that similar symptoms were described in a number of individuals with raised hair copper levels. These were symptoms of affective disorders, with individuals showing varying degrees of anxiety, depression, and sleep disorders as well as other problems. Serum and urine assessment for raised copper levels rarely showed abnormal levels. Chelation therapy using dextropenicillamine occasionally elicited a prompt reduction of symptoms. 24-hr urine output of copper during chelation therapy was generally proportional to the level of copper in hair analysis. The cases are discussed of 6 26–40 yr old females who had symptoms ranging from severe suicidal depression to insomnia; all had increased copper levels. It is postulated that since significantly raised hair copper levels are rare in most other geographical areas, there must be high levels of copper in domestic water supplies of the area in which the medical practice operated. (40 ref).

559. Otto, D. & Reiter, L. (1984). **Developmental changes in slow cortical potentials of young children with elevated body lead burden.** Sixth International Conference on Event-Related Slow Potentials of the Brain (EPIC VI): Normal and aberrant development (1981, Lake Forest/Chicago, Illinois). *Annals of the New York Academy of Sciences,* 425, 377–383.
Reviews current conceptions concerning the neurophysiology and neuroanatomy of evoked and slow potentials and data on the CNS effects of lead exposure and proposes a developmental model of the contingent negative variation (CNV) that accounts for the observed data. The proposed model suggests that slow surface-positive potentials in very young children may reflect axodendritic inhibitory processes. As the cortex matures, the locus of inhibitory activity shifts deeper to axosomatic connections. Negative slow potentials observed in older children, therefore, are presumed to reflect the surface negative (dendritic depolarization), depth positive (somatic hyperpolarization) dipole as the neurophysiological substrate of the CNV. Although the model is based on preliminary data and is speculative, its implications merit consideration. Positive shifts observed in very young children during the CS–UCS interval suggest why previous investigators have had great difficulty in eliciting CNV in Ss younger than 5 yrs of age. (39 ref).

560. Otto, D. et al. (1982). **Effects of low to moderate lead exposure on slow cortical potentials in young children: Two year follow-up study.** *Neurobehavioral Toxicology & Teratology,* 4(6), 733–737.
A follow-up study of slow cortical potentials in 28 35–95 mo old children with elevated blood lead (PbB) histories was conducted 2 yrs after initial evaluation (C. S. Milar et al; 1980, 1981). An age by PbB interaction was again observed wherein slow-wave voltage varied as a linear function of PbB with the slope of the function dependent on age. Results suggest that the observed alterations in CNS function are persistent, despite a significant decrease in mean PbB across time and indicate a need to reconsider the currently accepted 30 μg/dl threshold for undue lead absorption in children. (14 ref).

561. Perino, Joseph. (1973). **The relation of subclinical lead levels to cognitive and sensorimotor ability in preschool Black children.** *Dissertation Abstracts International,* 34(5-B), 2315-2316.

562. Perino, Joseph & Ernhart, Claire B. (1973). **The relation of subclinical lead levels to McCarthy scale performance in black preschool children.** *Proceedings of the 81st Annual Convention of the American Psychological Association, Montreal, Canada,* 8 , 721-722.
Determined the relation of blood lead levels to cognitive and sensorimotor functioning for 80 urban Black 3–5 yr olds. Lead levels ranged from .01 to .07 mg/100 ml of blood. The multiple regression as a general analytic system revealed a significant negative functional relation between lead level and general cognitive ability on the McCarthy Scales of Children's Abilities. Verbal and perceptual abilities and parental education were also significantly related in a negative direction. Lead levels were not significantly related to parental intelligence, birth order, birth weight, number of siblings, type of home, or time in home. It is concluded that the criteria for lead poisoning warrant reexamination.

563. Perino, Joseph & Ernhart, Claire B. (1974). **The relation of subclinical lead level to cognitive and sensorimotor impairment in black preschoolers.** *Journal of Learning Disabilities,* 7(10), 616-620.
Studied 80 3–5 yr old Black preschool children to determine the relation of blood lead levels to cognitive and perceptual-performance functioning. Results show that Ss' lead levels were below the criteria set for lead poisoning, but a regression formula revealed that the relationship was significant; as lead level increased, general cognitive, verbal, and perceptual abilities decreased. Lead levels were not related significantly to parental intelligence, birth order, birth weight, or number of siblings. It was, however, related to the educational level of the parents. It is concluded that the criteria set for lead poisoning warrant reexamination. (15 ref).

564. Pihl, R. O. & Parkes, M. (1977). **Hair element content in learning disabled children.** *Science,* 198(4313), 204–206.
Hair samples from 31 learning disabled and 22 normal 3rd and 4th grade children were analyzed for content of 14 elements. Ss had been selected according to their scores on the Pupil Rating Scale, Peabody Picture Vocabulary Test, and Metropolitan Achievement Test subtests of Reading, Spelling, Mathematics Computation, and Mathematics Problem Solving. Significant group differences were determined and a discriminant function was completed that separated the groups with 98% accuracy. Elevated lead and cadmium content in the learning disabled group is viewed as being of particular importance.

565. Pueschel, Siegfried M.; Cullen, Susan M.; Howard, Rosanne B. & Cullinane, Marie M. (1978). **Pathogenetic considerations of pica in lead poisoning.** *International Journal of Psychiatry in Medicine,* 8(1), 13–24.
An important factor associated with lead poisoning in children is the habit of eating nonfood substances, a condition termed pica. In a search for underlying mechanisms involved in the pathogenesis of pica, the present study compared the parental, environmental, and clinical characteristics of 92 children, found previously to have increased lead burden, with those of 92 matched controls. Results support the hypothesis that in many families, failure of normal mother–child interaction, paternal deprivation, culturally-dependent

maternal oral interests, and significant stress factors in the home where abundant lead-containing material is available would be etiologically related to the development of pica in lead poisoning. Other factors which have been thought to be associated with pica, nutritional deficiencies and maladaptive behavior pattern, are discussed. It is concluded that a multifocal treatment approach would be the most effective. (46 ref).

566. Raghavan, M. V.; Abrol, B. M. & Pujara, K. K. (1975). **Problems encountered in measurement of human tympanic membrane using time averaged holography.** *Journal of the All-India Institute of Speech & Hearing,* 5–6, 28–34.
Reports on methods adopted in an attempt to eliminate difficulties occurring in the use of time-averaged holography to measure the vibration of human tympanic membrane. Stability of the object required mounting all components on heavy bases in a 3-walled acoustic chamber, cushioning the holographic set-up, and conducting experiments at times when ground and air vibrations were low. Spraying the tympanic membrane with aluminum powder suspended in ether produced a more suitable coating than quick drying paints. A ratio of 2:1 between the intensities of the reference beam and the object beam gave the best time-averaged holograms. Other factors affecting the quality of holograms are discussed.

567. Raiten, Daniel J. (1984). **An evaluation of the role of nutrition in developmental disabilities.** *Dissertation Abstracts International,* 45(6-B), 1734–1735.

568. Ratcliffe, J. M. (1977). **Developmental and behavioural functions in young children with elevated blood lead levels.** *Journal of Epidemiology & Community Health,* 31(4), 258–264.
Blood lead levels in 465 preschool children living near a lead works, particularly those children with fathers employed at the lead works, showed evidence of increased exposure. 47 of them took part 3 yrs later in a follow-up study of their developmental and behavioral functions. The children were aged between 4 and 5½ yrs and were closely matched for age, sex, social class, parental education, area, and length of residence. Only 3 children had moved since their blood lead levels had been examined at 2 yrs of age; these levels ranged between 18 and 64 µg/100 ml. None of the children had clinical symptoms of plumbism. No statistically significant differences were found on developmental and behavioral scores (Griffith's Mental Developmental Scales and the Frostig Developmental Test) when the children were divided into 2 groups of less than and greater than 35 µg/100 ml. The differences in scores were of the same order as those between boys and girls, which were themselves generally not significant. Behavioral ratings did not differ. The variations in developmental skills were generally found to be more related to age and schooling; neither these factors nor the difference in sex was related to blood lead levels. (35 ref).

569. Rimland, Bernard & Larson, Gerald E. (1983). **Hair mineral analysis and behavior: An analysis of 51 studies.** *Journal of Learning Disabilities,* 16(5), 279–285.
Summarizes 51 studies on the relationship between hair mineral levels and various aspects of human behavior that covered a wide range of behaviors: learning disabilities, retardation, hyperactivity, criminality and delinquency, behavior disturbances, autism, schizophrenia, anorexia, hypoglycemia, fatigue, anxiety, allergy, senility, phenylketonuria, and giftedness and intelligence. High levels of certain minerals, especially Pb and Cd, and low levels of other minerals, especially K and Na, tend to be associated with undesirable behavior. There is a need for vigorous attempts to eliminate sources of environmental exposure to heavy metals and for further study of the role of mineral excesses and deficiencies in human health and behavior. (42 ref).

570. Ross, W. Donald; Emmett, Edward A.; Steiner, John & Tureen, Robert. (1981). **Neurotoxic effects of occupational exposure to organotins.** *American Journal of Psychiatry,* 138(8), 1092–1095.
Gave 22 chemical workers (mean age 37 yrs) neurological, psychiatric, and neuropsychological examinations and placed them in 1 of 2 groups according to their degree of exposure to trimethyltin chloride. Other chemicals to which they had been exposed were dimethyltin dichloride and methyl chloride. Specific and nonspecific symptoms of intoxication of the CNS showed a greater frequency in the highly exposed group, including cycles of depression and destructive rage, each lasting a few hours. These observations should alert diagnosticians to this type of occupational exposure. (15 ref).

571. Ross, W. Donald; Gechman, Arthur S.; Sholiton, Marilyn C. & Paul, Howard S. (1977). **Need for alertness to neuropsychiatric manifestations of inorganic mercury poisoning.** *Comprehensive Psychiatry,* 18(6), 595–598.
Summarizes case study findings on 9 individuals who were found to have significant urine levels of inorganic mercury. All of them worked in hospital laboratories and had been exposed to the mercury while working with Van Slyke blood gas apparatus. A checklist of 19 neuropsychiatric symptoms and 3 clinical signs was completed for each patient. Simple counts of the total number of symptoms and signs manifested by each patient were made and rank-ordered. Ranking was also done with respect to urine mercury levels, and a rank-order correlation coefficient was found to be positive and significant. Discussion centers around the need to consider possible occupational exposure problems in diagnosing patients with psychiatric difficulties. (10 ref).

572. Ross, W. Donald & Sholiton, Marilyn C. (1983). **Specificity of psychiatric manifestations in relation to neurotoxic chemicals.** *Acta Psychiatrica Scandinavica,* 67(Suppl 303), 100–104.
Previous impressions of specificity of psychiatric manifestations in relation to particular chemical intoxications were confirmed by comparisons of the symptoms and signs of 2 groups of individuals. Nine 22–33 yr old laboratory technicians exposed to inorganic mercury had "erethism" and xenophobia in addition to nonspecific features of CNS poisoning. 12 male chemical workers with heavy exposure to organotins, in contrast to 10 counterparts with light or no exposure, more frequently presented a unique alternation between outbursts of rage and deep depression, the latter lasting from a few hours to a few days. The more heavily exposed Ss also had a greater number of nonspecific symptoms from neurotoxins. (3 ref).

573. Routh, Donald K.; Mushak, Paul & Boone, Lois. (1979). **A new syndrome of elevated blood lead and microcephaly.** *Journal of Pediatric Psychology,* 4(1), 67–76.
Determined the blood lead levels of 100 children seen at an outpatient clinic for developmental and learning disabilities in a rural Southern state. One child with moderately elevated blood lead and 9 with minimally elevated blood lead were identified; 7 of these 10 children were microcephalic, a markedly and significantly higher rate of microcephaly than in the remainder of the clinic sample. Most of the children suffering from the lead-microcephaly syndrome were Black, and a majority had birth weights under 2,500 gm, suggesting the possibility that prenatal exposure to lead might have caused their microcephaly and developmental handicaps. (29 ref).

574. Rummo, Judith H. (1974). **Intellectual and behavioral effects of lead poisoning in children.** *Dissertation Abstracts International,* 35(6-B), 3035-3036.

METALLIC ELEMENTS

575. Ruth, Richard I. (1987). **Family organization and cohesion and low-level lead exposure.** *Dissertation Abstracts International,* 47(11-B), 4663.

576. Sachs, Henrietta K.; Krall, Vita & Drayton, Mary A. (1982). **Neuropsychological assessment after lead poisoning without encephalopathy.** *Perceptual & Motor Skills,* 54(3, Pt 2), 1283–1288.
100 children, most of whom were over 9 yrs of age, who were lead-poisoned in early childhood and treated before the onset of encephalopathy were given neuropsychological tests (e.g., the Halstead-Reitan Neuropsychological Test Battery for Children), along with 28 unaffected siblings. No difference was found for the 2 cohorts on the battery of tests. (13 ref).

577. Schauss, Alexander G. (1987). **Advances in Alzheimer's disease research: Recent reports on the entry, source, and cellular activity of aluminum and aluminosilicates.** *International Journal of Biosocial Research,* 9(1), 31–34.
Discusses 3 studies on the entry, source and cellular mechanism of aluminum and silicon in characteristic senile dendritic-neuritic plaques related to Alzheimer's disease: D. P. Perl and P. F. Good (1987), A. M. Coriat and R. D. Gillard (1986), and T. L. MacDonald et al (1987). The role of the nasal-olfactory mucosa as primary entry site, the leaching of aluminum from cooking vessels, and competition between magnesium and aluminum near microtubules are examined.

578. Schottenfeld, Richard S. & Cullen, Mark R. (1984). **Organic affective illness associated with lead intoxication.** *American Journal of Psychiatry,* 14(11), 1423–1426.
Notes that psychiatrists treating patients with depression or nonspecific somatic complaints seldom think of lead intoxication as a possible cause and that, because occupational exposure to lead is so common, these disturbances may often be associated with lead intoxication. 30 males and 1 female (22–65 yrs) who presented with excess levels of lead in the blood (defined as higher than 40 µg/dl) received psychiatric testing and neuropsychological evaluations. 17 Ss reported at least 1 nonspecific symptom (e.g., fatigue, irritability) often found in pure psychiatric disturbances. 14 Ss demonstrated significant neurophysiological deficits, such as abnormalities in visual-motor coordination and rapid motor control. Four Ss were found to have organic affective disturbance associated with lead intoxication. Neuropsychiatric disturbances that have been reported with chronic exposure to lead are reviewed, and it is noted that the condition of these Ss improved after removal from exposure. The case of a 30-yr-old White male is presented to illustrate the complex interplay between lead intoxication and psychosocial factors in leading to a major depressive episode. (13 ref).

579. Selbst, Steven M.; Henretig, Fred M. & Pearce, Jennifer. (1985). **Lead encephalopathy: A case report and review of management.** *Clinical Pediatrics,* 24(5), 280–285.
Reports the case of an 8-yr-old Black female with known sickle cell anemia who presented initially with findings suggestive of vaso-occlusive crisis but who deteriorated rapidly and was found to have severe lead poisoning. S's home was found to contain an enormous amount of peeling leaded paint. Chelation therapy was instituted, and S had no further seizures 1.5 yrs after her acute encephalopathy. (18 ref).

580. Shaheen, Sandra J. (1984). **Neuromaturation and behavior development: The case of childhood lead poisoning.** *Developmental Psychology,* 20(4), 542–550.
Presents a rationale for the study of the role of neuromaturation in cognitive and behavioral development. Early childhood lead poisoning is discussed in terms of physiological mechanisms and known cognitive sequelae. 18 children, 4–6 yrs old, with past histories of lead poisoning, were compared to matched controls on a 6-factor cognitive and neuromotor battery that included the WPPSI and the PPVT. A developmental hypothesis that specific cognitive sequelae of lead poisoning would depend on and vary with the age of the child at the time of lead ingestion was tested. Previous findings in the literature on asymptomatic childhood lead poisoning, which cited either language-linguistic or visuospatial skill decrements in nonoverlapping populations, were elucidated. When the performances of Ss who had suffered early (before 24 mo), middle (24–36 mo), and late (after 36 mo) exposure were compared on language-linguistic and spatial factors in this sample, significant differences were suggested. Ss who experienced increased lead consumption showed reductions in 3 motor and visual-motor skills. This finding illustrates the differential effects of interruptions in maturational processes on cognitive behavior as a function of age. Although the interaction of maturational and environmental events is acknowledged, the results imply that more attention to the structure-function relationship is needed in the study of behavior development and in the development of measures of cognitive functioning. (36 ref).

581. Shearer, T. R.; Larson, K.; Neuschwander, J. & Gedney, B. (1982). **Minerals in the hair and nutrient intake of autistic children.** *Journal of Autism & Developmental Disorders,* 12(1), 25–34.
Determined the concentrations of calcium, magnesium, zinc, copper, lead, and cadmium in scalp hair samples from 12 autistic children (mean age 8.4 yrs) and 12 nonautistic controls. A lower concentration of cadmium in the hair of autistic Ss marked the only statistically significant difference between the groups; this difference is probably not physiologically significant. The nutrient intake of autistic Ss was found to be adequate. (23 ref).

582. Silva, Phil A.; Hughes, Pauline; Williams, Sheila & Faed, James M. (1988). **Blood lead, intelligence, reading attainment, and behaviour in eleven year old children in Dunedin, New Zealand.** *Journal of Child Psychology & Psychiatry & Allied Disciplines,* 29(1), 43–52.
Conducted a study of blood lead levels and intelligence, reading, and behavior problems, using 579 11-yr-old children assessed as part of an 11-yr follow-up of a Dunedin multidisciplinary health and developmental study. Results suggest that when social, environmental, and background factors were considered, raised blood lead was associated with a small but significant increase in children's general behavior problems as reported by both parents and teachers. Results apply especially to inattention and hyperactivity.

583. Sine, Larry F. (1984). **The relationship of mercury to cognitive, affective and perceptual motor functioning in a normal sample in Hawaii.** *Dissertation Abstracts International,* 45(1-B), 366–367.

584. Smith, Marjorie. (1985). **Recent work on low level lead exposure and its impact on behavior, intelligence, and learning: A review.** *Journal of the American Academy of Child Psychiatry,* 24(1), 24–32.
Reviews epidemiological studies of the association of low levels of lead with the behavior, IQ, and educational attainment of children, with particular reference to the role of social factors in the relationship and the development of methodology designed to cope with confounding factors. Issues discussed include markers of exposure to lead, sample selection, outcome measures, and possible dose-related effects of lead. It is concluded that body lead levels in children act as a marker for socially disadvantaged factors and that when these factors are controlled adequately, adverse effects cannot be attributed to lead with any certainty, although they may exist. If there are any effects of lead at these levels, they are small and may not be detectable with existing methods of data collection and statistical analysis. (27 ref).

585. Smith, Marjorie et al. (1983). **The effects of lead exposure on urban children: The Institute of Child Health/ Southampton Study.** *Developmental Medicine & Child Neurology,* 25(5, Suppl 47), 54 p.
Studied the associations between levels of tooth lead (TL), behavior, intelligence, and other psychological skills in 4,105 British children (aged 6-7 yrs). Ss were assessed on an 8-test battery; TL was estimated from chemical analysis of Ss' shed teeth. 403 Ss, selected on the basis of their TL content and SES, were studied more intensively; these Ss were classified into 6 groups—high, medium, and low TL levels and manual and nonmanual labor families. Ss' parents were interviewed in their homes regarding parental interest/attitudes to education, family characteristics and relationships, early history of the S, and S's physical environment. Ss were then studied in the school setting. Results show that intelligence and psychological measures were strongly related to social factors. TL level was linked to a variety of factors in the home, including cleanliness and maternal smoking. Overall, it is concluded that improved social conditions would probably result in lower lead levels in young children. (64 ref).

586. Smith, Philip J. (1979). **Short-term memory scanning is related to memory span and mercury exposure.** *Dissertation Abstracts International,* 40(5-B), 2413.

587. Smith, Philip J. & Langolf, Gary D. (1981). **The use of Sternberg's memory-scanning paradigm in assessing effects of chemical exposure.** *Human Factors,* 23(6), 701-708.
Evaluated the utility of a binary classification task in assessing the neurotoxic effects of elemental mercury, using S. Sternberg's (1966) memory-scanning paradigm. 26 mercury cell chlor-alkali workers (mean age 38 yrs) were tested on 2 occasions. The RT paradigm provided reliable, stage-specific measures of cognitive functioning. In the 2 stages studied, processing times were found to increase significantly with increasing levels of exposure to mercury. The stage-specific nature of the measures used permits the inference that mercury has a locus of effect in the CNS. (14 ref).

588. Sohler, Arthur; Kruesi, Marcus & Pfeiffer, Carl C. (1977). **Blood lead levels in psychiatric outpatients reduced by zinc and vitamin C.** *Journal of Orthomolecular Psychiatry,* 6(3), 272-276.
Determined blood lead levels by the Hessel method in 1,113 psychiatric outpatients. Lead values ranged from 3.8 to 53 mcg% with a mean of 15.6 mcg%. Approximately 6% had lead levels above 25 mcg%. A therapeutic regimen of zinc and ascorbic acid significantly decreased the blood lead level. This treatment also lowered blood copper levels. The heavy metal burden of a number of hyperactive and autistic children was alleviated resulting in clinical improvement. It is concluded that vitamin C and zinc may be an attractive alternative to chelation therapy in the treatment of chronic lead intoxication. The real triad in hyperactivity may be excess lead and copper in zinc-deficient patients. (15 ref).

589. Sohler, Arthur; Pfeiffer, Carl C. & Papaioannou, Rhoda. (1981). **Blood aluminum levels in a psychiatric outpatient population: High aluminum levels related to memory loss.** *Journal of Orthomolecular Psychiatry,* 10(1), 54-60.
An examination of 400 outpatients (aged 10-79 yrs) revealed a positive relation between serum aluminum levels and age and memory loss. Previous studies have demonstrated the neurotoxicity of aluminum in animals and suggested that elevated aluminum levels play a role in senile dementia and Alzheimer's disease. (14 ref).

590. Stark, Alice D.; Quah, Ruth F.; Meigs, J. Wister & Delouise, Edward R. (1982). **Relationship of sociodemographic factors to blood lead concentrations in New Haven children.** *Journal of Epidemiology & Community Health,* 36(2), 133-139.
Examined blood-lead concentrations (BLCs) in 377 1-72 mo old Black, White, and Hispanic Ss. Characteristics associated with increased BLCs were those that tended to impair the ability of a family to provide the necessary care and supervision for an S. Risk factors produced different effects on the various race groups. (19 ref).

591. Stellern, John; Marlowe, Mike; Cossairt, Ace & Errera, John. (1983). **Low lead and cadmium levels and childhood visual-perception development.** *Perceptual & Motor Skills,* 56(2), 539-544.
Investigated possible relationships of lead and cadmium levels to childhood visual-perceptual development, using 25 6-12 yr olds experiencing learning problems. Hair-metal concentrations of lead and cadmium were analyzed. Ss were also administered the Bender Visual Motor Gestalt Test. Lead and cadmium levels correlated significantly and negatively with age-deviations of Bender errors. A continuing reexamination of lead and cadmium levels is needed because levels previously thought harmless may be associated with decrements in childhood visual-perceptual development. (22 ref).

592. Stock, Alfred & Jaensch, E. (1983). **Nothing new under the sun: Experiences with mercury poisoning.** *Journal of Orthomolecular Psychiatry,* 12(3), 202-207.
In this translation of the 1st author's 1926 article, personal experiences with mercury intoxication are recounted. Symptoms began with periodic light headaches and weak dizziness that increased to continuous nervous unrest and irritability. Intellectual exhaustion, depression, lack of energy, increased need for sleep, trembling of stretched fingers, stabbing pains, and slight vesicles on the inner sides of arms and the upper half of legs appeared before diagnosis. Illness of colleagues led to the discovery of mercury in the air of the laboratory. Fresh air and replacement of amalgam fillings led to improvement.

593. Struempler, Richard E.; Larson, Gerald E. & Rimland, Bernard. (1985). **Hair mineral analysis and disruptive behavior in clinically normal young men.** *Journal of Learning Disabilities,* 18(10), 609-612.
Investigated whether hair minerals may be predictive of significant behavioral criteria using hair samples from the nape of the necks of a nonclinical sample of 40 male, White US Navy recruits. Ss' scores on the Armed Forces Qualification Test, which assesses mental ability; information on their reading grade level and highest year of education; and in-service behavior, including demerits during training and premature discharge from the Navy, were examined. Atomic absorption spectroscopy was used to determine Ss' hair levels of copper, iron, magnesium, zinc, lead, cadmium, aluminum, and calcium. Findings reveal significant relationships between the behavioral criteria and the mineral measures. Hair cadmium levels were significantly related to both demerits and reading ability. The 3 Ss with the highest cadmium levels all displayed serious behavior difficulties in recruit training. Ss with high hair magnesium levels tended to earn excessive demerits and to be poor readers. Results support the hair mineral/behavior relationships previously reported for clinically diagnosed cases. (28 ref).

594. Thatcher, R. W. et al. (1983). **Intelligence and lead toxins in rural children.** *Journal of Learning Disabilities,* 16(6), 355-359.
Measures of hair lead content, intelligence (the WISC-R or the WPPSI), school achievement (Wide Range Achievement Test), and motor impairment (the Purdue Pegboard Test) were obtained from 149 5-16 yr old public school children. Hair lead concentration significantly discriminated 4 groups of Ss (gifted, normal, low, and very low achievers) and significantly predicted IQ scores, independent of group classifications. Regression analyses showed a significant negative correlation between lead and intellectual functioning, even in the normal-to-gifted IQ range. Results demonstrate a continuous

inverse relationship between intelligence and relatively low levels of body lead in which the higher levels of cognitive function are affected before any signs of gross motor impairment are observed. (32 ref).

595. Thatcher, R. W.; McAlaster, R. & Lester, M. L. (1984). **Evoked potentials related to hair cadmium and lead in children.** Sixth International Conference on Event-Related Slow Potentials of the Brain (EPIC VI): Normal and aberrant development (1981, Lake Forest/Chicago, Illinois). *Annals of the New York Academy of Sciences,* 425, 384–390.
Examined the sensory EPs of 149 5–16 yr olds to delineate electrophysiological correlates of cadmium and lead. Analysis of hair samples and EPs showed that there were significant relationships between hair lead and cadmium and EP peak measures. While the direction of significant effects was the same for cadmium and lead, there were differences in the topographic distribution of these effects: Lead was more strongly related to the EP measures obtained from the central than from the posterior derivations, while the reverse was true for cadmium. (19 ref).

596. Triebig, Gerhard & Schaller, Karl-Heinz. (1982). **Neurotoxic effects in mercury-exposed workers.** *Neurobehavioral Toxicology & Teratology,* 4(6), 717–720.
39 industrial workers exposed to mercury and 123 nonexposed Ss were assessed through neuropsychiatric examination, psychological testing, and measurement of blood and urine mercury levels. There was a significant mild degree of slowing of sensory nerve conduction velocities, but no dose–effect relationship was found. Significant correlations were found between duration of exposure and decrease of short-term memory, but no effects on intelligence, somatic disorders, vigilance, or mood were observed. Results indicate that mercury does not cause disorders in CNS function if the biological threshold limit values (50 μg Hg/l blood and/or 200 μg Hg/l urine) are not exceeded. (16 ref).

597. Uzzell, Barbara P. & Oler, Jacqueline. (1986). **Chronic low-level mercury exposure and neuropsychological functioning.** *Journal of Clinical & Experimental Neuropsychology,* 8(5), 581–593.
Investigated the effects of chronic low-level exposure to inorganic mercury by comparing the neuropsychological performances of 13 female dental auxiliary workers (mean age 41.15 yrs) with elevated head mercury levels (as measured by an X-ray fluorescence technique) with those of 13 workers (mean age 40.77 yrs) with no measurable mercury levels. Ss with elevated mercury levels scored significantly less well on 2 of 8 measures of neurological functioning. Findings suggest that chronic subtoxic levels of inorganic mercury appear to produce mild changes in short-term nonverbal recall and heightened distress generally, and particularly in categories of obsessive compulsion, anxiety, and psychoticism, without alterations in general intellectual functioning, attention, verbal recall, and motor skills. (48 ref).

598. Valciukas, José A. et al. (1978). **Central nervous system dysfunction due to lead exposure.** *Science,* 201(4354), 465–467.
Used performance tests to assess CNS dysfunction in 90 workers at a secondary lead smelter. Correlations between test scores and zinc protoporphyrin levels, a biological indicator of lead toxicity, were statistically significant. This correlation should prove to be useful in current efforts to evaluate effects of lead exposure.

599. Waldron, H. A. (1978). **Lead and human behaviour.** *Journal of Mental Deficiency Research,* 22(1), 69–78.
A review of the literature on the effects of blood lead levels on human behavior indicates that there is little evidence that levels below about 2.0 μmol/l cause an untoward neuropsychiatric effect. Between 2.0 and 3.0 μmol, results are conflicting; but those deviations from normality tha are not, most likely stem from subclinical neuronal damage that has been described by R. G. Feldman et al (1973). With blood lead levels in excess of 3.0 μmol/l, and particularly with prolonged exposure, neuropsychiatric effects are undoubtedly noted, increasing in frequency the closer the child is toward developing clinical signs of frank intoxication and encephalopathy. The need for investigating the possibility that intrauterine exposure to lead may be causally related to the development of mental retardation is stressed. (42 ref).

600. Winneke, Gerhard & Kraemer, Ursala. (1984). **Neuropsychological effects of lead in children: Interactions with social background variables.** *Neuropsychobiology,* 11(3), 195–202.
The authors summarize previous studies by the 1st author and colleagues (1982, 1983) investigating neuropsychological effects of lead concentrations in 167 school children from 22 cities. Tooth lead levels were the principal indicator of long-term cumulative lead exposure. From a comprehensive sample of neuropsychological outcome measures (including the WAIS and the Bender Gestalt Test), only a few significant findings emerged, namely lead-related deficits of visual-motor integration and of reaction performance but not of general intelligence. Without exception, the observed lead effects were small compared to those of social background. An interesting interaction was found between lead exposure and social background for visual-motor integration and for reaction performance: For both these measures, but not for intelligence, the degree of association between performance deficit and lead exposure was more pronounced in socially disadvantaged than in those from a more middle-class background. This finding was discussed within a transactional model of development. The common practice of simply controlling the effects of confounding social factors by analysis of covariance or related techniques is considered doubtful in this context. (42 ref).

601. Yamins, Janice G. (1977). **The relationship of subclinical lead intoxication to cognitive and language functioning in preschool children.** *Dissertation Abstracts International,* 37(8-B), 4176.

602. Yule, William; Urbanowicz, Marie-Anne; Lansdown, Richard & Millar, Ian B. (1984). **Teachers' ratings of children's behaviour in relation to blood lead levels.** *British Journal of Developmental Psychology,* 2(4), 295–305.
Teachers rated the behavior of 166 6–12 yr olds whose blood lead levels had been previously determined on the Conners Teachers' Rating Scale and the Teacher Rating Scale B(2). Ss were also assessed on the WISC-R, Neale Analysis of Reading Ability—Form A, Vernon Graded Word Spelling Test, and Vernon Graded Arithmetic-Mathematics Test. Results are consistent with those reported by H. L. Needleman et al (1979) in that they indicate a relationship between difficulties in attention and increased blood lead levels over the normal range of blood lead values. Teacher ratings of hyperactivity were significantly related to lead levels, independent of Ss' CA. The scale devised by Needleman et al was significantly related to WISC-R Full Scale IQ, although it appeared to be more sensitive than the teacher rating scales because it tapped behaviors related to attention rather than wider behavioral categories. (37 ref).

603. Zuckerman, Craig H. (1984). **Clinical utility of trace elements analysis for the prediction of diagnostic category and academic achievement in learning disabled and educable mentally retarded children.** *Dissertation Abstracts International,* 45(3-B), 1055.

Animal Research

604. Alfano, Dennis P. (1983). **Postnatal lead exposure and the cholinergic system: Effects on cholinergically mediated behaviors and cholinergic development and plasticity in the hippocampus.** *Dissertation Abstracts International,* 44(3-B), 949.

605. Alfano, Dennis P. & Petit, Ted L. (1985). **Postnatal lead exposure and the cholinergic system.** *Physiology & Behavior,* 34(3), 449–455.
Examined the possibility that the behavioral effects of early lead (Pb) exposure may be due to an underlying deficiency in cholinergic function. Long-Evans hooded rat pups were exposed to Pb for the 1st 25 postnatal days via the maternal milk. Dams were fed either 4.0% $PbCO_3$ (High Pb), 0.4% $PbCO_3$ (low Pb), or a Na_2CO_3 control diet. Beginning at 65 days of age, analysis showed that exposure to both levels of Pb impaired passive avoidance acquisition and produced lower rates of spontaneous alternation. In both Pb exposed groups, physostigmine (0.05 and 0.075 mg/kg) improved passive avoidance acquisition, increased the rate of spontaneous alternation, and lowered open-field activity scores. Scopolamine (0.4 mg/kg) impaired passive avoidance acquisition, lowered the rate of spontaneous alternation, and increased open-field activity scores in control Ss. Scopolamine (0.2 and 0.4 mg/kg) improved passive avoidance acquisition in both Pb exposed groups and decreased open-field activity scores in the High Pb group. Behavioral response of the Pb-exposed Ss may be interpreted as responses characteristic of cholinergically deficient animals. (48 ref).

606. Alfano, Dennis P. & Petit, Ted L. (1981). **Behavioral effects of postnatal lead exposure: Possible relationship to hippocampal dysfunction.** *Behavioral & Neural Biology,* 32(3), 319–333.
A review of previous evidence suggests the possibility of hippocampal involvement in the behavioral changes observed following postnatal lead (Pb) exposure. To further assess this possibility, Long-Evans hooded rat pups were exposed to inorganic Pb from postnatal Days 1 to 25 via the maternal milk. Mothers were fed diets containing either 4.0% $PbCO_3$, 0.4% $PbCO_3$, or a 2.2% Na_2CO_3 control diet throughout this period. Ss were tested at maturity in 4 situations considered sensitive to hippocampal dysfunction. Exposure to Pb resulted in delayed acquisition of the radial 8-arm spatial maze but produced no changes in either susceptibility to audiogenic seizures or acquisition and performance of a 2-way active avoidance response. Pb-exposed Ss also performed deficiently on a DRL-20 schedule of operant reinforcement, although significant variation was observed between control litters on this task. Other forms of CNS alterations have been observed to result from early Pb exposure, and alternative explanations for these behavioral changes are suggested. (65 ref).

607. Alfano, Dennis P.; Petit, Ted L. & LeBoutillier, Janelle C. (1983). **Development and plasticity of the hippocampal-cholinergic system in normal and early lead exposed rats.** *Developmental Brain Research,* 10(1), 117–124.
Long-Evans hooded rat pups were exposed to Pb for the 1st 25 postnatal days through maternal milk; dams were fed either 4% $PbCO_3$ or a Na_2CO_3 control diet. At 30 and 115 days of age, Ss' brains were processed for acetylcholinesterase activity. Results indicate that a decrease in neuroanatomical plasticity may be a critical brain mechanism underlying learning deficits observed following Pb exposure. Findings suggest that the reduced degree of cholinergic plasticity observed in the dentate gyrus following Pb exposure may provide a paradigm for evaluating the mechanisms related to the recovery of brain function and the processes of learning and memory formation. (36 ref).

608. Ali, M. M.; Murthy, R. C. & Chandra, S. V. (1986). **Developmental and longterm neurobehavioral toxicity of low level in-utero cadmium exposure in rats.** *Neurobehavioral Toxicology & Teratology,* 8(5), 463–468.
Assessed the developmental and behavioral toxicity of gestational exposure to low levels of cadmium (Cd) in Wistar-derived rats. Significant decreases in birth weight and growth rate were observed. Cd exposure had no effect on the ontogeny of physical landmarks, surface and air righting reflexes, and visual placing, but a significant hyperactivity and delay in the development of cliff aversion and swimming behavior were observed. Marked decreases in locomotor activity and shuttlebox performance were evident at 60 but not 90 days of postnatal life. Apomorphine-induced hyperactivity was not affected in these Ss at either age. Data indicate that Cd exposure during the critical periods of development might result in developmental and behavioral deficits with long-term implications for adult behavior.

609. Ali, M. Mohamed et al. (1983). **Effect of low protein diet on manganese neurotoxicity: I. Developmental and biochemical changes.** *Neurobehavioral Toxicology & Teratology,* 5(3), 377–383.
Studied the effect of concurrent low protein diet (10% casein) and manganese ion exposure (3 mg/ml drinking water) on growing rats (Fo generation—90 days), rehabilitated (Fo low to normal protein diet—28 days), and F1 generation pups (weaned). Mn exposure had no significant effect on growth pattern, brain weight, or brain and plasma protein contents in either dietary groups. The diet regimen had no significant effect on the accumulation of Mn in brain in any of the groups studied, but levels were higher in the F1 pups than in the parent (Fo) generation. In the F1 pups, Mn exposure had no effect on eye opening in either dietary group and delayed the development of startle reflex in low protein fed group only, but the air righting reflex development was delayed in both the dietary groups, the effect being more marked in the low protein fed group. These changes reflect the early neurotoxic effect of Mn. (46 ref).

610. Anderson, Brenda J. et al. (1985). **Prenatal exposure to aluminum or stress: I. Birth-related and developmental effects.** *Bulletin of the Psychonomic Society,* 23(1), 87–89.
12 sperm-positive female rats in 1 of 2 experimental conditions either ingested aluminum hydroxide or were stressed (via mild electric shock) during gestation. Birth-related effects, such as stillborn pups, aborted litters, and cannibalism, were found for Ss in the 2 experimental conditions, but not for 4 controls. Significantly lower weights (through 70 days of age) were associated with aluminum-exposed offspring that had been maintained with an aluminum-exposed mother until weaning. (21 ref).

611. Anderson, Brenda J. et al. (1985). **Prenatal exposure to aluminum or stress: II. Behavioral and performance effects.** *Bulletin of the Psychonomic Society,* 23(6), 524–526.
Presents results of shock-elicited aggression and learned helplessness testing of 129 offspring of Holtzman rats exposed to stress, aluminum, or a control condition during gestation. Compared to controls, aluminum- and stress-exposed Ss displayed significantly more aggressive responses. However, aluminum-exposed Ss spent significantly less time in contact with the target rod during aggression testing and had significantly longer latencies than did stress-exposed Ss during the escape-training phase of the learned helplessness study. Results indicate that the prenatal treatments produced lasting behavioral effects, including the disruption of a response inhibition/direction mechanism in the aluminum-exposed Ss. (6 ref).

612. Angell, Norman F. (1979). **Operant behavior of rats exposed before or after weaning to low levels of lead.** *Dissertation Abstracts International,* 40(4-B), 1607.

METALLIC ELEMENTS

613. Baraldi, Mario et al. (1985). **Neurobehavioral and neurochemical abnormalities of pre- and postnatally lead-exposed rats: Zinc, copper and calcium status.** 14th Congress of the Collegium Internationale Neuro-Psychopharmacologicum: Perinatal actions of psychotropic drugs and environmental chemicals and their behavioral effects in later life (1984, Florence, Italy). *Neurobehavioral Toxicology & Teratology,* 7(5), 499–509.
Using an experimental model of pre- and postnatal intoxication of female Wistar rats exposed to a low amount of lead (1 mg/kg/day), in parallel with behavioral anomalies, the authors observed slight changes in cerebral dopaminergic and gamma-aminobutyric acid (GABA)ergic receptors. A new finding was that there was a markedly increased number of opiate receptors in the hypothalamus (and other brain areas) in parallel with a decrease of beta-endorphin and an increase of met-enkephalin. Therefore, low levels of lead intoxication that could be pertinent to humans seem to induce neurotoxic effects that may be responsible for the behavioral anomalies in rats and possibly in children. (83 ref).

614. Barrett, J. & Livesey, P. J. (1985). **Low level lead effects on the learning and extinction of passive avoidance in the rat.** *Australian Journal of Psychology,* 37(1), 1–13.
In 5 replications of an experiment, 160 male Wistar rat pups were exposed to lead from birth to weaning through their dams ($n = 20$), who were fed diets containing 0, 0.2, 0.4, or 1% by weight metallic lead. Mean blood-lead levels of pups at weaning were 4, 24, 36, and 52 µg/100 mls of blood, respectively. Results of a passive avoidance learning trial indicate that experimental pups exhibited a developmental delay in the acquisition and retention of passive avoidance learning. Results are interpreted in terms of an altered stress response in lead-loaded pups, with experimental Ss maintaining the juvenile stress response of mobility rather than adopting the adult freezing response. The possibility that this effect was a result of hippocampal damage is explored. (49 ref).

615. Barrett, J. & Livesey, P. J. (1985). **Low level lead effects on activity under varying stress conditions in the developing rat.** *Pharmacology, Biochemistry & Behavior,* 22(1), 107–118.
Two experiments with 56 nursing Wistar albino rats studied whether lead ingestion by nursing rats would affect the way offspring ($n = 488$) reacted to the stress-inducing properties of the test environment both as juveniles and mature rats. Nursing dams were either exposed to diets with 0, 0.2, 0.4 or 1% by weight of metallic lead or they and their offspring served as controls. The pups' mean blood-lead levels at weaning were 4, 25, 36, and 55 µg/100 ml of blood, respectively. The stress factor for the pups was varied by (1) changing the test apparatus (i.e., forcing them to occupy an open field or allowing them to be a free agent in the start box of a T-maze); (2) testing the pups under a longitudinal and a cross-sectional experimental design to vary familiarity with the apparatus; and (3) comparing behavior in the presence or absence of noise. Reactivity was assessed by examining the inter- and intrasession pattern of ambulations and defecations. Analysis revealed that lead-treated pups demonstrated the greater response to stress. This response was generally dose related, although recovery was dependent on the test applied and the measures taken. Findings provide a conceptual framework to account for varied results across previous studies. (29 ref).

616. Barrett, J. & Livesey, P. J. (1983). **Lead induced alterations in maternal behavior and offspring development in the rat.** *Neurobehavioral Toxicology & Teratology,* 5(5), 557–563.
Studied whether lead ingestion by nursing rats would affect dam–pup interaction. 16 albino Wistar dams were exposed to lead-containing diets with 0.0, 0.2, 0.4, or 1.0% by weight. Mean blood-lead levels of pups at weaning were 3, 19, 40 and 57 µg/100 ml of blood, respectively. Maternal behavior was assessed by videotaping behavior for complete 24-hr periods on alternate days from birth to weaning. Data reveal that lead-affected dams nursed for longer periods than normal and offspring were slower to explore their environment. It is concluded that altered maternal behavior is related to delays in pup development and that the functional isolation of experimental pups from their environment may be the antecedent to altered behavior in maturity. (38 ref).

617. Baumeister, Alan A. (1982). **An investigation of the effects of chronic low-level prenatal lead exposure on behavioral development, general activity, and learning in neonatal and adult rats.** *Dissertation Abstracts International,* 42(11-B), 4594–4594.

618. Bernuzzi, Viviane; Desor, Didier & Lehr, Paul R. (1986). **Effects of prenatal aluminum exposure on neuromotor maturation in the rat.** *Neurobehavioral Toxicology & Teratology,* 8(2), 115–119.
Pregnant Wistar rats were treated orally with $AlCl_3$ from the 8th day of gestation to parturition to determine its influence on the neuromotor development of the young. Results indicate that aluminum, at the doses tested (160 and 200 mg/kg), had no effect on food intake, the weight of females, or their maternal behavior. Preweaning mortality was significantly increased in the treated dams' young. Surviving pups showed a delay in neuromotor development as well as a weight delay during the 1st postnatal week.

619. Bondy, Stephen C.; Tilson, H. A. & Walsh, T. J. (1985). **Effects of triethyl lead on hot-plate responsiveness and biochemical properties of hippocampus.** *Pharmacology, Biochemistry & Behavior,* 22(6), 1007–1011.
Male Fischer 344 rats treated with a single dose of triethyl lead chloride (TEL; 7.9 mg/kg, subcutaneously) showed a transient increase in latencies to lick the hind paw during hotplate testing. The time course of TEL-induced antinociception was temporally associated with depressed binding capacity of benzodiazepine receptor sites and reduced levels of Substance P. Both of these changes appeared to be confined to the hippocampus and were not apparent in the cortex or striatum of treated Ss. Lead levels within the brain were higher than blood levels 1 wk after TEL injection. (21 ref).

620. Booze, Rosemarie M. (1985). **Preferential vulnerability of the immature hippocampus of triethyl lead: A probe of behavioral and neural development.** *Dissertation Abstracts International,* 45(11-B), 3459.

621. Booze, Rosemarie M.; Mactutus, Charles F.; Annau, Zoltan & Tilson, Hugh A. (1983). **Neonatal triethyl lead neurotoxicity in rat pups: Initial behavioral observations and quantification.** *Neurobehavioral Toxicology & Teratology,* 5(3), 367–375.
94 offspring of 12 Fischer-344 dams were administered on Postpartum Day 5 either a sham injection, 15% ethanol, or 3 or 6 mg/kg of triethyl lead (TEL) via sc injection (20 µl). Small, but significant, weight reductions of 6 and 13% for the 3- and 6-mg/kg TEL-dosed pups, respectively, were observed (Days 14–30). Early sensory deficits of TEL Ss as indicated by impaired olfactory discrimination on Day 7 and decreased incidence of nipple attachment on Day 9 were accompanied by fine whole-body tremor (Day 10). While these effects were transitory, activity evaluations demonstrated persistent hypoactivity in high dose TEL males (Days 15, 22, 24, 26, and 29). Passive avoidance acquisition was not affected by TEL (Day 18). However, 72- and 144-hr tests of passive avoidance retention (Days 21 and 25) suggested alterations in affective behavior: hypoactivity in high-dose TEL males and hyperactivity in low-dose TEL females. A reduction in number, but not magnitude, of startle responses occurred as a function of TEL exposure. The single Postnatal Day 5 injection of TEL thus produced transitory effects possibly reflecting direct TEL

pharmacological activity, as well as apparent long-term effects suggesting potential permanent alterations in behavioral function. (37 ref).

622. Bornhausen, M. & Hagen, U. (1984). **Operant behaviour performance changes in rats after prenatal and postnatal exposure to heavy metals.** *IRCS Medical Science: Psychology & Psychiatry,* 12(9–10), 805–806.
Differential reinforcement of high rates of responding was significantly impaired in Wistar Neuherberg rats prenatally exposed to methylmercury chloride (.01 or .05 mg/kg by gastric intubation) but not by postnatal treatments. Similar results were obtained using lead acetate and thallium sulphate but not cadmium chloride. Findings indicate a functional impairment after exposure to heavy metals that is not apparent when other methods are used. (4 ref).

623. Bourg, Wendy J.; Nation, Jack R. & Clark, Donald E. (1985). **The effects of chronic cobalt exposure on passive-avoidance performance in the adult rat.** *Bulletin of the Psychonomic Society,* 23(6), 527–530.
Tested 16 male Sprague-Dawley rats for acquisition and retention of step-down passive avoidance (SPA) following exposure to either distilled water contaminated with cobalt chloride or uncontaminated distilled water. Results show that exposure to 20 mg cobalt/kg/day for 57 days produced significantly greater SPA latencies during retention testing in cobalt-treated Ss relative to controls. Analyses of SPA acquisition data, analgesic-tolerance test results, and body weights produced no significant group differences. Significant accumulations of cobalt were detected in blood, brain, and left testis of treated Ss. Results are attributed to cobalt-induced disturbances in neurochemistry, particularly gamma-aminobutyric acid (GABA) transmission. (16 ref).

624. Brady, Kathleen; Herrera, Yolanda & Zenick H. (1975). **Influence of parental lead exposure on subsequent learning ability of offspring.** *Pharmacology, Biochemistry & Behavior,* 3(4), 561-565.
Assessed CFE rat pups' learning ability following the exposure of one or both parents to lead acetate (Pb) from 30 to 90 days of age. At that time, parents were mated to yield 4 groups: Group Pb-Pb, both parents had received Pb; Group Pb-N, only the mother had received Pb; Group N-Pb, only the father had received Pb; and Group N-N, the control parents. Mothers were continued on their respective treatments throughout gestation and nursing. Testing of offspring began at 30 days of age, employing a black–white discrimination water T-maze. Results reveal that the 3 Pb groups made more errors than the controls but did not differ from one another. However, offspring in group Pb-Pb had longer swimming times than those in Groups Pb-N and N-Pb, who, in turn, had longer swimming times than Group N-N. Thus dual parental exposure was more severe than single parental exposure, which, however, still exerted a detrimental effect compared to control performance. (17 ref).

625. Burdette, Linda J. (1983). **The effects of asymptomatic lead exposure during different developmental stages in rats: Behavior and electrophysiology.** *Dissertation Abstracts International,* 44(5-B), 1628.

626. Burdette, Linda J. & Goldstein, Robert. (1986). **Long-term behavioral and electrophysiological changes associated with lead exposure at different stages of brain development in the rat.** *Developmental Brain Research,* 29(1), 101–110.
Assessed the behavioral and electrophysiological impairments exhibited by adult male rats as a function of the developmental stage during which lead exposure occurred. 48 Wistar dams were given either a lead acetate (0.3%) or a control drinking solution during Days 16–23 of gestation or during Days 1–8 or 9–16 of nursing. The temporal and spatial activity patterns exhibited by gestationally exposed offspring in the open field between 42–45 days of age were distinguished from all other groups by the absence of a decrement in peripheral field activity across days and by increased exploration of the center field. Lead selectively reduced 6–7 Hz energy in the hippocampus, independent of the developmental stage of exposure. It is suggested that the identification of toxic consequences depends on the function assessed and the developmental stage during which lead exposure occurred.

627. Burright, Richard G. et al. (1982). **Effect of amphetamine and cocaine on seizure in lead treated mice.** *Pharmacology, Biochemistry & Behavior,* 16(4), 631–635.
Lead administration (0.5% lead acetate) from conception increased the proportion of seizures in 21-day-old mice. Total duration of observed seizures was also increased. Ss from the low brain-weight line more frequently exhibited seizures than either mice from the high brain-weight line or the Binghamton heterogeneous stock. Lead administration from conception through testing increased the probability and duration of transcorneally induced electroconvulsive seizures of 21-day-old Ss within all 3 genotypes, and both cocaine and amphetamine injections 15 min prior to ECS reduced the number of Ss exhibiting seizures as well as the duration of seizures in both lead treated and control Ss. (17 ref).

628. Burright, Richard G.; Engellenner, William J. & Donovick, Peter J. (1983). **Lead exposure and agonistic behavior of adult mice of two ages.** *Physiology & Behavior,* 30(2), 285–288.
42 male heterogeneous stock (HET) mice were exposed to a 0.5% lead acetate solution when they were either 65 or 330 days of age. 15 wks later they were paired with same age (young or old) water control HET mice and tested for aggression. All pairs of younger Ss (60–70 days old) fought, and 6 out of 11 pairs of older Ss (aged 320–335 days) exhibited agonistic behavior. Although not all pairs of Ss that fought achieved dominance when dominant–subordinate relationships were established, the younger Ss exposed to lead typically were subordinate. In contrast, older Ss exposed to lead were always dominant. Differences in agonistic behavior patterns also were noted, with younger Ss displaying more frequent and longer bouts of fighting than the older ones. (32 ref).

629. Bushnell, Philip J. (1978). **Behavioral toxicology of lead in the infant rhesus monkey.** *Dissertation Abstracts International,* 39(5-B), 2560.

630. Bushnell, Philip J.; Bowman, Robert E.; Allen, James R. & Marlar, Rickey J. (1977). **Scotopic vision deficits in young monkeys exposed to lead.** *Science,* 196(4287), 333–335.
10 rhesus monkeys were reared on diets designed to produce blood lead concentrations of 14 (untreated), 55, or 85 mcg/100 ml for the 1st yr of life. 18 mo later, blood lead levels were normal in all Ss. At this time, however, visual discrimination performance in the 85 mcg group was impaired under dim light relative both to their own performance under bright light and to the performance of the other groups under all light levels used. Results reflect a deleterious, enduring impairment of scotopic visual function (night blindness) as a result of early lead intoxication.

631. Commissaris, Randall L. et al. (1982). **Behavioral changes in rats after chronic aluminum and parathyroid hormone administration.** *Neurobehavioral Toxicology & Teratology,* 4(3), 403–410.
Fischer-344 male and Sprague-Dawley female rats were administered parathyroid hormone (PTH, 17.5 IU twice/week) and dietary aluminum (0.2%, as $AlCl_3$), PTH alone, $AlCl_3$ alone, or vehicle for 12 wks (Protocol I). Sprague-Dawley male rats received aluminum (0.1% as $AlCl_3$ in the diet) or control diet for 11 mo (Protocol II). Protocol I Ss were tested

METALLIC ELEMENTS

for rotarod performance, locomotor activity, and shuttle-box avoidance behavior. Rotarod performance was not impaired by any of the treatments of Protocol I. Fischer rats showed increased locomotor activity only in response to PTH. Sprague-Dawley females receiving $AlCl_3$ or PTH with $AlCl_3$ had reduced locomotor activity relative to matched controls. Acquisition and extinction of shuttle-box avoidance in Fischer rats were unaffected by 5 wks of Protocol I treatments, but dietary $AlCl_3$ impaired retention. This retention deficit was not observed in the group treated with PTH plus $AlCl_3$. 10 wks of Protocol I treatment increased trials to acquisition for Fischer rats treated with $AlCl_3$, while PTH alone decreased trials to extinction. In Sprague-Dawley females, PTH increased trials for retention of shuttle-box avoidance. Protocol II Ss were tested for locomotor activity and shuttle-box avoidance behavior. Dietary $AlCl_3$ in these Ss decreased locomotor responses and slowed the acquisition of avoidance. (40 ref).

632. Cory-Slechta, Deborah A. (1986). **Prolonged lead exposure and fixed ratio performance.** *Neurobehavioral Toxicology & Teratology,* 8(3), 237–244.
Male Long-Evans hooded rats were chronically treated via drinking water with 50 or 500 ppm sodium acetate or lead acetate from weaning. Behavioral testing on an FR schedule of reinforcement began at 55 days of age. A series of increasing ratio values was studied. The lower exposure level was without effect at any ratio value. The 500-ppm concentration decreased response rates over the 1st 15–20 sessions of FR5 and FR25, after which rates reached control levels. Changes in response rate derived primarily from longer interresponse times and decreased running rates. Zinc protoporphyrin levels resulting from 500-ppm exposure differed from controls even after 1 mo and continued to increase over 8 mo of exposure. Comparison of these data to previous studies of FI performance suggests that FR response rates are less sensitive than FI rates to disruption by lead.

633. Costa, L. G. & Fox, D. A. (1983). **A selective decrease of cholinergic muscarinic receptors in the visual cortex of adult rats following developmental lead exposure.** *Brain Research,* 276(2), 259–266.
Examined the effects of low-level developmental Pb exposure (Postnatal Days 0–21) on the binding of [^{3}]quinuclidinylbenzilate (QNB) and on acetylcholinesterase (AChE) activity in the retina, superior colliculus, lateral geniculate nucleus, and visual cortex (VC) of female Long-Evans rats at Days 21 and 90. Large decreases in [^{3}H]QNB binding and AChE activity were found only in the VC of Pb-exposed Ss and were related to a decrease in the density but not in the affinity of the muscarinic receptors. Results suggest that the long-term effects of developmental Pb exposure are due to a direct action of Pb on VC cholinergic neurons. (35 ref).

634. Crapper, D. R. & Dalton, A. J. (1973). **Aluminum induced neurofibrillary degeneration, brain electrical activity and alterations in acquisition and retention.** *Physiology & Behavior,* 10(5), 935–945.
Studied neurofibrillary degeneration (NFD) in 8 cats. From the results it is concluded that in the early stages of an aluminum induced dementia model a positive correlation exists between the occurrence of NFD in hippocampus, entorhinal, and neocortex and the rate of conditioned avoidance response acquisition. Quantitative measurements from appropriate electronmicrographs indicate that the density of microtubules in a region of NFD is profoundly reduced. At the stage in the encephalopathy in which short-term retention and acquisition are impaired the EEG and averaged visual evoked potentials were normal. Observations suggest that a nonelectrical activity of neurons, important to the learning-memory mechanism, may be altered by the effects of aluminum chloride. The disorganization of the dendritic microtubular system is postulated to alter dendroplasmic flow and supports the hypothesis that the translocation of synaptically active agents by the cytoplasmic streaming mechanism may subserve a component of the associative learning mechanism. (26 ref).

635. Crapper, D. R. & Dalton, A. J. (1973). **Alterations in short-term retention, conditioned avoidance response acquisition and motivation following aluminum induced neurofibrillary degeneration.** *Physiology & Behavior,* 10(5), 925–933.
Theorized that aluminum chloride induced neurofibrillary degeneration may provide a useful model for the study of a human dementia process. This possibility was assessed in 9 adult cats trained to perform on a delayed-response task, a conditioned avoidance task, visual and temporal discrimination tasks, and a motivational task involving rewarding intracranial electrical stimulation. After an initial asymptomatic period, short-term retention and acquisition of a conditioned avoidance response were selectively impaired. The associated ultrastructural abnormalities plausibly implicate the cytoplasmic streaming mechanism in the cellular substrate for some retention and acquisition phenomena. (16 ref).

636. Cuomo, Vincenzo et al. (1984). **Behavioural and neurochemical changes in offspring of rats exposed to methyl mercury during gestation.** *Neurobehavioral Toxicology & Teratology,* 6(3), 249–254.
On Day 8 of gestation, pregnant Sprague-Dawley rats were intubated with 8 mg/kg of methyl mercury (MM). At 15 days of age, stereotyped sniffing was elicited by a challenge dose of apomorphine (1 mg/kg) only in pups prenatally exposed to MM. At 22 days of age, the stereotyped behavior induced by apomorphine (.5–1 mg/kg) was significantly potentiated in MM-pretreated Ss, and there was a significant increase of ^{3}H-spiroperidol binding sites in striatal membranes. It is suggested that behavioral alterations in response to apomorphine resulted from an enhancement of dopamine binding sites induced by MM. (32 ref).

637. Cutler, Margaret G. (1977). **Effects of exposure to lead on social behaviour in the laboratory mouse.** *Psychopharmacology,* 52(3), 279–282.
Provided mother mice with water or a 0.1% lead acetate solution as their only drinking fluid within 24 hrs after the birth of their litters, and the offspring received this fluid or water from the time of their weaning. Examination, by ethological techniques, of encounters at 8 wks between same-sex pairs of unfamiliar Ss from the same treatment group showed that frequency and duration of social and sexual investigations were significantly lower in the lead-treated Ss.

638. Czech, Donald A. & Faubert, Patricia. (1986). **Triethyl lead attenuates feeding and drinking, and induces a conditioned taste aversion, in adult rats.** Society for Neuroscience Annual Meeting (1985, Dallas, Texas). *Neurobehavioral Toxicology & Teratology,* 8(6), 627–630.
Studied the effects of triethyl lead (TEL) on ad lib feeding and drinking in 32 adult male Sprague-Dawley rats. Ad lib food and water intakes were measured over 10 days after subcutaneous injection of 1, 4, or 7 mg/kg body weight TEL. Consumption of both was significantly reduced at the 2 higher doses of TEL. In a conditioned taste aversion paradigm, the same doses of TEL were given and a dose-related reduction of intake of a saccharin solution was seen. Acute exposure to the trialkyl form of lead produced hypophagia and hypodipsia in adult rats within 1 to 3 days of exposure that lasted for about 2 wks at the highest dose. The results suggest that ingestive behavior can be attenuated by TEL exposure.

639. Czech, Donald A. & Hoium, Ellen. (1984). **Some aspects of feeding and locomotor activity in adult rats exposed to tetraethyl lead.** *Neurobehavioral Toxicology & Teratology,* 6(5), 2660.
Injected 2 groups of male Sprague-Dawley rats ($N = 21$) with a dose of tetraethyl lead (TTEL [7 mg/kg, ip]) that depressed

food intake. One group served as a control to replicate this effect. Ss in the 2nd lead group were food-yoked to Ss in a placebo group. Food intake of Ss in group 2 was maintained at or near the level of their yoked control via intragastric intubation. Food loads did not maintain body weights at control levels; however, locomotor activity level in both lead-treated groups was significantly elevated above controls during normophagic periods when body weights approximated control levels as well as during hypophagic, low-body-weight periods. Results suggest that activity shifts are not mediated in a simple way by factors linked to reduced food intake. Two additional experiments were conducted in which TTEL-exposed Ss were challenged with 2-deoxy-dextro-glucose and insulin, either during their hypophagic phase or during a later recovered (normophagic) period. Feeding in response to glucoprivic challenge was similar to that of controls under both conditions. (24 ref).

640. Czech, Donald A.; Schmidt, James C. & Stone, James M. (1976). **Effect of tetraethyl lead on food and water intake in the rat.** *Pharmacology, Biochemistry & Behavior,* 5(4), 387–389.
Studied the effect of tetraethyl lead (TEL) on food and water intake in 96 male Sprague-Dawley albino rats. Ss received 1, 4, 7, 10, or 13 mg/kg TEL in peanut oil, or a peanut oil placebo, via either intragastric (ig) intubation or ip injection. For food intake, route of administration was a significant factor and, compared to baseline levels, food intake was significantly depressed at dosage levels of 7, 10, and 13 mg/kg for both ip and ig administration. Further, the time course of food intake differed significantly across route of administration. Water intake was significantly depressed at 7, 10, and 13 mg/kg, but route of administration was not a critical factor. Results are discussed in relation to clinical and experimental data on lead intoxication, and are viewed as severely limiting the utility of employing food and/or water as motivational variables in assessment of behavioral effects linked to TEL poisoning. (23 ref).

641. Day, H. D. & Hupp, Eugene W. (1979). **Effects of co-insults of methyl mercury and gamma radiation on the open-field, sexual, and conditioned-avoidance behavior of the albino rat.** *Psychological Record,* 29(2), 275–285.
243 male Sprague-Dawley rats were assigned to 6 treatment groups in which they received 4.5 or 9 kr total body radiation, 4 or 8 mg/kg methyl mercuric chloride (MMC), and co-insults of 4.5 kr radiation with 4 mg/kg MMC or 9 kr with 8 mg/kg MMC. A control group received neither radiation nor MMC. MMC insult preceded the radiation insult by 7 days. Treatment effects were determined by examining open-field, sexual, and conditioned-avoidance behavior, beginning 60 to 105 min after irradiation or sham irradiation. The open-field tests showed no effects of mercury alone, but a significant reduction of activity was produced by both levels of radiation administered as single insults. The sexual performance of Ss receiving MMC and radiation as single insults was disrupted by low and high levels of both treatments. In the open-field and sexual-behavior tests, there was a consistent though statistically insignificant tendency for the co-insult treatment groups to show fewer disruptive effects than were shown by the radiation-alone groups. Controls exhibited more correct conditioned-avoidance responses than all experimental conditions except for 8 mg/kg MMC treatment, but the test did not distinguish between other treatment levels. (17 ref).

642. DeHaven, Diane L. (1983). **Effects of triethyl tin on operant, ingestive and avoidance behaviors.** *Dissertation Abstracts International,* 43(9-B), 3065.

643. DeHaven, Diane L.; Krigman, Martin R.; Gaynor, Jeffrey J. & Mailman, Richard B. (1984). **The effects of lead administration during development on lithium-induced polydipsia and dopaminergic function.** *Brain Research,* 297(2), 297–304.
Results of a study of the effects of lead administration during development on lithium-induced polydipsia (LIP) and dopaminergic function among Long-Evans rats confirm previous findings that the treatment of rats with lead during discrete time periods of development will result in at least 1 apparently permanent change in pharmacological responsiveness—an increase in LIP. This occurs when lead is administered during the 1st 19 days of life, and even after a single dose of lead at either Day 5 or 15 of life. (21 ref).

644. de Rossett, Sarah E. (1982). **Effects of lead on spontaneous alternation, reactivity, and intracranial self-stimulation.** *Dissertation Abstracts International,* 42(7-B), 3024.

645. Dolinsky, Z. S. et al. (1981). **Behavioral effects of lead and *Toxocara canis* in mice.** *Science,* 213(4512), 1142–1144.
Adult male Binghamton mice were administered the common parasite *Toxocara canis* or lead or both. The parasite clearly altered performance on tests of exploration, activity, learning, and motor coordination; behavioral effects in Ss receiving lead alone were less general. Consequences of *Toxocara* administration appeared attenuated in Ss receiving both agents. Parasite larvae were found in the CNS of all infected mice.

646. Dolinsky, Zelig S.; Burright, Richard G. & Donovick, Peter J. (1983). **Behavioral changes in mice following lead administration during several stages of development.** *Physiology & Behavior,* 30(4), 583–589.
98 male Binghamton Heterogenous mice were assigned to 1 of 4 groups defined by a 2 × 2 factorial in which the only available drinking fluid was either lead (L) or water from the time of mating to birth or from birth to the end of the experiment. Three groups received a 0.5% lead acetate solution either at the time they were mated (Group 1), when pups were discovered (Group 2), or throughout the experiment (Group 3). Controls received water throughout. The effects on activity were assessed in an open field or a running wheel when Ss were 25 and 55 days old. Aspects of agonistic behavior were also examined. Ss in Group 2 appeared most affected in the open field and in running wheels. Both the direction and degree of this effect were influenced by the specific test situation and measures as well as by the age of S when tested. For example, Ss in Group 2 crossed the most squares in the open field at both ages. However, this group was less active during their 1st day in the running wheels when 25 days old, but not when 55 days old. In general, activity of Ss in Group 1 was least affected by administration of lead, but the effects of continued exposure to lead (Group 3) were not simply additive. In contrast to measures of activity, agonistic testing at 60 days of age showed that all groups that had been or were being exposed to lead displayed a shorter latency to fight when compared to controls. (24 ref).

647. Domer, Floyd R. & Llera, Juan-Carlos. (1978). **Blood-brain barrier permeability changes caused by lead exposure and amphetamine in mice.** *Research Communications in Psychology, Psychiatry & Behavior,* 3(2), 101–108.
Changed the drinking water of pregnant CD-1 mice to 0.5% sodium acetate or 0.5% lead acetate from the time of delivery of the offspring. The pups were weaned at 21 days of age and maintained on the same drinking solutions. Body weight, locomotor activity, and blood–brain barrier (BBB) permeability were evaluated when the mice were 35–45 days of age. The lead-exposed mice were smaller and hyperactive relative to the sodium-exposed controls. The BBB permeability was also increased, but not significantly. When amphetamine sulfate (3 mg/kg ip) was given, the BBB permeability was significantly decreased in the lead-exposed mice. It is suggested that this contributes to the amphetamine activity in the treatment of hyperactive children. (25 ref).

METALLIC ELEMENTS

648. Domer, Floyd R. & Wolf, Carlos L. (1979). **Drugs, lead and the blood-brain barrier.** *Research Communications in Psychology, Psychiatry & Behavior,* 4(2), 135–148.
CD-1 mice were exposed from birth to either .5% sodium acetate or lead acetate in drinking water. Locomotor activity evaluation after weaning showed that lead-exposed Ss were hyperactive. Amphetamine and caffeine decreased activity, whereas methylphenidate and pemoline increased it. It is concluded that lead-induced hyperactivity is not a valid model for evaluating drugs for use in children with hyperactivity or minimal brain dysfunction. (2½ p ref).

649. Donald, J. M.; Cutler, M. G.; Moore, M. R. & Bradley, M. (1986). **Effects of lead in the laboratory mouse: II: Development and social behaviour after lifelong administration of a small dose of lead acetate in drinking fluid.** *Neuropharmacology,* 25(2), 151–160.
Investigated the effect of a 0.13% lead acetate solution as drinking fluid on breeding BK:W mice. Although there was no significant effect on the numbers of live or dead births or on weight of pups at 1 day, the appearance of fur was delayed and the body weights at 21 days and 31–38 wks were smaller than in controls. On weaning, the treated Ss received 0.13% lead acetate as drinking fluid. Concentrations of lead in bone and brain were markedly raised above control levels at 18 and 34 wks, being greatest at 34 wks. Behavior of the treated Ss in social encounters was shown by ethological procedures to differ from that of controls. The most consistent change after treatment was enhancement of social and sexual investigation, seen in females at 26–27 wks when encountering male partners, in isolated males at 32–33 wks encountering male partners, and in group-housed males and females in single sex encounters at 17–18 wks. At 17–18 wks, duration of this behavior was increased in treated females in the 1st 3 min and in treated males in the final 5 min of the 20 min period of observation. Behavioral changes in juvenile Ss at 6–7 wks occurred only during the final 5 of the 20 min observation. At 3–4 wks only a marginal difference in behavior was detectable, this being in the treated females. Results indicate that behavioral effects of lead differed between males and females and between juveniles and adults. (49 ref).

650. Donald, J. M.; Cutler, M. G. & Moore, M. R. (1987). **Effects of lead in the laboratory mouse: Development and social behaviour after lifelong exposure to 12 μM lead in drinking fluid.** *Neuropharmacology,* 26(4), 391–399.
Examined the effects of chronic exposure to 12 μM lead, from conception onwards, on development and social behavior in laboratory mice. Lead was administered as .25% solution of lead acetate in the drinking fluid. This level of exposure did not affect reproductive success, but caused decreased birthweight and retarded early development in offspring of treated dams. Effects on exploratory behavior, social investigation, aggression, and nonsocial activity are described.

651. Donald, J. M.; Cutler, M. G. & Moore, M. R. (1986). **Effects of 1.2 μM lead in the laboratory mouse: Developmental and behavioural consequences of chronic treatment.** *Neuropharmacology,* 25(12), 1395–1401.
Examined the behavior of mice treated pre- and postnatally with lead and of control mice by ethological analysis of social encounters between pairs of unfamiliar mice of similar treatment groups in a neutral cage. Evidence of enhanced reactivity to the test situation was seen in treated males at age 3–4 wks by increased social investigation, at 7–8 wks by decreased immobility, and at 18–19 wks by an increased duration of exploratory behavior. However, when encountering females at 30–31 wks, the treated males showed more immobility than did the controls. Treated females at 3–4 wks showed a decreased frequency of exploratory behavior and increased immobility, but at 7–8 and 18–19 wks they showed enhancement of social and sexual investigation.

652. Donovick, Peter J. & Burright, Richard G. (1986). **Short term lead exposure, age and food deprivation: Interactive effects on wheel running behavior of adult male mice.** *Experimental Aging Research,* 12(3), 163–168.
Studied interactive effects of short-term lead exposure, age, and food deprivation on wheel-running behavior of Binghamton Heterogeneous Stock male mice—aged 75 days (44 Ss), 220 days (24 Ss), and 365 days (18 Ss). Ss were maintained on food and either water or a 0.5% lead-acetate drinking solution for 3 wks prior to placement in cages with attached running wheels. Mice were kept on their assigned sources of fluid while in the cages for 6 days, and food deprivation was instituted on Days 3 and 4. Results indicate that age, lead exposure, and food deprivation interact significantly in affecting wheel-running behavior, suggesting that slight changes in environmental and dietary factors can combine with the effects of aging to significantly affect performance.

653. Driscoll, Janis W. & Stegner, Steven E. (1976). **Behavioral effects of chronic lead ingestion on laboratory rats.** *Pharmacology, Biochemistry & Behavior,* 4(4), 411–417.
Conducted 4 experiments with 146 rats. Ss continuously exposed to lead acetate solutions were tested on a visual discrimination reversal problem, on the open field, and in 2 shuttle avoidance situations. High lead intake produced slower acquisition of the visual discrimination problem but had no effect on reversal performance. High lead intake also reduced activity on the open field and improved performance on both shuttle avoidance problems. Results indicate that the effects produced by exposure to lead may involve an increase in responsiveness to aversive situations. (21 ref).

654. Driscoll, Janis W. & Stegner, Steven E. (1978). **Lead-produced changes in the relative rate of open field activity of laboratory rats.** *Pharmacology, Biochemistry & Behavior,* 8(6), 743–747.
In 2 experiments, 4 groups of female albino rats, continuously exposed to 1 of 2 lead acetate solutions, ad lib water, or a limited amount of water, were tested for 3 daily 5-min periods in the open field. The effects of treatment on activity, relative to Ss drinking ad lib water, depended on the concentration of the lead acetate solution. Ss exposed to a 10^{-4}M lead acetate solution showed increased overall activity, while Ss exposed to a 10^{-2}M lead acetate solution showed changes in the relative rate of activity. Activity was not affected by limiting the amount of water consumed. Findings illustrate the importance of recording activity in a manner that allows assessment of changes in activity as well as absolute level. (16 ref).

655. Dyer, Robert S.; Eccles, Christine U. & Annau, Zoltan. (1978). **Evoked potential alterations following prenatal methyl mercury exposure.** *Pharmacology, Biochemistry & Behavior,* 8(2), 137–141.
Pregnant Long-Evans hooded rats were given either 0 or 5 mg/kg methyl mercury by gastric intubation on Day 7 of gestation. Female offspring were implanted with recording electrodes 60 days after birth and had their cortically recorded visual evoked potentials studied at 4 different flash intensities. Mercury-exposed Ss had higher P1–N1 and N1–P2 amplitudes and shorter P2 and N2 latencies than controls. Data provide evidence that a single ingestion of methyl mercury by pregnant rats is sufficient to produce long-term alterations in CNS activity. (15 ref).

656. Dyer, Robert S. & Howell, William E. (1982). **Triethyltin: Ambient temperature alters visual system toxicity.** *Neurobehavioral Toxicology & Teratology,* 4(2), 267–271.
78 male Long-Evans hooded rats with chronically implanted electrodes were administered either triethyltin (TET; 6 mg/kg) or saline, and maintained in either a warm (30°C) or cool (22°C) environment for the next 7 hrs. Visual evoked re-

sponses (VERs) were recorded during this 7-hr period and at regular intervals for the next 2 wks. TET increased VER peak latencies. Findings indicate that toxicant-induced alterations in core temperature are potential determinants of other toxicant-induced effects. (18 ref).

657. Eccles, Christine U. & Annau, Zoltan. (1982). **Prenatal methyl mercury exposure: II. Alterations in learning and psychotropic drug sensitivity in adult offspring.** *Neurobehavioral Toxicology & Teratology,* 4(3), 377–382.
93 male Long-Evans rats that had been exposed in utero to 5 or 8 mg/kg of methyl mercury administered as a single dose on either Day 8 or 15 of gestation were tested as adults in 2 operant tasks. In 1 task, Ss were trained on 2-way avoidance to a criterion of 10 consecutive avoidances. Following acquisition, Ss' behavior was extinguished and 24 hrs later retrained to the previous criterion. Ss treated with 8 mg/kg on Day 8 of gestation required significantly more trials to reach criterion during reacquisition than controls. Ss treated on Day 15 with either 5 or 8 mg/kg took significantly more trials to reach criterion during acquisition than controls; and of the 8 mg/kg group, 55% failed to reach criterion. Ss treated with 8 mg/kg on Day 8 of gestation acquired a 10-sec DRL task at the same rate as controls. When challenged with dextroamphetamine, the treated Ss were less disrupted at the higher dose (1.0 mg/kg) than controls, suggesting a shift in the dose–response curve for this drug. Activity measures taken simultaneously with the DRL session confirmed this shift. Results suggest that a single prenatal exposure to methyl mercury can affect learning and drug sensitivity of the adult animal and that mercury exposure in late gestation has more deleterious consequences on learning ability than early exposure. (12 ref).

658. Eccles, Christine U. & Annau, Zoltan. (1982). **Prenatal methyl mercury exposure: I. Alterations in neonatal activity.** *Neurobehavioral Toxicology & Teratology,* 4(3), 371–376.
42 pregnant Long-Evans rats were intubated with 0, 5, or 8 mg/kg of methyl mercury on Day 8 or 15 of gestation. In litters that were delivered, the mercury treatment did not affect litter size or weight gain of the pups in the preweaning period. Methyl mercury content of the 1-day-old rat brains was directly related to both the dose and time of treatment. Results indicate that neonatal activity measures can be used as sensitive indicators of low prenatal neurotoxic exposures. (23 ref).

659. Elsner, Jürg. (1986). **Testing strategies in behavioral teratology: III. Microanalysis of behavior.** *Neurobehavioral Toxicology & Teratology,* 8(5), 573–584.
After having been tested in a standard behavioral teratology battery, a random sample of male offspring of rat dams exposed to methylmercury starting 2 wks prior to pairing until weaning were further tested in a wheel-shaped activity monitor and in an operant conditioning paradigm (spatial alternation). In the activity monitor, a significant interaction between locomotion and radial-activity-monitor compartments and a significant increase in stereotyped locomotion were observed. Significant increases in unresponded trials and response latency, as well as session-to-session variation of these measures, were detected during the spatial-alternation schedule. These observations are interpreted as an indication of a reduced attention and behavioral stability, induced by the schedule challenge. This interpretation is compared with the signs of minimal brain dysfunction in schoolchildren.

660. Elsner, Jürg; Hodel, Beat; Suter, Kurt E.; Oelke, Dieter et al. (1988). **Detection limits of different approaches in behavioral teratology, and correlation of effects with neurochemical parameters.** *Neurotoxicology & Teratology,* 10(2), 155–167.
Treated rat dams by gavage with 5 doses of methylmercury during gestation. Offspring were subjected to a routine developmental and behavioral testing battery. Random samples were further investigated using a variety of techniques. The following effects were noted in ascending dose sensitivity order: delayed vaginal opening, increased and more variable passiveness in spatial alternation, impaired swimming behavior, increased glial fibrillary acidic protein concentration in the cerebellar vermis, increased auditory startle amplitude, decreased intertrial interval pokes in the visual discrimination test, increased percentage of visits in passive area of figure-8 activity monitor, increased path iteration frequencies, decreased local activity in the wheel-shaped activity monitor, decreased locomotor activity in the 2-compartment monitor, increased cerebellar vermis weight, and decreased S-100 protein in the hippocampus.

661. Elsner, Jürg; Suter, Kurt E.; Ulbrich, Beate & Schreiner, Gerd. (1986). **Testing strategies in behavioral teratology: IV. Review and general conclusions.** *Neurobehavioral Toxicology & Teratology,* 8(5), 585–590.
Synthesizes the studies of K. E. Suter and H. Schön, G. Schreiner et al, and J. Elsner (all, 1986) in which 3 laboratories collaborated to evaluate test concepts used for testing in behavioral teratology. Rat dams were treated orally with methylmercury starting 2 wks prior to pairing until weaning of their offspring. In the 1st laboratory, reproduction parameters were assessed in the dams, and all offspring were subjected to developmental and behavioral tests. A random selection of these Ss was tested by multiparametric automated techniques in the other 2 laboratories. Both the developmental and behavioral testing battery, as well as the automated techniques, showed some significant effects in the offspring even at the low dose, where no reproduction effects had been noted. To obtain optimal information, it is proposed to combine both approaches for routine testing.

662. Engellenner, William J.; Burright, Richard G. & Donovick, Peter J. (1986). **Lead, age and aggression in male mice.** *Physiology & Behavior,* 36(5), 823–828.
Investigated factors contributing to changes in social behavior and dominance relationships as induced by lead exposure in 60- and 540-day-day Binghamton Heterogeneous male mice. The impact of 11 wks of ingestion of a 0.5% lead acetate solution on Ss' agonistic behavior was examined. Similar-aged Ss were paired for aggression testing. Younger Ss, regardless of fluid history, fought more vigorously than older Ss. However, when Ss of similar fluid history were paired together, lead ingestion decreased the latency to fight only in older Ss. Regardless of their prior fighting history, when lead-treated Ss fought similar-aged controls, the lead-exposed Ss in younger pairs were typically subordinate; in older pairs, lead-exposed Ss were dominant. (44 ref).

663. Feeney, Dennis M. et al. (1979). **Detection of the effects of lead exposure by visual evoked response latency.** *Physiological Psychology,* 7(2), 143–145.
Studied visual evoked responses (VER) in 26 male CD offspring of mother rats exposed to lead acetate. All measurements were taken by experimenters uninformed regarding treatment assignment. The latency of the P2 component was significantly shorter for the lead-exposed Ss than for the controls. It is suggested that VER latencies may be a sensitive index of subclinical effects of lead on brain, long after discontinuation of lead exposure and when blood levels are normal. (13 ref).

664. Flynn, Eleanor R. (1979). **Neurochemical and behavioral effects of prenatal lead ingestion: Brain lead content, brain calcium, activity level and maze learning.** *Dissertation Abstracts International,* 39(12-B), 6183.

665. Fox, D. A.; Wright, A. A. & Costa, L. G. (1982). **Visual acuity deficits following neonatal lead exposure: Cholinergic interactions.** *Neurobehavioral Toxicology & Teratology,* 4(6), 689–693.

METALLIC ELEMENTS

Clinical reports of children poisoned by lead describe long-term alterations in the spatial resolution properties of the visual system. The present studies examined whether low-level neonatal exposure to lead would alter the spatial resolution limit, visual acuity, in the adult rat. To examine possible mechanisms of action (and an additional stressor) the effects of scopolamine were studied in the psychophysical procedure. [^{3}H]Quinuclidinyl benzilate (QNB) binding was analyzed in retina, superior colliculus, lateral geniculate nucleus, and visual cortex. Neonatal Long-Evans hooded rats were exposed to Pb (Days 0–21) via the milk of dams drinking 0.2% Pb acetate. Visual acuity was 1.8 c/deg in controls compared to 1.3 c/deg in Pb-exposed Ss. Scopolamine caused dose-dependent decreases in spatial resolution, with decreases at higher spatial frequencies being greater in the Pb group. Positive controls revealed the effects to be centrally mediated. A decrease in QNB binding was found only in the visual cortex. Results suggest that long-term effects of developmental Pb exposure may be directly on the visual cortex. (36 ref).

666. Geist, Charles R. & Balko, Stanley W. (1980). **Effects of postnatal lead acetate exposure on activity and emotionality in developing laboratory rats.** *Bulletin of the Psychonomic Society,* 15(5), 288–290.
At 21 days of age, 3 groups of female hooded rats were exposed to lead at concentrations of 0, 25, or 50 ppm provided ad lib in the acetate form for 35 days in the drinking water. No significant differences were found in food consumption, lead acetate or water consumption, and weight gain. When Ss were tested in an open-field task, no significant differences were found in either the duration or frequency of grooming or rearing behavior, or the number of squares traversed. However, significant differences in emotionality were observed. Ss receiving 50 ppm lead acetate exhibited markedly greater emotionality when compared with Ss receiving either 25 or 0 ppm lead acetate. Results indicate that postnatal lead exposure may affect some elements of emotional behavior, while having little effect on activity. (19 ref).

667. Geist, Charles R.; Balko, Stanley W.; Morgan, Martha E. & Angiak, Robert. (1985). **Behavioral effects following rehabilitation from postnatal exposure to lead acetate.** *Perceptual & Motor Skills,* 60(2), 527–536.
Exposed 3 groups of 21-day-old male Sprague-Dawley rats to either untreated or lead-acetate-treated (25 or 50 ppm) drinking water for 40 days. When tested for spontaneous alternation, Ss receiving both amounts of lead acetate exhibited significantly reduced rates of alternation below those of untreated controls. Immediately subsequent to testing, lead was removed from the diet of the experimental groups and water was substituted for 70 days, at which time all Ss were tested on the problems of the Hebb-Williams closed-field maze-learning task. No significant differences between groups were found in the time taken to traverse the maze enclosure, in the number of squares traversed, or in the total number of error zones entered over the 12 test problems, although significantly increased latencies to leave the start box were noted for Ss previously exposed to lead acetate. Data indicate that some deficits produced by postweaning lead acetate exposure may be reversible and not persist beyond a period of rehabilitation. (25 ref).

668. Geist, Charles R. & Mattes, Ben R. (1979). **Behavioral effects of postnatal lead acetate exposure in developing laboratory rats.** *Physiological Psychology,* 7(4), 399–402.
At 23 days of age, 3 groups of male albino Sprague-Dawley rats were exposed to lead at concentrations of 0, 25, or 50 ppm provided ad lib, in the acetate form, for 35 days in drinking water. When tested on the problems of the Hebb-Williams maze, Ss receiving both 50 and 25 ppm displayed significantly impaired learning ability when compared to water-fed controls in the total number of error zones entered over the 12 test problems. The time taken to traverse the maze enclosure, however, was significantly reduced only in the group receiving 50 ppm. None of the overt manifestations characteristic of lead poisoning were observed. It is concluded that learning deficits can be produced in weanling rats at exposure levels similar to those that cause encephalopathy in developing neonates. (28 ref).

669. Geyer, Mark A.; Butcher, Richard E. & Fite, Kenneth. (1985). **A study of startle and locomotor activity in rats exposed prenatally to methylmercury.** Conference Proceedings of the National Center for Toxicological Research et al: Design considerations in screening for behavioral teratogens: Results of the collaborative behavioral teratology study (1985, Cincinnati, Ohio). *Neurobehavioral Toxicology & Teratology,* 7(6), 759–765.
Examined the permanence of developmental abnormalities from prenatal methylmercuric chloride (MMC) in the offspring of Sprague-Dawley albino rats exposed on Days 6–15 of gestation to 0, 0.25, 1.25, 2.5, or 5.0 mg/kg MMC. The effects of MMC on reproduction and early physical development were examined together with tests of negative geotaxis, righting, pivoting, swimming, locomotor activity in an open field, and startle responses to either tactile or acoustic stimuli. It was found that no live offspring were produced by females treated with 5.0 mg/kg MMC. Offspring from the 2.5 mg/kg dose group displayed impaired performance on almost all preweaning measures and continuing abnormalities on longitudinal tests of locomotor activity in an open-field and startle response performance. (11 ref).

670. Golter, Marianne & Michaelson, I. Arthur. (1975). **Growth, behavior, and brain catecholamines in lead-exposed neonatal rats: A reappraisal.** *Science,* 187(4174), 359–361.
Daily oral administration of lead to newborn Sprague-Dawley rats had no adverse effect on their body growth, although lead-treated rats were more active than age-matched controls. Endogenous levels of brain dopamine were unchanged, whereas norepinephrine was increased, suggesting a possible relationship between lead exposure during earliest developmental periods, increased motor activity, and brain norepinephrine, and not brain dopamine as previously postulated.

671. Harry, Gaylia J. (1982). **Neurotoxicological effects of postpartum exposure to triethyl tin bromide.** *Dissertation Abstracts International,* 42(12-B, Pt 1), 4966.

672. Hartwell, Stuart I. (1986). **Validation of laboratory versus field avoidance behavior of schooling fathead minnows to heavy metal blends relative to acute toxicity during long term exposure.** *Dissertation Abstracts International,* 46(8-B), 2545–2546.

673. Hastings, Lloyd; Cooper, Gary P.; Bornschein, Robert L. & Michaelson, I. Arthur. (1977). **Behavioral effects of low level neonatal lead exposure.** *Pharmacology, Biochemistry & Behavior,* 7(1), 37–42.
Male Long-Evans rats exposed to lead via maternal milk were tested at various stages of development on a number of behavioral tasks. Beginning at parturition, the dams were given either tap water, 0.02%, or 0.10% lead acetate in the drinking water. Pups from all 3 groups were weaned to normal chow and tap water at 21 days of age. The mean lead concentration of the dam's blood and of neonatal (20 days of age) brain and blood were all below 50 μg/100 ml. No significant differences were found between the high lead-exposed group and controls in general as measured by wheel running over a 21-day period beginning at 30 days of age. However, there was a significant difference in wheel running behavior during the 1st 3 hrs of testing. Both lead-exposed groups displayed significantly less aggressive behavior as measured by the shock-elicited aggression test. Low-level lead exposure had no discernible effect on the acquisition and subsequent

reversal of a successive brightness discrimination task. Lead exposure under these conditions appears to affect some aspects of emotional behavior, while having little effect on general activity or cognitive function. (26 ref).

674. Hellberg, Jan & Hellström, Jonas. (1977). **Changes in scotopic flicker fusion intensity (CFFI) in squirrel monkeys exposed to methyl mercury.** *Psychological Research Bulletin, Lund U.,* 17(12), 12 p.
Tested critical flicker fusion intensity (CFFI) in 7 squirrel monkeys (*Saimiri sciureus*) that were administered oral doses of methyl mercury (MeHg) until clinical signs developed. Flicker rate was held constant, and intensity was systematically varied within the thresholds for scotopic (dark) vision. Results show that an increase in CFFI was correlated with toxic blood levels of MeHg. In an early stage these increases were reversible; later, the increases became irreversible but appeared well in advance of conventional clinical signs.

675. Holloway, William R. & Thor, Donald H. (1988). **Social memory deficits in adult male rats exposed to cadmium in infancy.** *Neurobehavioral Toxicology & Teratology,* 10(3), 193–197.
Infant rats were injected sc with 0, 1, or 2 mg Cd/kg on Day 5 or 6 after birth. In adulthood (150 days of age) Ss in both experiments who received the 2 mg/kg dose failed to learn the identity of a strange rat in a social recognition test. Results with Ss in the 1 mg/kg group were less consistent; in Exp I, they failed to learn the identity of a stranger; in Exp II, they behaved like controls. The level of investigation of a strange rat did not differ among the experimental groups, indicating Cd did not cause a performance deficit. The 2 mg/kg dose of Cd had no effect on body weight in Exp I and a small (6.98%), but significant, depressant effect on body weight in Exp II.

676. Holloway, William R. & Thor, Donald H. (1988). **Cadmium exposure in infancy: Effects on activity and social behaviors of juvenile rats.** *Neurotoxicology & Teratology,* 10(2), 135–142.
Administered single injections of cadmium chloride (0, 1, 2, 3, or 4 mg/kg) on Day 5 or 6 to infant rats. Ss receiving the 3 and 4 mg/kg doses had high mortality rates at weaning; survivors were extremely underweight and were not used in postweaning tests. Males receiving 2 mg/kg were more active after weaning than littermates who had received 0 or 1 mg/kg doses, and on Day 29 they engaged in significantly more play with a nontreated partner than did Ss in other groups. The effect of exposure was also evident when males were tested with similarly treated Ss on Day 44: Ss with 2 mg/kg had higher pinning frequencies than 0 or 1 mg/kg Ss. Females in the 1 and 2 mg/kg groups did not have increased activity or play.

677. Holloway, William R. & Thor, Donald H. (1987). **Low level lead exposure during lactation increases rough and tumble play fighting of juvenile rats.** *Neurotoxicology & Teratology,* 9(1), 51–57.
Lactating Long Evans hooded rats were given distilled water alone or with 0.067% lead chloride as their sole source of drinking fluid from Days 1–21 of lactation. Activity, social investigation, and rough and tumble play fighting behaviors of the offspring were observed. When paired with a group-housed stimulus animal on Day 26, lead-treated Ss had increases in 2 measures of play fighting and in social investigation. When tested with a scopolamine-treated, nonplayful stimulus on Day 36, increased crossover frequencies were observed in lead-treated Ss. Results indicate that social interactive behaviors of juvenile rats are effective tools in the assessment of exposure to toxic substances early in development.

678. Hughes, J. A.; Rosenthal, E. & Sparber, S. B. (1976). **Time dependent effects produced in chicks after prenatal injection of methylmercury.** *Pharmacology, Biochemistry & Behavior,* 4(5), 507-513.
In Exp I methylmercury dicyandiamide (MMD) (0.05–10 mg/kg egg) injected into the yolk sac of fertilized White Leghorn chicken eggs prior to incubation produced a dose-related decrease in the percentage of chicks hatched. With dosage fixed at 0.5 or 5.0 mg/kg egg and injections made on Days 0, 7, or 14 of incubation, hatches were 90, 68, and 75%, respectively, for the low dose and 63, 13, and 18% for the high dose. In Exp II, in contrast to results obtained from Ss hatched from eggs injected on Day 0 of incubation, Ss hatched from eggs injected with 0.5 or 5.0 mg/kg on Day 7 or 14 were not different from controls in a detour learning situation. Administration of labeled methylmercury revealed that maximum brain radiolabel in embryos injected on Day 0 was 10% of that seen with eggs injected on Day 7 but twice that seen with eggs injected on Day 14. It is concluded tentatively that a period of maximum sensitivity to the behavior effects exists prior to Day 7 and that the mechanism of embryolethality is different from that producing the functional deficits. (28 ref).

679. Hughes, John A. (1973). **Developmental and behavioral effects of methyl mercury in mice.** *Dissertation Abstracts International,* 34(5-B), 2077-2078.

680. Hughes, John A. & Annau, Zoltan. (1976). **Postnatal behavioral effects in mice after prenatal exposure to methylmercury.** *Pharmacology, Biochemistry & Behavior,* 4(4), 385-391.
Injected CFW mice with methylmercury hydroxide (1, 2, 3, 5, or 10 mg/kg as mercury) on Day 8 of gestation. Ss treated with 3, 5, or 10 mg/kg averaged one-third fewer pups than controls. Pups from these treated Ss weighed less than controls, and the weight differences persisted through weaning but were no longer significant at 56 days of age. Ss exposed to methylmercury in utero showed significant differences from controls in their behavior in a 2-way active avoidance shuttlebox and in a punishment situation, but not when tested in an open field, a water escape runway, or a conditioned suppression paradigm. Neither the mothers nor progeny of the Ss exposed prenatally to methylmercury showed behavioral deficits. (36 ref).

681. Hughes, John A. & Sparber, Sheldon B. (1978). **d-Amphetamine unmasks postnatal consequences of exposure to methylmercury *in utero*: Methods for studying behavioral teratogenesis.** *Pharmacology, Biochemistry & Behavior,* 8(4), 365–375.
Pregnant Sprague-Dawley rats were given various doses of methylmercury (MM) at 3 stages of gestation (Days 0, 7, or 14). Administration of 56 or 27% of the dose given on the 1st day (Day 0) of pregnancy to 7- or 14-day pregnant rats, respectively, resulted in equivalent concentrations of MM in 19-day-old fetuses and 1-day and 1-wk-old neonates. A single 5 mg/kg oral dose on Day 0, or its equivalent on Days 7 or 14, of gestation did not produce any signs of toxicity in pregnant Ss or their offspring. Operant (autoshaped) behavior showed sex-related differences to the disrupting influence of dextroamphetamine (DAM); females were significantly more sensitive than males. Moreover, both males and females whose mothers were treated with MM on Days 0 or 7 of pregnancy were significantly less affected by DAM when compared with controls. Offspring born to Ss given MM on Day 14 of pregnancy did not show a differential effect of DAM. It is concluded that early prenatal exposure to low doses of MM can result in behavioral consequences subtle enough to require unmasking of the effects with psychotropic drugs. Additionally, periods may exist during development when the embryo or fetus is most susceptible to behavioral or func-

METALLIC ELEMENTS

tional teratogenic effects of exposure to chemical insult. (51 ref).

682. Hupp, E. W. & Day, H. D. (1980). **Methylmercuric chloride poisoning in the pigtailed macaque monkey (*Macaca nemestrina*).** *Psychological Reports,* 46(3, Pt 2), 1023–1029.
Six male pigtailed macaque monkeys were injected with 6.4 or 4.8 mg/kg methylmercuric chloride in acute or fractionated dose schedules. Aphagia and adipsia occurring for several days after injection were followed by a period of apparent normality. The high-acute dose led to grossly observable sensorimotor symptoms that appeared 26 days following treatment and that were followed by death 1 wk later. A 3-stage response to mercury poisoning is proposed. (8 ref).

683. Inouye, Minoru; Murao, Koji & Kajiwara, Yuji. (1985). **Behavioral and neuropathological effects of prenatal methylmercury exposure in mice.** *Neurobehavioral Toxicology & Teratology,* 7(3), 227–232.
Studied the offspring of 50 C3H/HeN mice that were orally administered a single dose of 20 mg/kg methylmercuric chloride on 1 of Days 13–17 of pregnancy and 10 nontreated controls. Newborn Ss were foster mothered, but the weaning rate was low. Long-term behavioral impairment was manifest in the offspring of every treated group. The righting movement was mildly disturbed when Ss were dropped from about 40 cm high, tail position was low during walking, and some Ss showed strong flexion of the hind limbs when held by the tail. Spontaneous locomotor activity was also reduced. At 10–12 wks of age, Ss were sacrificed, and the brain was histologically examined. Results show that for prenatally treated Ss, brain weight was reduced, the nucleus caudatus putamen was slightly reduced in size leaving the lateral ventricles dilated, and cerebellar folial patterns were slightly simplified. These neurobehavioral symptoms and pathological changes tended to be comparatively more severe in Ss treated on Days 13 and 14 of pregnancy than those of the other groups, but the differences were small. (26 ref).

684. Jason, Kathryn M. (1978). **Effects of neonatal exposure to lead on behavioral and neurochemical development in the rat.** *Dissertation Abstracts International,* 39(3-B), 1190.

685. Johnson, Gail V. & Jope, Richard S. (1986). **Aluminum increases cyclic AMP in rat cerebral cortex *in vivo*.** *Life Sciences,* 39(14), 1301–1305.
Reports that in vivo concentrations of adenosine 3',5'-monophosphate (cyclic AMP) were elevated in the cerebral cortex of male Sprague-Dawley rats administered aluminum citrate via diet or injection. Aluminum treatment altered the response of cortical cyclic AMP to the administration of pilocarpine and of apomorphine. It is proposed that the neurotoxicity of aluminum may be due to altered protein phosphorylation as a consequence of the chronic elevation of cyclic AMP.

686. King, G. A.; de Boni, U. & Crapper, D. R. (1975). **Effect of aluminum upon conditioned avoidance response acquisition in the absence of neurofibrillary degeneration.** *Pharmacology, Biochemistry & Behavior,* 3(6), 1003-1009.
Aluminum has been shown in previous experiments to induce neurofibrillary degeneration in cats but not rats. Cats develop a progressive encephalopathy in which an early manifestation is impaired learning/memory performance. In the present 3 experiments, at brain aluminum concentrations of 5–6 times that found in cat, 74 male hooded and Wistar rats demonstrated an initial transient weight loss and acquisition deficit immediately following intracranial injection. However, Ss did not develop a progressive encephalopathy or a chronic learning deficit. (16 ref).

687. Klein, Stephen B. & Atkinson, Elizabeth J. (1973). **Mercuric chloride influence on active-avoidance acquisition in rats.** *Bulletin of the Psychonomic Society,* 1(6-B), 437-438.
Administered sublethal doses of mercuric chloride for 14 days to 11 25-day-old female Sprague-Dawley rats. Although there was no impairment in either general appearance or escape behavior, mercury poisoning produced significant deficits in active-avoidance learning. Results indicate that behavioral impairments can occur as a consequence of low doses of mercury administration in the absence of gross physical abnormalities.

688. Klein, Stephen B.; Barter, Marie J.; Murphy, Arthur L. & Richardson, John H. (1974). **Aversion to low doses of mercuric chloride in rats.** *Physiological Psychology,* 2(3-A), 397-400.
In contrast to the detrimental influence of low mercury doses observed in prior research, mercuric chloride had no significant effect on either emotional behavior in the open field or on aversive conditioning of 24 adult and 24 juvenile Sprague-Dawley rats in the 1-way shuttlebox. Results also show that mercuric chloride had no obvious physiological effect as indicated by the absence of significant differences between experimental Ss and the 24 controls. However, the data indicate that adult male and female Ss were capable of reducing their intake of a solution containing mercury. This aversion to low doses of mercury developed in the apparent absence of any gross physiological and behavioral impairment. Juvenile Ss were able to develop an aversion to sugar water containing mercury but exhibited a difficulty in maintaining their aversion.

689. Koltes, Karen H. (1984). **Temporal patterns and environmental responses in the three-dimensional structure and activity of the Atlantic silverside, *Menidia menidia* (L.).** *Dissertation Abstracts International,* 44(7-B), 2041.

690. Krulík, R.; Farská, I. & Prokeš, J. (1977). **Distribution of rubidium in the organism.** *Neuropsychobiology,* 3(2–3), 120–128.
After administration of ^{86}RbCl (0.5 mM/kg, ip) to male mice, maximum levels in the liver and kidneys were attained in the 1st hr, but in the brain not for 24 hrs. The Rb^+ half-time in the tissues was about 170 hrs. With peroral administration, tissue ribidium levels at 3 days were higher than after ip injection. Rubidium did not affect sodium levels in rats, but lowered potassium levels. Cesium led to an increase in tissue rubidium levels, while diuretics had no significant effect on them. The erythrocyte saturation rate was correlated to the species, but there were no differences in vitro between young and old individuals in both human Ss and experimental animals, or between healthy humans and manic-depressive patients. Rubidium was not displayed from erythrocytes by the presence of high potassium concentrations in the medium.

691. Krulík, R.; Farská, I. & Prokeš, J. (1977). **Effect of rubidium, lithium and cesium on brain ATPase and protein kinases.** *Neuropsychobiology,* 3(2–3), 129–134.
Studied the effect of rubidium, lithium and cesium on the adenosine triphosphatase (ATPase) and cyclic adenosine monophosphate (cAMP) protein kinase in male Wistar rat brain. It was demonstrated that rubidium could replace potassium in the Na^+K^+-ATPase system, whereas lithium and cesium had no effect on this enzyme activity in the absence of potassium. K^+-dependent ATPase was activated by even low rubidium concentrations; lithium and cesium inhibited it. Rubidium, lithium, and cesium did not affect cAMP protein kinase. (15 ref).

692. Kutscher, Charles L.; Sembrat, Melanie; Kutscher, Cheryl S. & Kutscher, Nancy L. (1985). **Effects of the high methylmercury dose used in the Collaborative Behavioral Teratology Study on brain anatomy.** Conference Proceedings of the National Center for Toxicological Research et al: Design considerations in screening for behavioral teratogens: Results of the collaborative behavioral teratology study (1985, Cincinnati, Ohio). *Neurobehavioral Toxicology & Teratology,* 7(6), 775–777.
Pregnant albino Charles River rats were injected with 0, 6, or 10 mg/kg of methylmercuric chloride (MMC) on Days 6–9 of gestation. Ss given the 10 mg/kg dose failed to deliver young or produced stillborn. External morphology was normal for offspring given either the 0 or 6 mg/kg dose. Brains of 21- or 90-day-old offspring were sectioned at 3 criterion locations and examined to measure intrastructural distances and abnormalities. It was found that MMC produced hydrocephalus, decreased thickness of cerebral cortex in the parietal section, and increased thickness of hippocampus in the occipital section. With these exceptions, the brains of mercury-treated offspring showed normal development. (16 ref).

693. Lacz, Joseph P. (1979). **Behavioral and neurochemical alterations associated with neonatal lead encephalopathy models.** *Dissertation Abstracts International,* 39(9-B), 4299.

694. Lanthorn, Thomas & Isaacson, Robert L. (1978). **Effects of chronic lead ingestion in adult rats.** *Physiological Psychology,* 6(1), 93–95.
Adult male Long-Evans rats were given lead (0.27%) in their drinking water and compared with pair-fed controls on several behavior problems: spontaneous alternation and 2 learning problems with 3 reversals in each. The lead-treated Ss had reduced rates of spontaneous alternation and difficulty in changing behavior when the cues signaling reward and nonreward were reversed. In addition, Ss without much handling showed exaggerated responsiveness. These changes are similar to but less extreme than those seen in neonates treated with lead. The development of a peripheral absorption barrier may account for the reduced sensitivity of adults to lead poisoning relative to similar poisoning with younger Ss.

695. Laties, Victor G. & Evans, Hugh L. (1982). **Effects of methylmercury on operant behavior.** *Neurobehavioral Toxicology & Teratology,* 4(6), 683–688.
Experimental observations on methylmercury's effects on the behavior of pigeons illustrate how operant techniques can be used to investigate long-lasting consequences of a toxic insult. Over 21 mo, methylmercury (2 mg/kg/day) disturbed the ability of Ss to discriminate the amount of behavior that they had emitted; data show an increase in the variability of run lengths, a decrease in mean run length, and a decrease in the proportion of runs that met the requirement for reinforcement. It is argued that operant procedures are the best means of investigating the effects of chronic exposure to toxic agents. (30 ref).

696. Laughton, Watson; Sawchenko, Paul & Gold, Richard M. (1977). **Effects of gastric acidity on food intake in rats.** *Physiology & Behavior,* 18(5), 991–992.
Intragastric infusion of hydrochloric acid lowered 12 female Charles River CD rats' intragastric pH but failed to produce any increase or decrease in food intake. Conversely, infusions of base (aluminum and magnesium hydroxide) increased pH without altering food intake.

697. Levin, Edward D. (1985). **The long-term effects of developmental lead exposure on learning and memory in monkeys.** *Dissertation Abstracts International,* 46(2-B), 462.

698. Levin, Edward D. & Bowman, Robert E. (1983). **The effect of pre- or postnatal lead exposure on Hamilton search task in monkeys.** *Neurobehavioral Toxicology & Teratology,* 5(3), 391–394.
Rhesus monkeys were exposed to low, chronic levels of lead acetate either pre- or postnatally. Ss were tested as juveniles on a spatial memory test, the Hamilton search task (HST). Ss exposed prenatally to lead did not show a deficit, while those exposed postnatally showed a significant deficit on the HST. The deficit was not apparent until the Ss were required to meet the most strict criterion, suggesting that the impairment may have been due to the memory rather than the learning components of the task. The fact that the deficit was seen more than 3 yrs after the end of lead exposure indicates that the lead-induced cognitive effect is quite long-lasting and perhaps permanent. (21 ref).

699. Levin, Edward D. & Bowman, Robert E. (1986). **Scopolamine effects on Hamilton search task performance in monkeys.** *Pharmacology, Biochemistry & Behavior,* 24(4), 819–821.
Administered G. V. Hamilton's (1911) search task, a test of spatial memory, to adult monkeys after administration of scopolamine bromide. Three monkeys had been exposed to lead during development, and 2 were controls. The task consisted of opening 8 boxes for food reinforcement. Ss had to remember which boxes had already been opened and avoid them to obtain the remaining reinforcements. Percent correct response, openings-to-repeat, trials per session, repetitive index, and response latency were measured. There were no significant lead-related effects. Significant scopolamine-induced deficits were detected with 4 of the measures. Low doses of scopolamine (1–3 μg/kg) did not affect response accuracy, but 15 and 30 μg/kg caused impairments. (10 ref).

700. Levin, Edward D. & Bowman, Robert E. (1986). **Long-term lead effects on the Hamilton Search Task and delayed alternation in monkeys.** *Neurobehavioral Toxicology & Teratology,* 8(3), 219–224.
Exposure of 5 rhesus monkeys to lead during the 1st yr after birth resulted in cognitive deficits when the Ss were tested as adults (5–6 yrs of age). A pronounced lead-related deficit was detected in the test of delayed spatial alternation (DSA), and a much less robust effect was detected in the Hamilton search task. Both tests are seen as providing a behavioral criterion challenging enough to elicit a deficit in lead-treated Ss while still being within the capabilities of the controls. The lead-induced deficit in DSA was most pronounced after short intertrial delays, suggesting that the effect may have been due to deficits in strategy or attention. The lose-shift type of error accounted for most of the lead-related DSA deficit, indicating that the lead-treated Ss perseverated on an alternation strategy even when it was not rewarded. Results indicate that exposure to lead during the 1st yr after birth can result in long-term and possibly permanent cognitive deficits.

701. Levin, Edward D.; Bowman, R. E.; Wegert, S. & Vuchetich, J. (1987). **Psychopharmacological investigations of a lead-induced long-term cognitive deficit in monkeys.** *Psychopharmacology,* 91(3), 334–341.
Investigated pharmacological manipulations of the cholinergic (ACh) and dopaminergic (DA) transmitter systems in 5 rhesus monkeys (*Macaca mulatta*) with a long-term lead-induced cognitive deficit on delayed spatial alternation (DSA). The deficit persisted throughout the 2 yrs of this experiment. The ACh antagonist, scopolamine (.001, .005, and .015 mg/kg), caused a dose-related decline in performance in both groups. Significant amelioration of the lead-induced DSA deficit was achieved by chronic treatment with the DA agonist, levodopa (15 mg/kg/day). After withdrawal from levodopa, the lead-related deficit reappeared. Improvement in performance of the lead-treated group was also seen after chronic amphetamine (0.2 mg/kg/day) administration, but this effect was not significant.

METALLIC ELEMENTS

702. Levin, Edward D.; Schneider, Mary L.; Ferguson, Sherry A.; Schantz, Susan L. et al. (1988). **Behavioral effects of developmental lead exposure in rhesus monkeys.** *Developmental Psychobiology,* 21(4), 371–382.
Investigated possible antecedents of lead-induced cognitive dysfunction (LICD) by evaluating the behavioral effects of pulse-chronic lead exposure in 8 rhesus monkeys during the 1st 6 postnatal months. Lead-treated Ss exhibited significantly decreased looking behavior on a visual exploration test and significantly decreased muscle tonus and increased arousal or agitation on a behavioral assessment battery compared with nonexposed controls. No effects of lead exposure were seen on a Piagetian object permanence task. In addition to providing indices of behavioral dysfunction during postnatal lead exposure, results suggest that performance on these early behavioral tests may predict later LICD.

703. Levine, Tina E. (1978). **Conditioned aversion following ingestion of methylmercury in rats and mice.** *Behavioral & Neural Biology,* 22(4), 489–496.
12 male Sprague-Dawley rats (Exp I) and 11 CF1 mice (Exp II) were given a choice between a plain or methylmercury-adulterated fluid, after previous exposure to either a high or low concentration of methylmercury in the fluid. Ss exposed to the high concentration consumed very little of the solution in the choice situation. The low concentration had a less marked effect. There was no change in total fluid intake. Ss responded to the stimulus properties of the methylmercury in that aversion was maintained with shifts in position of the tubes, although no external cue was associated with the mercury solution. In mice, there was a stimulus generalization decrement demonstrated by increased consumption of methylmercury solution when a low concentration was substituted for the previously avoided high-concentration solution. In addition, a readily consumed low concentration was avoided by mice following exposure to a high concentration of methylmercury. (18 ref).

704. Lilienthal, Hellmuth; Winneke, Gerhard; Brockhaus, Arthur & Molik, Beate. (1986). **Pre- and postnatal lead-exposure in monkeys: Effects on activity and learning set formation.** *Neurobehavioral Toxicology & Teratology,* 8(3), 265–272.
17 rhesus monkeys were pre- and postnatally exposed to 0, 250, or 600 ppm lead acetate in the diet. Blood lead levels of the mothers were less than 1, 24.4, and 37.4 μg/100 g blood, respectively, while those of the offspring were substantially higher, at least in the early stages of development. At the age of 2–15 mo, Ss were tested for group activity levels in an unfamiliar environment. No substantial lead-related alterations of activity occurred either for group activity or for the activity of individual Ss. There were, however, significant dose-related impairments of pattern discrimination learning-set formation; in simple discrimination learning during the early training phases, deficits were seen in the high-lead group only. Emotional alterations of these Ss may account for this result, whereas true cognitive deficits are likely to underlie the impairment of learning-set formation seen in the low-lead group.

705. Lipman, J. J.; Colowick, S. P.; Lawrence, P. L. & Abumrad, N. N. (1988). **Aluminum induced encephalopathy in the rat.** *Life Sciences,* 42(8), 863–875.
24 male rats implanted with icv cannula were administered aluminum tartrate (ALT) or sodium tartrate (NaT). An early startle reaction, later joined by locomotor discoordination, was followed by locomotor and electrocorticographic seizures in chronically instrumented ALT Ss. When Ss were tested in a shuttlebox for estimation of learning and memory function 7–8 days after ALT injection, impairment of both active and passive avoidance was observed. When glucose uptake capacity of synaptosomes from brain areas of ALT and NaT Ss was sampled, striatal and cortical synaptosomes showed reduced uptake activity, striatal uptake was inhibited, and cortical uptake was reduced to 57% of control.

706. Livesey, D. J.; Dawson, R. G.; Livesey, P. J.; Barrett, J. et al. (1986). **Lead retention in blood and brain after preweaning low-level lead exposure in the rat.** *Pharmacology, Biochemistry & Behavior,* 25(5), 1089–1094.
Newborn male Wistar rats were exposed to lead from birth to 20 days of age through milk from dams fed diets containing 0, 0.25, 0.5, or 1.0% powdered lead. There was a direct relationship between lead levels in the blood and brain of the pups and the lead dosage received by their milk source. Lead retention in both tissues was still evident at 100 days of age, with the elevation of lead levels being higher in brain than in blood. There was mild growth retardation in the group with the highest lead burden and a significant retardation in behavioral development in all the lead-exposed groups.

707. Lorton, Dianne & Anderson, William J. (1986). **The effects of postnatal lead toxicity on the development of cerebellum in rats.** *Neurobehavioral Toxicology & Teratology,* 8(1), 51–59.
Examined and quantified the morphologic changes in the cerebellar cortex and Purkinje cell dendritic development following neonatal lead exposure in male hooded Long-Evans rat pups. Ss were given 600 mg/kg lead acetate every 24 hrs beginning 1 day after birth until an accumulated dose of 2,400 mg/kg was achieved. Results indicate that lead exposure resulted in a significant decrease in molecular layer width and in a reduction in the dendritic arborization of Purkinje cells in the cerebellum.

708. Lorton, Dianne & Anderson, William J. (1986). **Altered pyramidal cell dendritic development in the motor cortex of lead intoxicated neonatal rats: A Golgi study.** *Neurobehavioral Toxicology & Teratology,* 8(1), 45–50.
Male Long-Evans hooded neonate pups were given lead acetate beginning 1 day after birth until a cumulative dose of 2,400 mg/kg had been administered. Brain tissue analysis showed that neonatal lead exposure altered the dendritic development of pyramidal cells of the motor cortex. It is suggested that findings could explain many behavioral alterations associated with lead intoxication (e.g., hyperactivity, increased aggressiveness); reduced complexity of neocortical structures might be responsible for the diminished learning capacities and reduced adaptive behavioral patterns observed following lead poisoning.

709. Lucchi, L. et al. (1981). **Chronic lead treatment induces in rat, a specific and differential effect on dopamine receptors in different brain areas.** *Brain Research,* 213(2), 397–404.
There is now evidence that 2 classes of dopaminergic receptors are present in CNS of the rat: D_1, associated, and D_2, not associated with adenylate cyclase activity. Drugs that interact specifically with D_2 receptor are more capable of antagonizing the hyperkinetic behavior induced by lead exposure in the rat. They also have a beneficial effect in children with hyperkinetic disorders. The present study, using Sprague-Dawley rats, found that the dose of levo-sulpirid that causes sedation was lower in lead-intoxicated Ss than in controls. In lead-exposed Ss, D_2 receptors, measured by levo-[3-H]sulpiride stereospecific binding, were altered while D_1 receptors seemed to be unaffected. The impairment of D_2 receptors might explain the better capacity of substituted benzamides to improve the hyperkinetic behavior observed in lead exposed Ss. (30 ref).

710. Magos, Laszlo. (1982). **Neurotoxicity, anorexia and the preferential choice of antidote in methylmercury intoxicated rats.** *Neurobehavioral Toxicology & Teratology,* 4(6), 643–646.
In a series of experiments with Porton-Wistar rats, the 1st clinical signs of methylmercury intoxication was loss of appetite, which was restored by the administration of dimercap-

tosuccinic acid (DMSA). In female Ss that lost body weight as a result of methylmercury treatment, the anorexic effect of methylmercury was reversed even when DMSA was given in the drinking water. When intoxicated Ss had the choice between DMSA supplemented water (2.5 mg DMSA/ml) and tap water, they preferred DMSA. This preference was related to the severity of intoxication and was abolished after 1–2 days. (24 ref).

711. Marquis, Karen L. (1985). **The effects of neonatal lead exposure on the discriminative stimulus properties of apomorphine and pentobarbital in rats.** *Dissertation Abstracts International,* 45(12-B, Pt 1), 3781.

712. Massaro, Thomas F.; Miller, Gregory D. & Massaro, Edward J. (1986). **Low-level lead exposure affects latent learning in the rat.** *Neurobehavioral Toxicology & Teratology,* 8(2), 109–113.
Neonatal Wistar rats were administered intragastrically either lead acetate (50 mg/kg) or an equal molar solution of sodium acetate at Days 6, 9, 12, 15, and 18 postpartum. At 33 days of age, each S began a training sequence to develop maze-running skills. Ss within each treatment group—lead exposed (Pb), control vehicle (CV), and control nonhandled (CNH)—were assigned randomly to either latent learning or open-field testing groups. The former individually explored a symmetrical maze while satiated; the latter were exposed to an apparatus devoid of barriers. All Ss were then food deprived and appetitively tested in the latent learning maze. The Pb, CV, and CNH Ss naive to the maze did not differ in maze performance. The CV and CNH Ss that previously experienced the maze committed fewer errors than nonexperienced counterparts. Pb-treated Ss showed no evidence of a positive transfer effect of their earlier experience. (35 ref).

713. McFarland, Dennis J. (1979). **Effects of neonatal lead exposure on learning and performance in the rat.** *Dissertation Abstracts International,* 40(2-B), 970–971.

714. Mele, Paul C.; Bushnell, Philip J. & Bowman, Robert E. (1984). **Prolonged behavioral effects of early postnatal lead exposure in rhesus monkeys: Fixed-interval responding and interactions with scopolamine and pentobarbital.** *Neurobehavioral Toxicology & Teratology,* 6(2), 129–135.
Lead acetate dissolved in milk was administered to 12 rhesus monkeys throughout the 1st yr of life. The doses of lead administered were 0.9 mg/kg/day (high lead group), 0.3 mg/kg/day (low lead group), and no added dietary lead (control group). These doses resulted in mean blood lead concentrations over the 1st year of 65, 32 and 4 μg/dl for the high lead, low lead, and control groups, respectively. Lead administration was terminated at the end of the 1st yr, and blood lead concentrations fell steadily over the next 44 mo. The effects of prior lead exposure on an FI schedule of food presentation were examined beginning at 33 mo of age. Acquisition of the barpress response varied widely among Ss, and no group differences were observed. Throughout 20 sessions of responding under an FI 60 sec food schedule, lead-treated Ss had a significantly lower index of curvature (IC) than controls, indicating a less pronounced positively accelerated pattern of responding. The magnitude and consistency of this effect were directly related to the dose of lead administered. Sodium pentobarbital (2.5–10 mg/kg, im) decreased IC and increased response rate; these effects were not altered by lead treatment. Scopolamine HBr (0.01–0.04 mg/kg) decreased IC and response rate in a dose-dependent manner. The low dose of scopolamine did not alter the IC in the high lead group but decreased the IC in the control group. Lead treatment did not alter response rate, running rate, pause duration, or the reduction in responding produced by extinction. (36 ref).

715. Merigan, William H. et al. (1983). **Neurotoxic actions of methylmercury on the primate visual system.** *Neurobehavioral Toxicology & Teratology,* 5(6), 649–658.
Studied visual system consequences of exposure to methylmercury in 6 adult female monkeys (*Macaca nemestrina* and *M. arctoides*). Visual field measures, visual thresholds, and morphological examination were used to determine the nature and possible reversibility of alterations in vision. Visual field constriction (especially in the inferior-nasal field) was an early and apparently reversible indicator of methylmercury intoxication. Findings support the conclusion that macaques provide a close model of visual toxicity of methylmercury in humans. (18 ref).

716. Michaelson, I. Arthur & Sauerhoff, Mitchell W. (1973). **The effect of chronically ingested inorganic lead on brain levels of Fe, Zn, Cu, and Mn of 25 day old rat.** *Life Sciences,* 13(5), 417-428.

717. Molfese, Dennis L.; Laughlin, Nellie K.; Morse, Philip A.; Linnville, Steven E. et al. (1986). **Neuroelectrical correlates of categorical perception for place of articulation in normal and lead-treated rhesus monkeys.** *Journal of Clinical & Experimental Neuropsychology,* 8(6), 680–696.
Evaluated categorical perception of place of articulation contrasts in 15 rhesus monkeys (*Macaca mulatta*). The Ss had been chronically exposed to subclinical levels of lead, either from conception to birth or for 6 mo beginning at birth, or were never exposed to lead. The brain responses recorded from the right hemisphere of the normal control group discriminated between the categories of [dae] and [gae]. Categorical discriminations were also noted for Ss exposed to lead over only the left hemisphere. Postnatal exposure resulted in categorical discrimination associated with slower latency components, suggesting a less mature pattern than that obtained for prenatally exposed Ss. Results suggest that the neurocortical mechanisms associated with categorical perception of place information may differ between human and nonhuman primates and that early exposure to lead alters these processes. (51 ref).

718. Morrison, John H.; Olton, David S.; Goldberg, Alan M. & Silbergeld, Ellen K. (1975). **Alterations in consummatory behavior of mice produced by dietary exposure to inorganic lead.** *Developmental Psychobiology,* 8(5), 389–396.
Mice suckled by 6 CD-1 mothers given tap water and by 6 mothers given a 5 mg/ml lead acetate solution during lactation were given a choice between tap water and a lead acetate solution after lactation. All offspring demonstrated an immediate aversion to the lead acetate solution. The offspring from the mothers receiving lead acetate during lactation demonstrated a greater aversion to the lead acetate solution than did the offspring from mothers receiving tap water. In addition, the lead acetate offspring drank more total fluid (tap water plus lead acetate solution) after weaning than the control offspring. Results indicate both learned and unlearned changes in motivation for fluid following ingestion of lead via the mother's milk in infancy. (19 ref).

719. Morse, Philip A.; Molfese, Dennis L.; Laughlin, Nellie K.; Linnville, Steven E. et al. (1987). **Categorical perception for voicing contrasts in normal and lead-treated rhesus monkeys: Electrophysiological indices.** *Brain & Language,* 30(1), 63–80.
Evaluated categorical perception of voicing contrasts in 15 rhesus monkeys (*Macaca mulatta*), chronically exposed to subclinical levels of lead either from conception to birth, for approximately 6 mo postnatally beginning at birth, or never exposed to lead. Auditory evoked responses were recorded at 1 yr of age from scalp electrodes placed over the left and right hemispheres during stimulus presentation. A late component of the brain responses recorded from the right tempo-

METALLIC ELEMENTS

ral region of all Ss discriminated between stimuli in a categorical manner. Results suggest that the neurocortical mechanisms associated with categorical perception for voicing information may be similar across human and nonhuman primates. It is suggested that early exposure to lead alters these processes. (51 ref).

720. Munoz, Carmen; Garbe, Kurt; Lilienthal, Hellmuth & Winneke, Gerhard. (1988). **Significance of hippocampal dysfunction in low level lead exposure of rats.** *Neurobehavioral Toxicology & Teratology,* 10(3), 245–253.
Rats maternally and permanently exposed to lead (750 ppm in the diet as lead acetate) were tested in a radial arm maze and compared with controls and rats with ibotenic acid-induced neuronal depletion in the dorsal hippocampus. Lead-exposed groups showed an impairment in the acquisition performance of the spatial task while hippocampally damaged Ss did not.

721. Nation, Jack R.; Baker, Dorothy M.; Bratton, Gerald R.; Fantasia, Martha A. et al. (1987). **Ethanol self-administration in rats following exposure to dietary cadmium.** *Neurotoxicology & Teratology,* 9(5), 339–344.
Investigated the toxicologic effects of cadmium on stress reactions in 12 adult male rats. Ss were maintained on an ad lib diet containing cadmium or a control diet with no added cadmium. After 55 days of exposure to their respective diets, Ss were tested for fluid intake, using a nonchoice procedure that presented a 15% ethanol solution in the home cage for 5 days. Subsequently, all Ss were offered a 10% ethanol solution or tap water in a 3-bottle, 2-fluid choice test in the home cage. Results show that ethanol intake was greater for Ss exposed to cadmium on all tests of fluid consumption, and all Ss consumed more ethanol during the periods following termination of the stressor (avoidance extinction, postavoidance) than during the actual period of stress (avoidance acquisition). The effects of cadmium on stress reactivity, sensory processing, and metabolism are discussed.

722. Nation, Jack R.; Bourgeois, Anthony E. & Clark, Donald E. (1983). **Behavioral effects of chronic lead exposure in the adult rat.** *Pharmacology, Biochemistry & Behavior,* 18(6), 833–840.
Adult male Sprague-Dawley rats fed daily rations of lab chow laced with lead acetate were tested for operant responding and conditioned suppression. In Exp I, Ss receiving 10 mg/kg lead showed significantly lower response rates (leverpressing) than controls. Conditioned suppression performance was not different between groups. During retraining that followed a 42-day no-training period, lead-treated Ss showed greater percent of prior baseline responding than controls. The groups were not different on a test for stimulus control or appetitive resistance to extinction. In Exp II, separate lead-treated groups were chronically exposed to either 10, 5, or 1 mg/kg lead daily. Behavioral tests showed that while the lowest lead level occasioned higher rates of operant leverpressing relative to controls, the highest level again produced lower rates. On a retraining task administered after an interpolated 90-day no-training period, the 2 highest exposure groups were significantly above controls in percent of baseline responding, and there was evidence that the 5-mg/kg group was significantly superior to controls in terms of absolute response rate. (27 ref).

723. Nation, Jack R.; Baker, Dorothy M.; Taylor, Betty & Clark, Donald E. (1986). **Dietary lead increases ethanol consumption in the rat.** *Behavioral Neuroscience,* 100(4), 525–530.
When 36 male Sprague-Dawley rats fed either a diet containing 500 parts per million Pb (as lead acetate) or an unadulterated control diet for 50 days were offered a 15% ethanol (ETOH) solution in a nonchoice (1-bottle) test situation, Pb-diet Ss consumed greater amounts of the ETOH solution than did controls. In a subsequent choice (3-bottle, 2-fluid) test situation offering a nonpreferred ETOH solution or tap water as alternatives, Pb-diet Ss again ingested greater amounts of the ETOH solution. Findings are discussed in terms of possible Pb-induced increases in emotionality and the potential stress-reduction properties of ETOH. (23 ref).

724. Nation, Jack R.; Wellman, Paul J.; von Stultz, Jeannine; Taylor, Betty et al. (1988). **Cadmium exposure results in decreased responsiveness to ethanol.** *Alcohol,* 5(2), 99–102.
Adult male rats were maintained on a diet containing cadmium (Cd) or a control diet with no added Cd. Cd-treated adult males injected with ethyl alcohol, ip, regained the righting reflex significantly more rapidly than did controls.

725. Niklowitz, Werner J. & Yeager, David W. (1973). **Interference of Pb with essential brain tissue Cu, Fe, and Zn as main determinant in experimental tetraethyllead encephalopathy.** *Life Sciences,* 13(7), 897–905.
Found that after exposure of male New Zealand White rabbits to tetraethyllead, each analyzed brain area (frontal cortex, cerebellum, hippocampus) contained approximately 33 mg/gm lead. At the same time, there was a statistically significant loss in the same brain areas of the essential elements, copper, iron, and zinc. While the molar ratio between gain of lead and decrease of copper revealed an approximate proportionality of 1:1, the ratio between lead and iron was approximately 1:2. The decrease of zinc levels varied in these brain areas and was lowest in the inferior hippocampus. The potentiality of an interference of lead with essential trace metals of the brain, preferentially with the metal group of metalloenzymes, as the primary and dominant mechanism of the toxic action of lead in lead encephalopathy, is discussed. (21 ref).

726. Noland, Elizabeth A.; Taylor, Douglas H. & Bull, R. J. (1982). **Monomethyl- and trimethyltin compounds induce learning deficiencies in young rats.** *Neurobehavioral Toxicology & Teratology,* 4(5), 539–544.
Male Sprague-Dawley rat pups were exposed to monomethyltin trichloride (MMTC) and trimethyltin chloride (TMTC) via their dams' drinking water throughout gestation and postpartum until 21 days of age. At 11 days of age, Ss were tested for acquisition and extinction learning in an appetitive paradigm, and at 21 days for learning ability in a 1-trial swim escape test. At 11 days, Ss from dams exposed to 120 mg/l of tin as MMTC and to 1.0 mg/l as TMTC displayed statistically significant increases in acquisition time, while all dose groups (12, 40, 120 mg/l MMTC and 0.15, 0.5, 1.0 mg/l TMTC) displayed significant decreases in extinction learning ability as compared to controls. At 21 days of age, Ss exposed to 12 and 120 mg/l MMTC displayed higher escape times than controls, as did Ss exposed to 0.5 mg/l TMTC. (35 ref).

727. Null, David H.; Gartside, Peter S. & Wei, Eddie. (1973). **Methylmercury accumulation in brains of pregnant, non-pregnant and fetal rats.** *Life Sciences,* 12(2, Pt. 2), 65–72.

728. O'Kusky, J. R. & McGeer, E. G. (1985). **Methylmercury poisoning of the developing nervous system in the rat: Decreased activity of glutamic acid decarboxylase in cerebral cortex and neostriatum.** *Developmental Brain Research,* 21(2), 299–306.
Investigated the specific activities of glutamic acid decarboxylase (GAD) and choline acetyltransferase (ChAT) in 6 regions of the central nervous system (CNS) of 18 Sprague-Dawley rat pups following chronic postnatal administration of methylmercuric chloride (5 mg Hg/kg). Ss exhibited signs of neurological impairment that included visual deficits, ataxia, spasticity, and myoclonus. Preceding the onset of neurological impairment, diminished GAD activity was detected only in

the occipital cortex. In the cerebellum, thalamus, and spinal cord, GAD activities were normal throughout the experiment. No significant differences in ChAT activity were detected in any of the 6 regions. (44 ref).

729. O'Kusky, John R.; Boyes, Barry E. & McGeer, Edith G. (1988). **Methylmercury-induced movement and postural disorders in developing rat: Regional analysis of brain catecholamines and indoleamines.** *Brain Research,* 439(1–2), 138–146.
Administration of methylmercury (MeHg) sc to rats during early postnatal development resulted in movement and postural disorders by Days 22–24. Findings indicate altered metabolism in aromatic amine systems in the developing central nervous system (CNS) during the pathogenesis of MeHg-induced movement and postural disorder.

730. O'Kusky, John R.; Radke, James M. & Vincent, Steven R. (1988). **Methylmercury-induced movement and postural disorders in developing rat: Loss of somatostatin-immunoreactive interneurons in the striatum.** *Developmental Brain Research,* 40(1), 11–23.
Measured tissue concentrations of the neuropeptide somatostatin and the activities of glutamic acid decarboxylase in the central nervous system (CNS) of young rats, following chronic postnatal administration of methylmercuric chloride. With the 4th postnatal week, Ss exhibited signs of a mixed spastic/dyskinetic syndrome with visual deficits.

731. Oskarsson, Agneta; Ljungberg, Tomas; Ståhle, Lars; Tossman, Ulf et al. (1986). **Behavioral and neurochemical effects after combined perinatal treatment of rats with lead and disulfiram.** *Neurobehavioral Toxicology & Teratology,* 8(5), 591–599.
Pregnant Sprague-Dawley rats were treated with lead (0.25% in the drinking water), disulfiram (0.1 mmol/kg twice a week), or with both lead and disulfiram from Day 1 of pregnancy until parturition. After parturition, the offspring were exposed to lead via the milk of the dams; the disulfiram was given directly to the offspring. Two weeks after weaning, neither lead alone nor disulfiram alone caused significant effects in the behavior-activity measurements. However, the combination of the compounds increased home-cage activity and behavioral reactivity. Levels of dopamine were significantly increased in both the lead-treated and the lead-plus-disulfiram groups. Analyses revealed that the increased lead level in brain found after combined treatment with lead and disulfiram was associated with pronounced effects on behavior and on extracellular levels of neurotransmitters and amino acids in brain. This interaction should be taken into consideration when evaluating the health effects of environmental and occupational exposure of both lead and dithiocarbamate derivatives.

732. Overmann, Stephen R. (1976). **Behavioral effects of asymptomatic developmental plumbism in rats.** *Dissertation Abstracts International,* 37(2-B), 1010–1011.

733. Padich, Robert & Zenick, Harold. (1977). **The effects of developmental and/or direct lead exposure on FR behavior in the rat.** *Pharmacology, Biochemistry & Behavior,* 6(4), 371–375.
20 21-day-old female CD rats were exposed to daily doses of 750 mg/kg of lead acetate via a restricted water intake regimen for 70–80 days prior to mating. Treatment was then continued throughout gestation and nursing. At weaning, litters from half the treated and control mothers were placed on similar lead treatment regimens for the remainder of the experiment. This manipulation yielded 4 groups for testing: (a) developmental and direct postweaning exposure (Group Pb/Pb); (b) developmental exposure only; (c) direct exposure only; and (d) no exposure. Beginning at 42–49 days of age, offspring were shaped to barpress on an FR-20 reinforcement schedule, and 20 20-min sessions were conducted. Group Pb/Pb received significantly fewer reinforcements per minute across sessions than the other 3 groups and also took significantly longer to emit each 20-response block. Contrary to previous reports, it is suggested that rats may not be impervious to postweaning lead exposure, particularly when there is a history of developmental exposure. (20 ref).

734. Patton, Jim H. (1979). **The behavioral and physiological effects of administering lead to neonatal rats: A test of the model of childhood hyperactivity.** *Dissertation Abstracts International,* 39(11-B), 5635.

735. Rafales, Lee S. et al. (1979). **Drug induced activity in lead-exposed mice.** *Pharmacology, Biochemistry & Behavior,* 10(1), 95–104.
Three interrelated studies were conducted to examine the locomotor activity of lead-exposed CD-1 mice. The effects of lead were examined as a function of the dose and duration of exposure. Exposure during the 1st 3 wks occurred via the maternal milk supply. Exposure following weaning was achieved via the water supply. Ss received challenges with various pharmaceutical agents, including dextroamphetamine, methylphenidate, apomorphine, and phenobarbital. Spontaneous activity prior to injection and drug-induced activity were monitored. Lead-exposed Ss usually displayed spontaneous activity that was indistinguishable from that of the controls. In only one set of observations did lead exposure result in a modest increase in spontaneous activity. The drug-induced activity varied in a complex manner as a function of the magnitude and duration of the lead exposure. Depressed body weight, which was concurrent with high lead exposure (0.5%), was also a significant parameter affecting both the spontaneous and drug-induced activity. (26 ref).

736. Rice, Deborah C. (1987). **Methodological approaches to primate behavioral toxicological testing.** First Joint International Union of Toxicology and Italian Society of Toxicology Symposium: Behavioral toxicology: New experimental approaches (1986, Bari, Italy). *Neurotoxicology & Teratology,* 9(2), 161–169.
Investigated the effects of low-level developmental exposure to neurotoxicants in the cynomolgus monkey (*Macaca fascicularis*), using operant conditioning techniques to detect subtle defects. Such intellectual functions as learning, memory, adaptability, and distractibility were explored. Findings reveal impairment produced by lead similar to that observed in lead-exposed children; visual deficits produced by methylmercury were revealed by psychophysical techniques, in the absence of any obvious signs of toxicity.

737. Rice, Deborah C. & Karpinski, K. F. (1988). **Lifetime low-level lead exposure produces deficits in delayed alternation in adult monkeys.** *Neurobehavioral Toxicology & Teratology,* 10(3), 207–214.
Cynomolgus monkeys were dosed continuously from birth to age 200 days with 100, 50, or 0 µg/kg/day of lead. At 7 to 8 yrs of age, Ss were tested on a delayed alternation task. After each S learned the task, a delay was instituted between trials. Treated Ss were impaired in their ability to learn the alternation task but were not different from controls at short delay values (1 and 3 sec). At longer delay values (5 and 15 sec), treated Ss again exhibited impairment. Treated Ss were also more variable in their performance across sessions than were controls. Data are interpreted as indicative of spatial learning and short-term memory deficits in the lead-exposed Ss.

738. Richer, Connie A. (1984). **Classical conditioning, Fuller Brain Weight mice, and low-level neonatal lead exposure.** *Dissertation Abstracts International,* 45(5-B), 1620.

METALLIC ELEMENTS

739. Rius, R. A.; Lucchi, L.; Govoni, S. & Trabucchi, Marco. (1984). **In vivo chronic lead exposure alters [^{3}H]nitrendipine binding in rat striatum.** *Brain Research,* 322(1), 180–183.
Pregnant Sprague-Dawley rats received lead acetate solution (2.5 g/l; 1360 ppm lead) or sodium acetate as a control in their drinking water, and their offspring at 21 days received the same drinking solution as their mothers. Brain membrane analysis at 6 wks of age showed that in vitro, lead shared the action of calcium in enhancing [^{3}H]NDP binding, although it was more potent on a molar basis. In vivo, lead exposure through drinking water enhanced [^{3}H]NDP binding to crude synaptosomal membrane preparations. Findings indicate that the increased binding was due to the persistence of lead in the brain of treated Ss. (23 ref).

740. Roginski, Edward T. (1983). **The effect of neonatal lead treatment on rat brain enolase activity.** *Dissertation Abstracts International,* 44(3-B), 759.

741. Rosen, Jeffrey B.; Berman, Robert F.; Beuthin, Frederic C. & Louis-Ferdinand, Robert T. (1985). **Age of testing as a factor in the behavioral effects of early lead exposure in rats.** *Pharmacology, Biochemistry & Behavior,* 23(1), 49–54.
Long-Evans hooded rats received intraperitoneal injections of either 10 mg/kg lead acetate or equimolar sodium acetate daily for the 1st 20 days of life, and tests of performance on an 8-arm radial maze and a passive avoidance task were begun at either 25 or 90 days after birth. Findings indicate that lead-treated (LT) Ss did not perform significantly differently from controls (CTRs) on the radial arm maze at either age. Young LT Ss performed with significantly longer lick latencies than young CTRs on the passive avoidance task. Adult LT Ss performed with shorter food latencies than adult CTRs. Performance of a group of young Ss retested on the passive avoidance task at 150 days after birth was similar to their early performance. (31 ref).

742. Rosen, Jeffrey B.; Young, Alice M.; Beuthin, Frederic C. & Louis-Ferdinand, Robert T. (1986). **Discriminative stimulus properties of amphetamine and other stimulants in lead-exposed and normal rats.** *Pharmacology, Biochemistry & Behavior,* 24(2), 211–215.
Examined the discriminative stimulus properties of amphetamine (AMP) at progressively lower doses in 4 lead-exposed (10 mg/kg/day, ages 1–20 days) and 4 normal male Long-Evans rats. Generalization gradients of AMP (0.032–1.0 mg/kg), apomorphine (0.01–0.18 mg/kg), methylphenidate (0.1–10 mg/kg), and caffeine (1 mg/kg) to both high and low training doses of AMP were also determined. Under the high AMP training dose condition (1.0 mg/kg), generalization gradients of AMP were similar for lead-exposed and control Ss. When the training doses were progressively lowered, the lead-exposed Ss tended to require a higher range of AMP doses (0.24–0.49 mg/kg) than did controls (0.18–0.32 mg/kg) to maintain discriminative control. The minimal discriminable doses tended to be higher for lead-exposed Ss than for controls. Methylphenidate generalization gradients were different for lead-exposed and control Ss under the high AMP training condition but became similar under the low AMP training condition. No differences attributable to training dose or lead exposure were evident for apomorphine or caffeine. (24 ref).

743. Rosenthal, Eugene. (1974). **The effect of methylmercury dicyandiamide, administered during embryogenesis, upon the development of the young chicken.** *Dissertation Abstracts International,* 34(11-B), 5662.

744. Royalty, Joel; Taylor, G. T. & Korol, B. A. (1987). **The effects of prenatal exposure to methylmercury on aggressive behavior in the rat.** *Neurotoxicology & Teratology,* 9(2), 87–93.
Assessed the sensitivity of isolation-induced aggressive behavior to prenatal treatment of 6.0 mg/kg methylmercuric chloride (MMCl) by gavage on gestation days 6–9 in a subset of rats from the J. Adams et al (1986) collaborative behavioral teratology study (CBTS). 12 males and 12 females were assigned to each of 4 treatment conditions: high MMCl, low MMCl, vehicle control, and no treatment control. CBTS behavioral measures consisted of negative geotaxis, olfactory discrimination, auditory startle habituation, 1-hr activity, 23-hr activity, activity following pharmacological challenge, and visual discrimination learning. Auditory startle was the only CBTS behavioral measure that discriminated among prenatal treatment groups. Results suggest that tests of aggressive behavior should be considered in the formulation of behavioral screening paradigms.

745. Salvaterra, Paul; Lown, Bradley; Morganti, John & Massaro, Edward J. (1973). **Alterations in neurochemical and behavioural parameters in the mouse induced by low doses of methyl mercury.** *Acta Pharmacologica et Toxicologica,* 33(3), 177–190.
Studied the open field behavior of male Swiss-Webster mice after controlled single doses of methyl mercury (MeHg) (1, 5, 10 mg/kg) at varying times after intraperitoneal injection (1, 3, 72 hrs). In an effort to correlate behavioral and biochemical data, the effects of dose and time after dose on the levels of selected glycolytic pathway intermediates, alpha-glycerophosphate, adenine nucleotides, and phosphocreatine were monitored. A good correlation between brain biochemistry and behavioral effects of MeHg was observed: The dose-response relationship for the open field task correlated with alterations in levels of metabolic intermediates. At 1 and 3 hrs after administration of MeHg, when the levels of the metabolic intermediates were significantly different from those of controls, altered behavior was observed. At 72 hrs post administration, when the biological parameters were approaching control values, a return to normal behavior was observed. (48 ref).

746. Schalock, Robert L.; Brown, W. J.; Kark, R. A. & Menon, N. K. (1981). **Perinatal methylmercury intoxication: Behavioral effects in rats.** *Developmental Psychobiology,* 14(3), 213–219.
32 Sprague-Dawley rats were subjected to perinatal methylmercury intoxication (10 mg/kg) to determine the long-term behavioral effect of the mercury poisoning. Experimental and control Ss were evaluated at 110–140 days of age. ANOVAs revealed that, compared to controls, Ss treated with methylmercury demonstrated significant behavioral deficits characterized by hypoactivity and by reduced appetitive, escape, and avoidance learning. (12 ref).

747. Schmidt, James C. & Czech, Donald A. (1977). **Effect of tetraethyl lead and restricted food intake on locomotor activity in the rat.** *Pharmacology, Biochemistry & Behavior,* 7(6), 489–492.
Investigated the effect of tetraethyl lead (TEL) and restricted food intake on spontaneous locomotor activity in 80 male Sprague-Dawley albino rats. 40 Ss were injected ip with 4, 7, 10, or 13 mg/kg TEL in peanut oil, or a peanut oil placebo. 40 Ss were food yoked to TEL Ss as a control procedure to hold food intake constant between lead-treated and lead-free Ss. A comparison of pre- and posttreatment measures revealed significant decreases in food intake and increases in activity levels at dosages of 7, 10, and 13 mg/kg TEL. In addition, food intake and activity were significantly correlated in both lead-treated and yoked groups. The issue of factors associated with reduced food intake playing a role in observed activity level increases is raised. (15 ref).

748. Schnell, R. C.; Prosser, T. D. & Miya, T. S. (1974). **Cadmium-induced potentiation of hexobarbital sleep time in rats.** *Experientia,* 30(5), 528-529.
Attempted to determine the minimum effective dose of cadmium required to potentiate drug response and the peak time for this phenomenon. Cadmium was administered as the acetate salt to male Sprague-Dawley rats, while control rats received a volume-equivalent injection of saline. Eight control Ss and 33 Ss that were administered varying doses of cadmium acetate were monitored. In Exp I, the minimum dosage required to prolong hexobarbital sleep time was 2.0 mg/kg. In Exp II, the sleep times of all cadmium-dosed Ss were significantly prolonged when compared to controls. Implications for the issue of cadmium as an industrial pollutant are discussed. It is concluded that in any attempt to link contaminants with biological response and environmental exposure, the dose-response relationship between contaminant and specific biological changes must be established. (German summary).

749. Schreiner, Gerd; Ulbrich, Beate & Bass, Rolf. (1986). **Testing strategies in behavioral teratology: II. Discrimination learning.** *Neurobehavioral Toxicology & Teratology,* 8(5), 567-572.
Male and female Wistar rats exposed to methylmercury chloride prenatally via drinking water (1.5 and 5.0 mg/l) were tested in a microcomputer-directed learning task (visual discrimination reversal) at the age of 2 mo. Differences were observed between controls and high-dose Ss for several parameters, especially an increase in passivity and in response latency and a decrease in intertrial interval response rates in the methylmercury group. Females showed longer response latencies, and passivity scores were somewhat higher than in males.

750. Schwark, Wayne S.; Haluska, Marianne; Powell, Kelly & Blackshear, Pamela. (1983). **Lead intoxication and the amygdaloid kindling model of epileptogenesis in the adult rat.** *Neurobehavioral Toxicology & Teratology,* 5(3), 325-329.
Male Sprague-Dawley rats' exposure to 1% lead (in the form of lead acetate) in drinking water for periods up to 4 wks led to significant increases in lead content in the blood and various brain regions. Signs of lead intoxication, including behavioral depression, loss of body weight, and decreased hematocrit were produced by this treatment regime. The intensity and nature of behavioral convulsions as well as the rate of development of amygdaloid kindled seizures did not appear to be affected by lead intoxication. However, lead exposure during kindling led to significant increases in an electrographic aspect of the seizure, i.e., the afterdischarge duration. (31 ref).

751. Schwartz, Arthur S. & Marchok, Patricia L. (1975). **The influence of early lead exposure on morphine reinforcement in the rat.** *Drug & Alcohol Dependence,* 1(2), 97-102.
Investigated the effect of early lead burdens on morphine-seeking behavior in the albino rat. Several concentrations of lead acetate were administered to nursing mothers starting at 0, 7, or 14 days after birth, or provided directly to their 103 pups in the drinking water after weaning, so that lead exposure was continuous for 3 successive weeks in each group. The offspring were later tested for acquisition and maintenance of a goal-box preference based on morphine reinforcement. High lead burdens imposed before the 2nd wk of age resulted in a mild but significantly greater incidence of morphine-seeking responses, as well as retarded growth, compared with placebo-treated controls or Ss treated at a later age. Data support the proposition that lead, introduced at a critical stage of development via the lactating mother, increases the potency of morphine reinforcement as a result of changes in cerebral dopaminergic activity. This effect may be mediated directly by the high lead burdens in the offspring or indirectly by interfering with the mother's nursing capacity. (21 ref).

752. Shapiro, Martin M.; Tritschler, J. M. & Ulm, Ronald A. (1973). **Lead contamination: Chronic and acute behavioral effects in the albino rat.** *Bulletin of the Psychonomic Society,* 2(2), 94-96.
Trained 14 male albino rats on an operant discrimination and subjected them daily to a low level of lead contamination. Chronic contamination increased the variability of the discrimination behavior. Increased contamination produced an acute shift in the distribution of interresponse times.

753. Shih, Tsung-ming; Khachaturian, Zaven S. & Hanin, Israel. (1977). **Involvement of both cholinergic and catecholaminergic pathways in the central action of methylphenidate: A study utilizing lead-exposed rats.** *Psychopharmacology,* 55(2), 187-193.
The effects of methylphenidate (MPH) and the cholinergic agonists nicotine and oxotremorine were tested on the spontaneous multiple unit activity in the mesencephalic reticular formation of 2 groups of Sprague-Dawley rats. Data support previous evidence that MPH exerts its action in the CNS by a cholinergic pathway in addition to catecholaminergic pathways. Findings also indicate that chronic lead-exposure in rats results in cholinergic hypofunction and supersensitivity at central cholinergic receptor sites. This alteration of central cholinergic function may be partially attributed to the malnutrition observed in the lead-exposed animals.

754. Silbergeld, Ellen K. & Goldberg, Alan M. (1973). **A lead-induced behavioral disorder.** *Life Sciences,* 13(9), 1275-1283.
Exposed Charles River CD-1 mice to lead from birth by substituting solutions of lead acetate (2, 5, and 10 mg/ml) for the drinking water of mice 12 hrs after parturition. Controls received equal concentrations of sodium acetate. There were no deaths in mothers or offspring due to treatment, but growth and development were retarded in the lead-treated offspring. It has recently been suggested that lead exposure may account for some incidences of hyperactivity and retardation in children. Activity of offspring was measured between 40 and 60 days of age for 4 consecutive days. Treated Ss were more than 3 times as active as age-matched controls. These studies show that chronic ingestion of lead can produce a significant behavior disorder in mice.

755. Silbergeld, Ellen K. & Goldberg, Alan M. (1974). **Lead-induced behavioral dysfunction: An animal model of hyperactivity.** *Experimental Neurology,* 42(1), 146-157.
Developed an animal model of lead poisoning in which suckling CD-1 mice were exposed to lead acetate from birth indirectly through their mothers and then directly after weaning. For the 1st 60 days, no deaths of offspring occurred due to lead but growth and development were significantly retarded. Activity was measured between 40 and 60 days of age. Treated Ss were more than 3 times as active as age-matched controls. Treated and control Ss were given drugs used in the treatment and diagnosis of minimal brain dysfunction hyperactivity in children: dextro- and levoamphetamine, methylphenidate, phenobarbital, and chloral hydrate. Lead-treated hyperactive Ss responded paradoxically to all drugs except chloral hydrate: The amphetamines and methylphenidate suppressed hyperactivity, while phenobarbital increased levels of motor activity. Chloral hydrate was an effective sedative. Implications for the study of the central effects of lead poisoning and for the relationship between lead poisoning and minimal brain dysfunction hyperactivity are discussed. (42 ref).

756. Silbergeld, Ellen K. & Lamon, Joel M. (1982). **Effects of altered porphyrin synthesis on brain neurochemistry.** *Neurobehavioral Toxicology & Teratology,* 4(6), 635-642.
The effects of acute and chronic exposure to lead in Sprague-Dawley rats on porphyrin metabolism and on neurochemistry and behavior were compared to the effects associated with

METALLIC ELEMENTS

exposure to the "suicide" inhibitor of aminolevulinic acid dehydrase, succinylacetone. Assessment included neurochemical and behavioral measures of GABAergic function, seizure threshold, and hexobarbital sleeping time. Similarities in both porphyrinopathy and in associated neurotoxicity suggest an etiologic role for altered porphyrin synthesis in lead neurotoxicity. (53 ref).

757. Smith, Mark J.; Pihl, Robert O. & Farrell, Brian. (1985). **Longterm effects of early cadmium exposure on locomotor activity in the rat.** *Neurobehavioral Toxicology & Teratology,* 7(1), 19–22.
Investigated the hypothesis that changes in the frequency of specific behaviors, not assessed by the traditionally employed global measures of locomotor activity, may occur following exposure to cadmium ($CdCl_2$). 23 newborn male Sprague-Dawley rat pups were treated orally with either 1 mg/kg of $CdCl_2$ for 14 days or 10 mg/kg $CdCl_2$ for 1 day followed by 13 days of the treatment vehicle only. A control group of 14 male Ss received only the vehicle. At 50 days of age, Ss were observed in their home cage for 12 hrs, and the amount of time spent engaged in each of 8 separate categories of behavior was recorded. Subsequently, exploratory behavior in an open field was assessed. The single large dose of cadmium resulted in weight loss and a significantly slower growth rate but did not result in any significant changes in behavior. Ss administered the lower treatment dose exhibited significantly increased rearing in the home cage and significantly decreased inner square exploratory behavior in the open field. Implications of emotional hyporeactivity and physiological explanations that may account for the differences observed between the 2 treatment regimens are discussed. (23 ref).

758. Snowdon, Charles T. (1973). **Learning deficits in lead-injected rats.** *Pharmacology, Biochemistry & Behavior,* 1(6), 599-603.
56 weanling and 56 adult Sprague-Dawley rats injected with 1 of 3 concentrations of lead acetate for 37 days failed to demonstrate any learning impairments as measured by a Hebb-Williams maze series relative to water injected controls. Ss at the highest dose level showed clear symptoms of lead poisoning. 17 pregnant female Holtzman rats injected during pregnancy with an asymptomatic dose of lead acetate showed a 100% abortion rate, while 75% of 16 water injected controls delivered litters. 36 rat pups whose mothers were injected with asymptomatic doses of lead acetate throughout nursing developed more slowly, weighed less, and demonstrated learning deficits relative to 26 controls. It is concluded that behavioral and physiological effects of lead may be greatest during the earliest developmental stages. (20 ref).

759. Snowdon, Charles T. (1977). **A nutritional basis for lead pica.** *Physiology & Behavior,* 18(5), 885–893.
Lead pica is a behavioral phenomenon involving continued voluntary ingestion of a toxic substance. In 5 experiments, calcium deficiency produced an elevated proportion of lead ingestion in weanling CFE rats, while magnesium and zinc deficiency produced proportional levels of lead ingestion intermediate to control and calcium deficient Ss. Partial restoration of calcium did not eliminate the increased proportion of lead ingestion while full calcium restoration did. Calcium deficient Ss offered lead to drink gained more weight than deficient Ss not offered lead. Controls showed a reduction in novel solutions ingested following intubation of lead acetate, while calcium deficient Ss did not. Ss deficient in calcium, iron, and zinc also showed elevated proportional levels of quinine sulfate ingestion compared to controls, suggesting that a pica may be a general response to nutritional deficiency. The increased proportion of lead ingestion by calcium, zinc, and magnesium deficient Ss and the failure of calcium deficient Ss to form a learned aversion to lead acetate suggests that mineral deficiency may be a major factor in producing lead pica. (35 ref).

760. Snowdon, Charles T. & Sanderson, Blythe A. (1974). **Lead pica produced in rats.** *Science,* 183(4120), 92-94.
Results of a study with 97 Sprague-Dawley weanling rats show that Ss eating a low calcium diet voluntarily ingested lead acetate solutions in much greater proportions than did iron-deficient or control Ss. This increased ingestion occurred even with high concentrations of lead acetate, which normal Ss found extremely aversive. Chronic injections of lead acetate did not change lead ingestion, indicating an absence of behavioral regulation of body lead levels. Lead-injected females did show a significant increase in calcium ingestion, indicating that calcium deficiency may be 1 component of lead pica. (19 ref).

761. Sobotka, Thomas J. & Cook, Michelle P. (1974). **Postnatal lead acetate exposure in rats: Possible relationship to minimal brain dysfunction.** *American Journal of Mental Deficiency,* 79(1), 5-9.
Male Sprague-Dawley rats receiving oral doses of lead acetate during their 3-wk postnatal development exhibited pharmacobehavioral characteristics similar to those of the minimally brain-dysfunctioned child: altered responsiveness to amphetamine, poor learning performance, and alleviation of this poor performance by amphetamine treatment. Data suggest that prenatal lead exposure may be etiologically related to variants of minimal brain dysfunction.

762. Spence, Ian; Drew, Colleen; Johnston, Graham A. & Lodge, David. (1985). **Acute effects of lead at central synapses in vitro.** *Brain Research,* 333(1), 103–109.
Studied the acute effects of lead in the rat CNS on transmitter release at central synapses in vitro in the isolated hemisected spinal cord from newborn rats and on the transport of exogenous GABA, acetylcholine, and cis-3-aminocyclohexane carboxylic acid from slices of cerebral cortex from adult rats. Results indicate that under the appropriate conditions, lead can inhibit CNS synaptic function in a manner consistent with lead competing with calcium ions in transmitter-release processes, as has been established for acetylcholine release at peripheral synapses. The diffuse and nonspecific symptoms seen in cases of acute lead poisoning (e.g., arouseness, tremor, sleeping difficulties) may be attributable to its ability to reduce or alter uptake mechanisms at a number of central synapses. (22 ref).

763. Stineman, Carl H. (1980). **Studies on behavioral alterations and tissue distribution following cerium or platinum exposure in mice.** *Dissertation Abstracts International,* 41(2-B), 556.

764. Suter, Kurt E. & Schön, H. (1986). **Testing strategies in behavioral teratology: I. Testing battery approach.** *Neurobehavioral Toxicology & Teratology,* 8(5), 561–566.
Female rats were given drinking water containing 1.5, 5, or 15 mg/l methylmercury chloride from 2 wks prior to pairing until the end of the lactation period. The morphological, functional, and behavioral development of the offspring was assessed. Results demonstrate that a routine testing battery can detect behavioral effects in the offspring at a dose where no reproduction effects are observed.

765. Swartzwelder, H. S. et al. (1982). **Impaired maze performance in the rat caused by trimethyltin treatment: Problem-solving deficits and perseveration.** *Neurobehavioral Toxicology & Teratology,* 4(2), 169–176.
Either 7.0 mg/kg of trimethyltin (TMT) or 0.9% saline was injected into the gastric lumen of 18 male Long-Evans rats. Treated and nontreated Ss were tested subsequently on a series of maze problems. In comparison to controls, tin-treated Ss made markedly more errors on all but one of the maze patterns. The rate of error reduction across problems over the 10 daily trials was significantly retarded in hippocampal-lesioned Ss. In addition to these severe problem-solving defi-

cits, TMT-treated Ss often exhibited a characteristic pattern of perseverative behavior while running in the maze. The pattern was not unlike stereotypies associated with the psychomotor pathology observed following treatment with certain drugs. Parallels are noted between the TMT syndrome in rats and minimal brain dysfunction syndrome in humans. (29 ref).

766. Taylor, D. H. et al. (1982). **Low level lead (Pb) exposure produces learning deficits in young rat pups.** *Neurobehavioral Toxicology & Teratology,* 4(3), 311–314.
23 11-day-old Sprague-Dawley (CD strain) rat pups whose mothers were maintained on a 200 mg/l dosage of Pb acetate in their drinking water, from breeding and through gestation until the pups were weaned, exhibited differences in a learning paradigm as compared to 18 controls. No significant differences were noted between controls and experimentals with respect to acquisition rates, but there were significant differences between the 2 groups in extinction rates. Similar results were obtained in tests of 21 Ss whose dams had been maintained on a 400 mg/l dosage of Pb acetate. Data suggest that low-level Pb exposure can induce significant behavioral deficits in young rat pups. (14 ref).

767. Thorne, B. Michael et al. (1986). **Aluminum ingestion and behavior in the Long-Evans rat.** *Physiology & Behavior,* 36(1), 63–67.
32 adult Long-Evans male rats were fed ground rat chow containing either no added aluminum, low aluminum (1.5 g/kg), moderate aluminum (2.5 g/kg), or high aluminum (3.5 g/kg). There were no effects of aluminum on either body weight or mouse killing. There was an inverse relationship between brain aluminum and open-field activity. Elevated brain aluminum was correlated with relatively poor performance on a single-trial, passive-avoidance task and on a visual discrimination with reversal task. The high concentration of aluminum found in hippocampal tissue is discussed in relation to findings in patients with Alzheimer's disease. (24 ref).

768. Thorne, B. Michael; Cook, Art; Donohoe, Tim; Lyon, Steve et al. (1987). **Aluminum toxicity and behavior in the weanling Long-Evans rat.** *Bulletin of the Psychonomic Society,* 25(2), 129–132.
Studied muricidal behavior, weight changes, brain aluminum content, fluid intake, open-field activity, passive-avoidance learning, and learning of an 8-arm radial maze by 15 male Long-Evans hooded rats subjected as weanlings to 60 days of oral administration of aluminum hydroxide gel or tap water. Experimental apparatus and procedures are described. Results indicate that (1) the 2 groups did not differ significantly in neural incorporation of aluminum; (2) although the highest aluminum concentrations were found in the hippocampus, there was no evidence of cognitive impairment; and (3) aluminum exposure was associated with lower weight and initial fluid intake levels and slight changes in behavior. It appears that young rats are not as susceptible as are older rats to aluminum toxicity.

769. Tilson, Hugh A.; Mactutus, Charles F.; McLamb, Ronnie L. & Burne, Thomas A. (1982). **Characterization of triethyl lead chloride neurotoxicity in adult rats.** *Neurobehavioral Toxicology & Teratology,* 4(6), 671–681.
Five experiments, with 156 male Fisher-344 rats, examined the neurotoxic effects of triethyl lead chloride (TEL). The single lethal dose (LD_{50}) following sc administration was 11 mg/kg, while the LD_{50} after repeated exposure over 5 days was 14 mg/kg. TEL (1–2.5 mg/kg, sc) given for 5 days produced a phase of hyperexcitability and hyperactivity 1–2 wks postdosing, which was followed by hypoexcitability and hypoactivity at 3–4 wks. TEL increased hot plate and tail flick latencies during the 1st 2 wks following TEL exposure. An operant titration procedure indicated that TEL increased shock detection thresholds 2 wks after cessation of exposure.

TEL-exposed Ss performed better than controls in a 2-way shuttlebox avoidance task 3 wks after cessation of dosing, whereas flinch-jump thresholds of TEL-exposed Ss were not affected. Results indicate that TEL produces a profile of toxicity characterized by changes in reactivity or emotionality possibly similar to that of animals having lesions in limbic forebrain areas. (69 ref).

770. Vickers, Colin & Paterson, Anna T. (1986). **Two types of chronic lead treatment in C57BL/6 mice: Interaction with behavioural determinants of pain.** *Life Sciences,* 39(1), 47–53.
Male C57BL/6 mice were offspring of either untreated or lead-treated parents. Offspring of lead-treated parents were reared on 0.1% lead acetate (PbAc) until weaning and also given 0.5% PbAc to drink for 3 wks prior to testing (Pb2 group). Offspring of untreated parents were either given 0.5% PbAc to drink (Pb1 group) or maintained on tap water throughout (controls). Controls and lead-treated Ss were subdivided according to no confrontation (unfought) or confrontation with a trained aggressor mouse (defeated). All Ss were then given a hot-plate pain test. In untreated Ss, latencies were reduced after defeat. Lead treatment increased pawlick and escape latencies in most instances relative to the appropriate control group. Escape latencies were longer in the Pb2 group than in the Pb1 group. Treatment with naloxone of single-housed Pb2 unfought Ss abolished the analgesic effect of lead treatment.

771. Vitulli, William F. (1974). **Mercury effects from chronic and acute doses on fixed-interval operant behavior of female squirrel monkeys.** *Psychological Reports,* 35(1, Pt 1), 3–9.
Two adult female squirrel monkeys were trained on an FI-10 min schedule of food reinforcement until steady states were recorded. Chronic, sublethal ip doses of dimethylmercury (0.004 mg/kg) were then administered prior to each experimental session. Physiologically normal saline was administered during control sessions. Following the chronic series, 1 acute dose of mercury was administered to each S (16.16 mg/kg). As transitions between the chronic doses and the acute dose occurred, proportionate rate changes typical of the effects of VI scheduling were observed, even though the schedule contingencies remained constant. Results are explained as a function of sensory-motor disruptions due to the entrance of organic mercury into the brain and spinal cord.

772. Vorhees, Charles V. (1985). **Behavioral effects of prenatal methylmercury in rats: A parallel trial to the Collaborative Behavioral Teratology Study.** Conference Proceedings of the National Center for Toxicological Research et al: Design considerations in screening for behavioral teratogens: Results of the collaborative behavioral teratology study (1985, Cincinnati, Ohio). *Neurobehavioral Toxicology & Teratology,* 7(6), 717–725.
Pregnant Sprague-Dawley CD rats treated with 0, 2.0, or 6.0 mg/kg of methylmercuric chloride on Days 6–9 of gestation or left untreated as part of J. Buelke-Sam and colleagues' (1985) Collaborative Behavioral Teratology Study (CBTS) were assigned to either the CBTS or the present author and colleagues' (1979) Cincinnati test protocol after birth. Offspring assigned to the Cincinnati test system were evaluated for effects of physical and neurobehavioral development and behavior. It was found that several developmental and behavioral factors were significantly affected by the high dose. It is concluded that at the doses and exposure period used here, methylmercury was confirmed to be a potent behavioral teratogen using the Cincinnati test system and is in agreement with results obtained in the CBTS. (28 ref).

METALLIC ELEMENTS

773. Walbran, Bonnie B. & Robins, Eli. (1978). **Effects of central nervous system accumulation of tellurium on behavior in rats.** *Pharmacology, Biochemistry & Behavior,* 9(3), 297–300.
23 male Long-Evans rats were treated for 112 days with daily injections of 2 mg/kg potassium tellurite in Sorensen's phosphate buffer or with the buffer vehicle only. At sacrifice, the cerebral gray matter of the Ss treated with tellurite was grossly darkened. The presence of tellurium in cerebellum was confirmed by atomic absorption spectrophotometry. Growth of tellurite-treated Ss was significantly impaired when compared with controls. However, in a T-maze the activity level of tellurite-treated Ss was increased. On a simple delayed response task, the performance of tellurite-treated Ss was more consistent than that of buffer-treated Ss. (16 ref).

774. Walsh, Thomas J.; Schulz, David W.; Tilson, Hugh A. & Dehaven, Diane L. (1986). **Acute exposure to triethyl lead enhances the behavioral effects of dopaminergic agonists: Involvement of brain dopamine in organolead neurotoxicity.** *Brain Research,* 363(2), 222–229.
Acute exposure to triethyl lead chloride (7.88 mg/kg) enhanced the behavioral effects of both direct- and indirect-acting dopamine agonists in male Fischer 344 rats. Ss treated with lead 1 wk before testing exhibited an increased response to the motor stimulant effects of dextroamphetamine (1.25, 2, 3.15, and 5 mg/kg) and apomorphine (0.2, 0.5, 1.25, and 2 mg/kg). Data suggest that acute exposure to triethyl lead enhances the responsiveness of dopaminergic processes that contribute to locomotor activity. (34 ref).

775. Weiner, William J.; Nausieda, Paul A. & Klawans, Harold L. (1977). **Effect of chlorpromazine on central nervous system concentrations of manganese, iron, and copper.** *Life Sciences,* 20(7), 1181–1185.
Chronic administration of chlorpromazine (CPZ; 10 mg/kg/day, sc, for 10 days) produced alterations in trace metal concentrations in caudate nucleus, frontal cortex, and cerebellar hemisphere of 12 male guinea pigs. Compared to findings in 16 saline-treated controls, CPZ manganese concentration following chronic CPZ rose significantly in the caudate nucleus and cerebellar hemisphere, whereas iron concentration rose most significantly in the caudate nucleus. Copper content was decreased in all regions examined. The possible significance of increased manganese and iron in the caudate nucleus is discussed in relationship to the clinical problems of CPZ-induced dyskinesias. (29 ref).

776. Wisniewski, Henryk M.; Sturman, John A. & Shek, Judy W. (1982). **Chronic model of neurofibrillary changes induced in mature rabbits by metallic aluminum.** *Neurobiology of Aging,* 3(1), 11–22.
A slurry of aluminum powder injected into the brains of New Zealand rabbits produced neurofibrillary changes in neurons of the spinal cord and cerebrum. This chronic animal model of neurofibrillary changes, induced in a mature nervous system, will allow better investigations of alterations in biochemistry, pathology, behavior, and cognition. Results are discussed in terms of research suggesting that neurofibrillary changes impair some cognitive functions and possible implications for senile dementia of the Alzheimer type. (11 ref).

777. Wootten, V.; Brown, D. R.; Callahan, B. G.; Vetrano, K. et al. (1985). **Behavioral and biochemical alterations following *in utero* exposure to methylmercury.** Conference Proceedings of the National Center for Toxicological Research et al: Design considerations in screening for behavioral teratogens: Results of the collaborative behavioral teratology study (1985, Cincinnati, Ohio). *Neurobehavioral Toxicology & Teratology,* 7(6), 767–773.
Studied behavioral changes induced in utero by methylmercury (MeHg) at 0, 2, or 6 mg/kg with a noninvasive measure of patterns of effects in 1–35 day old Sprague-Dawley rats, using lipid peroxidation and acetylcholinesterase activity to compare effects in 4 brain regions. No changes in body or brain weights or other ancillary measures of growth and development occurred between 1 and 35 days. It is concluded that MeHg produced alterations in behavioral patterning that were not dose related, that Postnatal Day 12 appeared to be a critical period for behavioral pattern development, that observation of growth and development indices were less sensitive measures of subteratogenic insults than manifested behavioral aberrations, and that frequency of activity and dispersion of behaviors over time were less sensitive indicators of MeHg toxicity than behavioral patterns. (14 ref).

778. Wulff, V. J. & Mendez, Carlos. (1973). **The effect of manganous chloride and tetrodotoxin on Limulus lateral eye retinular cells.** *Vision Research,* 13(12), 2327-2333.
Manganese chloride dissolved in sea water at concentrations of 8–14 mM affected all of the measured parameters of horseshoe crab lateral eye retinular cells (e.g., membrane potential and effective input resistance). It is proposed that manganese ions reduce Ca^{2+} influx and the permeability of the retinular cell membrane. Tetrodotoxin reversibly blocked eccentric cell spike potentials but had no observable effects on those properties of retinular cells that were measured. (French, German, & Russian summaries).

779. Yamamoto, Bryan K. (1981). **Chronic dietary lead administration during different developmental stages: Activity changes and neurochemical correlates.** *Dissertation Abstracts International,* 42(5-B), 2123–2124.

780. Yokel, Robert A. (1983). **Repeated systemic aluminum exposure effects on classical conditioning of the rabbit.** *Neurobehavioral Toxicology & Teratology,* 5(1), 41–52.
Excessive aluminum exposure and accumulation has been implicated as the cause of 2 disorders that involve learning deficits (dialysis encephalopathy and Alzheimer's disease). To develop an animal model, 61 female New Zealand White rabbits were given 20 aluminum lactate injections (0, 25, 50, 100, 200, or 400 μmole/kg, sc) over 4 wks. Dose-dependent weight reductions were observed. When the baseline frequency of nictitating membrane extension (NME) was determined 2 wks later, differential classical conditioning of the NME was conducted. No treatment group differences were observed in frequency of baseline NME, amplitude of the response to shock, or shock threshold to produce NME, suggesting no aluminum effects on the Ss' ability to perform the response. All Ss developed the discrimination. The 2 highest dose groups acquired the CR less well than controls, as shown by a lower percent of CRs in the 2nd half of the conditioning sessions (80 and 74% of controls) and a greater latency to onset of the CR (327 and 310 msec vs 261 msec for controls). Results indicate that chronic systemic exposure of adult rabbits to aluminum results in learning deficits not due to sensory or motor impairment of the learned response. (33 ref).

781. Zenick, H. (1976). **Evoked potential alterations in methylmercury chloride toxicity.** *Pharmacology, Biochemistry & Behavior,* 5(3), 253-255.
Results from 30-day-old male offspring of Holtzman albino rats show decreased visual-cortex evoked-potential latencies in Ss from mothers exposed to methylmercury chloride (MMC) during either gestation or nursing, and in Ss exposed directly to MMC for 9 days after weaning. A similar, nonsignificant trend was observed in lateral geniculate potentials. It is suggested that the decreased latencies may be the result of compressed brain development.

782. Zenick, Harold. (1974). **Behavioral and biochemical consequences in methylmercury chloride toxicity.** *Pharmacology, Biochemistry & Behavior,* 2(6), 709-713.
Assessed the developmental periods during which exposure to methylmercury chloride (MMC) would result in permanent

learning deficits in Holtzman albino rats. In addition, the mercury (Hg) content of the brain at these different stages was measured. 280 offspring of 35 mothers were tested. Offspring (30 days of age) of mothers exposed during gestation and offspring exposed directly to MMC for 9 days after weaning exhibited the greatest learning deficits on a water escape T-maze. These deficits persisted through a retest session 21 days later. Biochemical analysis of brain Hg content indicated that Hg need not be present for these learning deficits to occur.

783. Zenick, Harold. (1974). **The behavioral, biochemical, and electrophysiological consequences of methylmercury chloride toxicity.** *Dissertation Abstracts International,* 35(2-B), 1102.

784. Zenick, Harold & Goldsmith, Marshall. (1981). **Drug discrimination learning in lead-exposed rats.** *Science,* 212(4494), 569–571.
Lead acetate (.02 or .05%) was administered to 12 female Long-Evans hooded rats throughout the lactation period, with half of the litters continuing on lead after weaning. Drug thresholds for dextroamphetamine (1 mg/kg, sc) were determined by using the drug-discrimination learning paradigm. All offspring exposed to lead were less sensitive to the stimulus properties of dextroamphetamine.

785. Zenick, Harold; Padich, Robert; Tokarek, Theresa & Aragon, Polly. (1978). **Influence of prenatal and postnatal lead exposure on discrimination learning in rats.** *Pharmacology, Biochemistry & Behavior,* 8(4), 347–350.
The 20 animals in this study were the offspring of CD Charles River dams, who, from 21–99 days of age, were exposed to 1,000 mg/kg of lead acetate via a daily restricted watering schedule with exposure continuing throughout gestation and nursing. Control dams received distilled water under the same watering schedule. Offspring were weaned at 21 days of age and did not receive lead treatment from that point. Testing began at 30 days of age with animals receiving 10 trials/day for 10 days on a brightness discrimination task conducted in a water-escape T-maze. This task was followed by a shape discrimination problem in the same apparatus. Results reveal that the lead-exposed pups made significantly more errors than the controls but had significantly shorter swimming times on both the brightness and shape dicrimination tasks. The failure to attend to relevant discriminative cues may account for the observed deficits in lead-exposed animals.

786. Zenick, Harold; Rodriquez, Ward; Ward, Jerry & Elkington, Brian. (1979). **Deficits in fixed-interval performance following prenatal and postnatal lead exposure.** *Developmental Psychobiology,* 12(5), 509–514.
10 female Charles River CD rats were exposed daily to 750 mg/kg of lead acetate via a restricted watering schedule for 70–80 days prior to mating and then throughout pregnancy and nursing (5 others were controls). At weaning, litters from half of the lead dams were placed directly on treatment for the duration of the experiment. These manipulations yielded 3 groups: Group Pb/Pb, offspring exposed during pre- and postweaning periods; Group Pb/C, offspring exposed only during preweaning periods: and Group C/C, control offspring. Beginning at 42–49 days of age, postnatal, offspring were shaped to barpress under an FI 1-min schedule and then given 20 sessions, each 45 min in length. Analyses revealed that Group Pb/Pb received significantly fewer reinforcements across sessions than the other 2 groups, which did not differ. When the Pb/Pb offspring did receive reinforcement, they exhibited the scalloped pattern of responding characteristic of FI schedules. (5 ref)

FOOD ADDITIVES

787. Ber, Abram. (1983). **Neutralization of phenolic (aromatic) food compounds in a holistic general practice.** *Journal of Orthomolecular Psychiatry,* 12(4), 283–291.
Discusses the neutralization of phenolic (aromatic) food compounds in a holistic general practice, by which allergic persons experienced the disappearance of symptoms such as arthritic pains, abdominal bloating, anxiety, autism, mental retardation, hyperactivity, dyslexia, insomnia, enuresis, respiratory allergies, headaches, and asthma. Phenolic exposure has been found to cause depressed serotonin, elevated histamine and prostaglandins, and abnormal complement and immune complex formation. A list of phenolic compounds and their therapeutic and diagnostic consequences is provided. (6 ref)

788. Dortch, Annie L. (1981). **A compilation of the literature relating to hyperactivity–hyperkinesis, learning disabilities and food additives.** *Dissertation Abstracts International,* 41(7-A), 3046.

789. Gilka, Libuse. (1983). **Hyperactivity, learning disabilities, GABA, inborn errors of metabolism, and modern environmental factors.** *International Journal of Biosocial Research,* 4(2), 85–98.
Discusses how food additives may influence hyperactivity and learning disabilities in children. Hyperactivity may be the only clinical manifestation of a hypersensitivity to foods or food additives. Inborn errors of metabolism characterized by an absence or reduction of an enzyme catalytic activity may affect brain functions by producing abnormality in the synthesis of proteins, neurotransmitters, or other metabolites or through an accumulation of normal metabolites to toxic levels. These disorders, such as phenylketonuria, may cause retardation; however, dietary restriction may prevent such retardation. General therapeutic principles for correcting inborn errors of metabolism include restoring the activity of the defective enzyme, dietary restrictions, replacement of the missing metabolite, and supplementation of vitamins. Hyperactivity in some children has been traced to a genetic glutamic acid decarboxylase (GAD) enzyme variation that results in a reduced formation of GABA—the neurotransmitter that inhibits action of the CNS. Various food additives may affect the GAD enzyme. Food additives that have been found to cause hyperactivity in some children include chlorine, artificial food dyes and flavorings, foods with salicylate groups, and sugar. Supplementation of the hyperactive child's diet with GABA, specific vitamins, Ritalin, or amphetamines is sometimes helpful. (43 ref)

790. Harley, J. Preston. (1978). **Hyperactivity and food additives: A bibliography.** *Catalog of Selected Documents in Psychology,* 8, 42–43. MS. 1691 (7 pp/paper: $4; fiche: $2).

791. Kavale, Kenneth A. & Forness, Steven R. (1983). **Hyperactivity and diet treatment: A meta-analysis of the Feingold hypothesis.** *Journal of Learning Disabilities,* 16(6), 324–330.
Reviews primary research investigating the hypothesis by B. F. Feingold (1975) that suggests diet modification can be an efficacious treatment for hyperactivity. The techniques of meta-analysis were used to integrate statistically the findings from 23 studies. The primary finding is that diet modification by removal of artificial additives is not an effective intervention for hyperactivity, as evidenced by the negligible treatment effects that are only slightly greater than those expected by chance. When the data were refined into groupings related to outcome and design variables, support was rendered for the primary finding. It is concluded that extant research has not validated the Feingold hypothesis and that diet modification should be questioned as an efficacious treatment for hyperactivity. (67 ref)

FOOD ADDITIVES

792. Mailman, Richard B. & Lewis, Mark H. (1981). **Food additives and developmental disorders: The case of erythrosin (FD&C Red #3), or guilty until proven innocent?** *Applied Research in Mental Retardation,* 2(4), 297–305.
Discusses studies evaluating the behavioral effects of Red Dye Number 3, which has been reported to alter neurotransmitter uptake or oubain binding; either effect would be sufficient to explain behavioral disturbances such as hyperkinesis and learning disabilities. Contrary to earlier reports by E. K. Silbergeld (1981) and W. J. Logan and J. M. Swanson (1979), R. B. Mailman et al (1980) found that the chemical nature of the compound caused biochemical artifacts that obfuscated interpretation of the previously cited biochemical data. Only extremely high doses of this color caused behavioral effects in rats. Since preliminary pharmacokinetic studies by D. M. Niedwiecki and Mailman (1981) suggested that the color would not enter the CNS readily, then it is probably not sufficiently neurotoxic to pose a human hazard. Results exemplify the necessity of considering basic principles of pharmacology and physiology before assigning neurotoxicity to a specific agent. (23 ref).

793. Mattes, Jeffrey A. (1983). **The Feingold diet: A current reappraisal.** *Journal of Learning Disabilities,* 16(6), 319–323.
The Feingold diet (B. F. Feingold, 1975)—eliminating artificial colorings, artificial flavorings, and salicylates—has been claimed, based on anecdotal evidence, to improve the learning and behavior of hyperactive children. A review of all published, completed controlled studies, however, indicates that the Feingold diet is probably not effective, except perhaps in a very small percentage of children. The positive results in a few studies have been inconsistent among studies and greatly outnumbered by negative results. Even among children whose parents feel the diet has helped them greatly, the improvement seems more often a placebo effect (e.g., due to the increased attention received by the child rather than a true effect of artificial colorings or flavorings). (30 ref).

794. Podell, Richard N. (1983). **Hyperactivity and diet.** *Behavioral Medicine Update,* 5(1), 27–32.
Reviews recent literature concerning the purported link between diet and childhood hyperactivity. Two important hypotheses are discussed: the Feingold hypothesis, which states that food additives and/or natural food salicylates can contribute to hyperactive behavior; and the food allergy hypothesis, which states that allergy-like sensitivity to common foods such as milk or wheat can provoke hyperactivity. It is concluded that evaluation of the diet–hyperactivity hypotheses remains incomplete in part because of methodological weaknesses in the research. Better experimental design might be accomplished through collaboration between research scientists and clinician-practitioners of the dietary treatment of hyperactivity. (23 ref).

795. Rimland, Bernard. (1983). **The Feingold diet: An assessment of the reviews by Mattes, by Kavale and Forness and others.** *Journal of Learning Disabilities,* 16(6), 331–333.
J. Mattes (1983), K. A. Kavale and S. R. Forness (1983), and other reviewers of the Feingold diet concluded that the diet is of little or no value as a means of reducing hyperactivity. The present author argues that such a conclusion is unwarranted, probably incorrect, and very likely damaging. This assessment is based on the limited value of the data analyzed in studies of the effectiveness of the diet in reducing hyperactivity. (21 ref).

796. Rimland, Bernard. (1984). **The Feingold diet: An assessment of the reviews by Mattes, by Kavale and Forness and others.** *Journal of Orthomolecular Psychiatry,* 13(1), 45–49.
Asserts that reviews of the Feingold additive-free diet, which suggest that the diet is of no or marginal value, are unwarranted, incorrect, and damaging. Previous studies of the Feingold diet are criticized for their small dosage levels, failure to recognize the role of S nutritional status, lack of control of relevant variables, arbitrary negative conclusions, and inadequate attention to animal in vitro studies. It is concluded, in congruence with the Feingold diet, that unnecessary pollutants (additives) should be removed from food supplies. (21 ref).

797. Thorley, Geoff. (1983). **Childhood hyperactivity and food additives.** *Developmental Medicine & Child Neurology,* 25(4), 531–534.
Comments on findings by a multidisciplinary panel of experts from the US National Institute ot Mental Health. The panel particularly addressed evidence by B. F. Feingold (1973, 1975) concerning the hypothesis that artificial food-colors produce adverse psychological reactions, such as hyperactivity. The author concludes that a standard series of tests should be devised and insisted upon before a product is approved, and that cognitive and behavioral effects in humans and animals should also be considered. (26 ref).

798. Trites, Ronald L. & Tryphonas, Helen. (1983). **Food additives: The controversy continues.** *Topics in Early Childhood Special Education,* 3(2), 43–47.
Evidence from controlled studies suggests that the early claims of widespread adverse behavioral effects of artificial additives in food were exaggerated. However, studies conducted to date have suffered from serious methodological flaws. Results of most studies indicate that among the children being studied (usually classified as hyperactive), there is a small group of adverse responders. Nothing is known about the characteristics of the adverse responders because valuable data that could have been obtained from physical examinations, psychological tests, pediatric allergy assessment, birth records, and family histories have not been reported. Well-controlled studies that collect these kinds of information are needed. Of particular importance are well-controlled investigations in preschool-age children, because this group may be physically the most vulnerable and because there is some evidence that it is easiest to demonstrate an adverse behavioral response in this group. (16 ref).

799. Walker, Mildred M. (1982). **Phosphates and hyperactivity: Is there a connection?** *Academic Therapy,* 17(4), 439–446.
Discusses H. Hafer's (1978) hypothesis that phosphates contribute to hyperactivity. An electronic device (the Zero Input Tracking Analyzer/Auxiliary Distraction Task) is described that quantitatively measures attention deficit disorders and may possibly be a valuable instrument for measuring the effects of phosphates on sensitive children. (9 ref).

800. Weiss, Bernard. (1982). **Food additives and environmental chemicals as sources of childhood behavior disorders.** *Journal of the American Academy of Child Psychiatry,* 21(2), 144–152.
B. F. Feingold (1973, 1975) postulated that many children who exhibit disturbed behavior improved on a diet devoid of certain food additives. Its validity has been examined by other researchers in controlled trials. The total evidence, although not wholly consistent, nevertheless suggests that the hypothesis is, in principle, correct. Such a conclusion poses difficult problems and new issues for etiology, treatment, toxicology, and regulation. (23 ref).

801. Wender, Esther H. (1986). **The food additive-free diet in the treatment of behavior disorders: A review.** *Journal of Developmental & Behavioral Pediatrics,* 7(1), 35–42.

Discusses problems in research design and summarizes research results of studies of the effectiveness of B. F. Feingold's (1975) food additive-free diet for the treatment of developmental/behavioral disorders in children. This diet was initially developed by Feingold for the treatment of aspirin sensitivity in adults and then extended by him to the management of hyperactivity and learning disability in children. The claimed therapeutic effects of this diet have been investigated in a number of well-designed studies that generally refute a causal association between food additives and behavioral disturbance in children. (30 ref).

Human Research

802. Brunner, Robert L.; Vorhees, Charles V. & Butcher, Richard E. (1981). **Food colors and behavior.** *Science,* 212(4494), 578–579.
Comments on the article by B. Weiss et al (1980) on the results of a study on the possible relationship between food colorings in the diet and behavior problems in children—the Feingold hypothesis. The present authors assert that the sample selection, methodology, and the single case showing a marked improvement make it impossible to derive a scientific generalization. (3 ref).

803. Buckley, Robert. (1977). **Hyperkinetic aggravation of learning disturbance.** *Academic Therapy,* 13(2), 153–160.
Charges that R. L. Sieben (1977) did not define the conditions he discussed and did not propose alternative therapeutic procedures. Hyperkinesis is not a cause of learning disability but can complicate it. Children sensitive to chemical elements in foods have hyperkinetic symptoms. Unlike the antigen-antibody mechanisms in allergy, the mechanism in food sensitivity is unknown and hence presumed by some physicians not to exist. Improved functioning in schoolchildren on the Feingold KP diet has been indicated by teacher ratings. Other research is cited to show that food additives have addictive effects. In hyperkinetics the hypothalamus does not perform its regulatory function. At least one-third of hyperkinetic children are believed to be sensitive to certain foodstuffs.

804. Chernick, Eleanor. (1980). **Effects of the Feingold diet on reading achievement and classroom behavior.** *Reading Teacher,* 34(2), 171–174.
Examined the classroom behavior and reading achievement of 13 6–12 yr old children placed on the Feingold diet and compared them with 6 control children. Assessments included the Gates-MacGinite Reading Tests, Wide Range Achievement Test, Matching Familiar Figures Test, and Connors Teacher Rating Scale. Reading achievement and classroom behavior were not significantly different after Ss' 6-mo diet. However, there was a significant change in personality that showed a low positive correlation with reading scores. A limitation of this study is recognized as the inability to monitor Ss' food intake. (13 ref).

805. Conners, C. Keith; Goyette, Charles H. & Newman, Elisa B. (1980). **Dose–time effect of artificial colors in hyperactive children.** *Journal of Learning Disabilities,* 13(9), 512–516.
Determined if those children apparently most reactive to food dyes could show a pharmacologic dose–time effect by using more sensitive laboratory instruments and observations than the relatively uncontrolled global instruments utilized in the present authors' 3 previous studies (1976, 1977, 1980). Ss were 9 children aged 5–10 yrs who had participated in the previous trials (with 1 exception); all Ss were on the Feingold diet and all satisfied *Diagnostic and Statistical Manual of Mental Disorders* criteria for hyperkinetic reaction or attentional deficit of childhood. Ss were tested in 2 sessions that began with a baseline period during which the S completed the learning task and activity measures. Two chocolate cookies were then distributed; these contained either 15 mg of artificial colors or placebo. Further learning tests were then conducted 45–180 min after cookie ingestion, with activity and rating measures obtained concurrently. Data fail to demonstrate a significant pharmacological dose–time effect between the active and placebo materials. Ss' activity level appeared to increase following ingestion of both kinds of material and then return gradually to baseline. (6 ref).

806. Cott, Allan. (1977). **A reply.** *Academic Therapy,* 13(2), 161–171.
Disputes R. L. Sieben's claim (1977) that no evidence exists to support nondrug treatment of learning disability. Successfully treated cases supply better evidence than poorly designed double-bind studies, and many parents in the Feingold Associations have indicated that their children were dramatically improved by the diet. Similar comments were made by parents whose children received the Doman Delcato treatment. It is also indicated that Sieben misrepresented the case made by nondrug therapies. Drugs like Ritalin and amphetamines, used in treating some learning disabled, have sedative effects on children but opposite effects on adults. Hence it may not be surprising that children with hypoglycemia become reactive after eating sugar but adults become depressed. An American Psychiatric Association report found no evidence that megavitamin therapy was effective in treating schizophrenia, but did not refer to the treatment of learning disability. Evidence is available that when lead is present in the hair there is interference with brain function.

807. del Ser, T.; Espasandin, P.; Cabetas, I. & Arredondo, J. M. (1986). **Trastornos de memoria en el síndrome del aceite tóxico (SAT). / Memory disturbances in the toxic oil syndrome.** *Archivos de Neurobiología,* 49(1), 19–39.
13 toxic oil syndrome (TOS) patients complaining of memory disturbances and 13 controls matched in sex, age and educational level were assessed with an extensive psychometric battery. (TOS cases were caused by consuming foods cooked in industrial rapeseed oil illegally sold as cooking oil). The IQ of the TOS Ss was slightly but significantly lower; the anxiety and depression levels significantly higher, and the errors in an attentional test more frequent. There were no differences between groups in short-term memory, but long-term memory, semantic memory, and information processing were impaired in TOS Ss, suggesting deficits in encoding and retrieval mechanisms. Memory disturbances in TOS patients are suggested to be central in origin.

808. Del Ser Quijano, T. (1985). **?Existen trastornos de memoria en el síndrome del aceite tóxico? Estudio caso-control de dos gemelas. / Are there memory disturbances in Toxic Oil Syndrome? A case-control study of one pair of twin girls.** *Archivos de Neurobiología,* 48(3), 124–132.
An extensive psychomotor test battery was administered to a 17-yr-old female who had 3 yrs earlier suffered toxic oil syndrome with severe neuromuscular involvement. Her healthy identical twin sister was also tested. The patient was found to be lower than her sister on 14 of 18 memory dimensions, higher on only one. She showed slightly higher IQ and performance scores. Both manifested slight depression; the control twin demonstrated higher anxiety. It appears that the memory deficits of the one twin may have been the result of the toxic oil syndrome. They were mild and secondary to retrieval process deficiencies.

809. Díez Manrique, J. F. et al. (1983). **Valoración de salud mental y neuroticismo en un grupo de afectados por el síndrome tóxico (S. T.). / Mental health and neuroticism evaluation in a group of patients with toxic-oil syndrome (T.O.S.).** *Actas Luso-Españolas de Neurología y Psiquiatría y Ciencias Afines,* 11(6), 453–458.

FOOD ADDITIVES

Examined the psychiatric manifestations of 43 patients (mean age 42.29 yrs) affected by TOS, using adaptations of the General Health Questionnaire and the Eysenck Personality Inventory. The results were compared with those obtained from 137 cardiac patients (mean age 49.82 yrs). It was found that both populations had similar scores on the instruments. (English abstract) (9 ref).

810. Etuk, Ezekiel M. (1986). **The influence of nutrition on hyperkinesis.** *Dissertation Abstracts International,* 47(5-B), 2159.

811. Feingold, Benjamin F. (1977). **A critique of "Controversial medical treatments of learning disabilities".** *Academic Therapy,* 13(2), 173–181.
Charges that R. L. Sieben (1977) has ignored, misrepresented, or misinterpreted available published evidence showing the value of the Feingold KP diet in treating learning disability. The dietary restrictions are not extensive; they include foods containing natural salicylates, artificial color and flavor, and the antioxidant preservatives. Criticism from food processors overlooks the fact that conventional tests for toxicity are not adequate or applicable in this field. Allergists have been prescribing similar diets for many decades. Although years of investigation will be needed to determine the effect of such dietary restrictions, the evidence now available is promising.

812. Ferguson, H. Bruce; Rapoport, Judith L. & Weingartner, Herbert. (1981). **Food dyes and impairment of performance in hyperactive children.** *Science,* 211(4480), 410–411.
Discusses several issues that were not directly addressed by J. M. Swanson and M. Kinsbourne (1980) but are essential to the proper interpretation of their results on the study of food dyes and impairment of performance in hyperactive children. For example, the label "hyperactivity" is widely applied and the criteria used by them are questionable. A reply by Swanson and Kinsbourne is included in the article.

813. Gross, Mortimer D.; Tofanelli, Ruth A.; Butzirus, Sharyl M. & Snodgrass, Earl W. (1987). **The effect of diets rich in and free from additives on the behavior of children with hyperkinetic and learning disorders.** *Journal of the American Academy of Child & Adolescent Psychiatry,* 26(1), 53–55.
39 11–17 yr olds in a summer camp were given the Feingold Diet, which eliminates artificial additives and salicylate-containing foods, for 1 wk, followed by administration for 1 wk of food containing those ingredients. The Ss' behavior was monitored by videotape for 4-min intervals at mealtime. All Ss were classified by public school psychologists as having moderate to severe learning disorders; 18 were also hyperkinetic, and 17 were taking medication for the latter condition. Three raters blind to the respective diets rated Ss' behavior for motor restlessness, disorganized behavior, and misbehavior. No significant differences were found in behaviors during Weeks 1 and 2, suggesting that the Feingold Diet has no beneficial effect on most children with learning disorders or on hyperkinetic children taking medication.

814. Holborow, Patricia; Elkins, John & Berry, Paul. (1981). **The effect of the Feingold diet on "normal" school children.** *Journal of Learning Disabilities,* 14(3), 143–147.
344 5–12 yr old children in 7 elementary schools followed the Feingold diet for hyperactivity for 2 wks. Teachers rated Ss before and after the diet using a questionnaire that incorporated the C. K. Connors et al (1976) hyperactivity factor items related to the normal or average child. Of the total sample, 8.5% improved by 5 points or more. Before-diet mean scores of Ss who improved were below the cut-off value for hyperactivity, indicating hyperactivity itself is not a necessary condition for improvement. Item-by-item analysis of the response showed that the behavior problems most likely to show improvement were distractability, attention span, fiddling, and demands for attention. Ss who ingested a great deal of additive rated significantly higher in behavioral problems than Ss receiving little additive. (28 ref).

815. Knapczyk, Dennis R. (1979). **Diet control in the management of behavior disorders.** *Behavioral Disorders,* 5(1), 2–9.
Describes 3 major diet-related conditions that lead to behavior disorders in school-age children: (1) hypoglycemia, (2) vitamin/mineral deficiencies, and (3) allergies to food substances or additives. It is stressed that public school personnel need to become aware of the complex relationship between the nutritional needs of students and the behavioral problems the students exhibit. (36 ref).

816. Lester, Michael L.; Thatcher, R. W. & Monroe-Lord, L. (1982). **Refined carbohydrate intake, hair cadmium levels, and cognitive functioning in children.** *Nutrition & Behavior,* 1(1), 3–13.
Measures of hair cadmium, intelligence (WISC-R, Wechsler Preschool and Primary Scale of Intelligence, and Wide Range Achievement Test), school achievement, and proportion of refined carbohydrate foods in a 1-day dietary sample were obtained from 184 5–16 yr old public school children. Regression analyses indicated that the proportion of refined carbohydrates in Ss' diets was positively related to hair cadmium and negatively correlated with intelligence and school achievement scores. Furthermore, the relationship between diet and cognitive functioning remained even after the effects of cadmium, age, sex, socioeconomic status, and race were regressed out. Results suggest that the consumption of foods low in nutrient density and high in sucrose may contribute significantly to childhood learning disorders. (66 ref).

817. Levy, Florence & Hobbes, Gary. (1978). **Hyperkinesis and diet: A replication study.** *American Journal of Psychiatry,* 135(12), 1559–1560.
Attempted to replicate an unpublished study by C. H. Goyette et al that found a significant challenge effect in a Group by Order by Challenge ANOVA of data from a study of hyperkinetic responses to dietary restriction of food additives. Data from 8 5-yr-olds who responded previously to the dietary restriction do not replicate the Goyette et al findings; however, the small sample size and the use of a symptom rating scale to measure small or transient effects may have accounted for the nonsignificant results. (7 ref).

818. López-Ibor, J. J. (1987). **Social reinsertation after catastrophes: The toxic oil syndrome experience.** *European Journal of Psychiatry,* 1(1), 12–19.
Reports that 6,000 victims of a toxic oil syndrome (brought about by adulterated olive oil) in Spain were referred for psychiatric help after showing signs of posttraumatic stress disorder, with the at-risk population being characterized as female, of low socioeconomic status (SES), and with a history of nervous disorders. The public repercussions of the disease and the specific administrative measures it provoked are discussed and evaluated because they paved the way for the creation of a minority group psychology that increased the social disability of these patients. A bio-psycho-social model is presented that indicates that the impact of an event for which an individual is not prepared unchains an exaggerated response that paves the way for the succeeding responses: exhaustion and chronic maladaptation.

819. López-Ibor, J. J.; Soria, J.; Cañas, F. & Rodriguez-Gamazo, M. (1985). **Psychopathological aspects of the Toxic Oil Syndrome catastrophe.** *British Journal of Psychiatry,* 147, 352–365.
In May 1981 a new disease, the toxic oil syndrome (TOS), caused by widespread food-poisoning appeared in Spain. Although TOS was not primarily a psychiatric condition, more than 6,000 TOS patients were referred to psychiatrists. These patients showed a well-defined reactive disaster syndrome,

vulnerability being associated with female sex, low income and class, and a personal history of nervous disorders. It is suggested that teams of psychologists and psychiatrists should play a significant role in managing the effects of major catastrophes. (41 ref).

820. Mattes, Jeffrey A. & Gittelman, Rachel. (1981). **Effects of artificial food colorings in children with hyperactive symptoms: A critical review and results of a controlled study.** *Archives of General Psychiatry,* 38(6), 714–718.
The "Feingold diet" (B. F. Feingold, 1975), which eliminates artificial food colorings, has been claimed to be beneficial to hyperactive children. Previous studies have yielded equivocal results. The present investigation sought to maximize the likelihood of demonstrating behavioral effects of artificial food colorings by (1) studying only children who were already on the Feingold diet and who were reported by their parents to respond markedly to artificial food colorings, (2) attempting to exclude placebo responders, and (3) administering high dosages (maximum 78 mg/day) of coloring. The design was a 4-wk double-blind crossover with order randomized; 11 children aged 4–13 yrs maintained on the Feingold diet were challenged with food coloring and placebo (one each week). Evaluations by parents, teachers, and psychiatrists and psychological testing yielded no evidence of a food coloring effect. (29 ref).

821. Mattes, Jeffrey & Gittelman-Klein, Rachel. (1978). **A crossover study of artificial food colorings in a hyperkinetic child.** *American Journal of Psychiatry,* 135(8), 987–988.
Investigated previous conflicting studies on the effect of a diet eliminating artificial food colorings on hyperkinetic symptoms in children. Dose-ranging and multiple crossover studies with a 10-yr-old boy who had been previously helped by the diet failed to support the contention that artificial food colorings are instrumental in inducing significant changes in hyperactive symptomatology. Methodological suggestions are noted. (8 ref).

822. O'Shea, James A. & Porter, Seymour F. (1981). **Double-blind study of children with hyperkinetic syndrome treated with multi-allergen extract sublingually.** *Journal of Learning Disabilities,* 14(4), 189–191, 237.
Investigated whether the hyperkinetic syndrome is due, in part, to certain foods, food colors, and inhalant allergens and, if so, whether it could be treated by specific immunotherapy sublingually. 14 5–13 yr olds were tested by the provocative intradermal and sublingual method, and an optimal or neutralizing dose was obtained that was included in a multiallergen extract for sublingual treatment. The study was conducted over a 6-wk period—3 wks of treatment with the allergen extract and 3 wks with a placebo. Each S's behavior was monitored weekly by parents, teacher, and a psychologist. Significant improvement was reported in 11 Ss during the 3 wks of treatment vs placebo. A case history of a 13-yr-old male is given. (5 ref).

823. Prinz, Ronald J.; Roberts, William A. & Hantman, Elaine. (1980). **Dietary correlates of hyperactive behavior in children.** *Journal of Consulting & Clinical Psychology,* 48(6), 760–769.
Investigated the effects of sugar in hyperactive children. Seven-day dietary records were obtained on 28 hyperactive 4–7 yr olds, and independent, reliable observations of hyperactive behaviors were made on each S. Amount of sugar products consumed, ratio of sugar products to nutritional foods, and ratio of carbohydrates to protein were all significantly associated with amounts of destructive-aggressive and restless behaviors observed during free play. In contrast, the percentage of S's diet containing additives or salicylates (i.e., foods not allowed by the Feingold diet) was not significantly correlated with observed hyperactive behavior. A partial correlation procedure used to rule out 3rd variables that could have produced a spurious correlation between sugar consumption and observed behavior did not diminish the original correlations. (44 ref).

824. Rapp, Doris J. (1978). **Does diet affect hyperactivity?** *Journal of Learning Disabilities,* 11(6), 383–389.
Notes that conflicting reports make it difficult to determine if foods, food coloring, or allergies are related to hyperactivity. 24 5–16 yr old hyperactive children were tested with sublingual foods and dyes followed by a 7-day diet omitting milk, wheat, egg, cocoa, corn, sugar, and food coloring, and by subsequent individual ingestion challenges with these same food items. More than 70% of the Ss had evidence of allergy in their personal and family history, as well as positive allergy skin tests. The sublingual dye, but not the sublingual mixed-food test, correlated well with repeated ingestion challenges. 12 Ss improved to a moderate or marked degree during the 7-day diet. A simple sublingual food-coloring test or a 1-wk experimental diet can be used to detect a subgroup of children hyperactive from specific food dyes or foods. Improvement persisted in Ss who avoided offending food dyes or foods for at least 12 wks. (22 ref).

825. Rippere, Vicky. (1983). **Food additives and hyperactive children: A critique of Conners.** *British Journal of Clinical Psychology,* 22(1), 19–32.
Reviews C. K. Conners's (1980) book, *Food Additives and Hyperactive Children,* which evaluates B. F. Feingold's (1975) additive and salicylate-free Kaiser-Permenente diet for the treatment of hyperactive children. It is argued that the studies as reported do not constitute a methodologically adequate test of Feingold's hypothesis that many hyperactive children are hypersensitive to artificial colors, flavors, other chemical additives, and naturally occurring substances in foods. It is argued, further, that Feingold's approach to the environmental etiology of childhood hyperactivity is too limited and may for this reason lead to a failure to discover and eliminate other possible environmental causes of this increasingly prevalent condition. (51 ref).

826. Rose, Terry. (1978). **The functional relationship between artificial food colors and hyperactivity.** *Journal of Applied Behavior Analysis,* 11(4), 439–446.
The presence of a functional relationship between the ingestion of artificial food colors and an increase in the frequency and/or duration of selected behaviors that are representative of the hyperactive behavior syndrome was experimentally investigated. Two 8-yr-old females, who had been on B. F. Feingold's (1975, 1976) K-P diet for a minimum of 11 mo, were the Ss studied. The experimental design was a variation of the BAB design (S. W. Huck et al, 1974), with double-blind conditions. This design allowed an experimental analysis of the placebo phases as well as challenge phases. Data were obtained by trained observers on out of seat, on task, and physically aggressive behaviors, as they occurred in the Ss' regular class setting. Results indicate (a) the existence of a functional relationship between the ingestion of artificial food colors and an increase in both the duration and frequency of hyperactive behaviors, (b) the absence of a placebo effect, and (c) differential sensitivity of the dependent variables to the challenge effects. (25 ref).

827. Roshon, Melinda S. (1986). **The relationship between sugar consumption, attention, activity level, and learning in children of preschool age.** *Dissertation Abstracts International,* 47(2-B), 803.

828. Rotton, James; Tikofsky, Ronald S. & Feldman, Hobart T. (1982). **Behavioral effects of chemicals in drinking water.** *Journal of Applied Psychology,* 67(2), 230–238.
In Exp I, 42 Ss (mean age 30.4 yrs) tracked a moving target and monitored lights after receiving sublingual drops that contained either water, sodium nitrate (4.5, 45, 450, or 4,500

FOOD ADDITIVES

ppm), or sodium fluoride (.1, 1, 10, or 100 ppm). Dosage levels equaled, exceeded, or fell below those of municipal waters. In Exp II, 20 females performed this task after receiving sublingual drops of the same test substances in a repeated measures design; dosage levels equaled or exceeded levels found in municipal waters by 100 or 500 times. Neither type nor amount of chemical affected primary task performance; however, after receiving sublingual drops in Exp I, Ss paid less attention to lights on their right. In Exp II, Ss made more errors and had longer response latencies after they received moderate and very high concentrations of test substances. It is concluded that challenge testing is a safe but effective technique for provoking and studying reactions to chemicals when combined with a sensitive measure of sensorimotor performance. (24 ref).

829. Ruch, Marcella W. (1980). **The role of food additives in the incidence of disruptive behavior of school boys in a residential setting.** *Dissertation Abstracts International,* 41(4-A), 1331.

830. Sallade, Jacqueline B. (1980). **Group counseling with children who have migraine headaches.** *Elementary School Guidance & Counseling,* 15(1), 87–89.
Examined the cumulative effects of 3 treatment modalities on frequency of migraine headaches among 8 middle-class children aged 8–11 yrs. Inclusion was limited to referrals showing symptoms of stress, tension, and migraines. Following baseline measurement, treatment proceeded in 3 6-wk phases. In Phase 1, artificial additives, preservatives, chocolate, cheese, and nuts were excluded from Ss' diets. In Phase 2, relaxation exercises were introduced. During the 3rd and final 6-wk period, nondirective group counseling was applied. The incidence of headaches decreased by 50% on average during relaxation training; it did not vary from baseline during the other 2 treatment phases. The merits of relaxation as a treatment intervention need to be studied further. (4 ref).

831. Schoenthaler, Stephen J.; Doraz, Walter E. & Wakefield, James A. (1986). **The impact of a low food additive and sucrose diet on academic performance in 803 New York City public schools.** *International Journal of Biosocial Research,* 8(2), 185–195.
Tested the effect of modifying selected nutritional policies on academic performance, attendance, and delinquency, by introducing a diet policy that lowered sucrose, synthetic food color/flavors, and 2 preservatives (BHA and BHT) over 4 yrs in 803 New York City public schools. Results show that the change was followed by a 15.7% increase in mean academic percentile ranking above the rest of the nation's schools on the same standardized tests. Each school's academic performance ranking was negatively correlated with the percentage of Ss who ate school food prior to the diet policy changes. After the policy transitions, the percentage of Ss who ate lunches and breakfasts within each school became positively correlated with that school's rate of gain.

832. Spring, Carl; Vermeersch, Joyce; Blunden, Dale & Sterling, Harold. (1981). **Case studies of effects of artificial food colors on hyperactivity.** *Journal of Special Education,* 15(3), 361–372.
Tested B. F. Feingold's (1976) hypothesis that synthetic food colors cause hyperactivity, using 6 8–13 yr old White males. Results from other diet challenges are reviewed, and it is concluded that evidence for Feingold's hypothesis is weak. (16 ref).

833. Swanson, James M. & Kinsbourne, Marcel. (1980). **Food dyes impair performance of hyperactive children on a laboratory learning test.** *Science,* 207(4438), 1485–1487.
36 male and 4 female children (average age 10 yrs) referred to a child development clinic for symptoms suggestive of hyperactivity were given a diet free of artificial food dyes and other additives for 5 days. 20 Ss had been classified as hyperactive on the Conners Rating Scale and were reported to have favorable responses to stimulant medication. A diagnosis of hyperactivity had been rejected for the other 20 Ss. Oral challenges with 100–150 mg doses of a blend of US Food and Drug Administration-approved food dyes or placebo were administered on Days 4 and 5 of the experiment. Paired-associate learning performance on the day the dye blend was given was impaired in hyperactive Ss, compared to performance after the placebo was given. The nonhyperactive Ss' performance was not affected by the dye challenge.

834. Thorley, Geoffrey. (1984). **Pilot study to assess behavioural and cognitive effects of artificial food colours in a group of retarded children.** *Developmental Medicine & Child Neurology,* 26(1), 56–61.
10 institutionalized children (mean age 139.9 mo; mean IQ 52; mean social age [Vineland Social Maturity Scale] 97.2 mo) were maintained on an additive-free diet for 2 wks, followed by 2 wks in which 2 high, consecutive doses of artificial food colors were administered orally in a placebo-masked, double-blind experimental design. Measures of short-term verbal learning and visuomotor skills and actometer measures of limb activity, together with behavioral rating scales completed by teachers and care staff, all indicated the absence of any adverse behavioral or cognitive effect. (French, German & Spanish abstracts) (20 ref).

835. Turman, Mary W. (1985). **A study of research on the effects of food additives on children's behavior as evidenced by the hyperactivity/learning disabilities syndrome.** *Dissertation Abstracts International,* 46(2-A), 401–402.

836. Weiss, Bernard. (1981). **Food colors and behavior: A response.** *Science,* 212(4494), 579.
Replies to the criticisms of R. L. Brunner et al (1981) of the present authors' (1980) study of the behavioral effects of food colorings in hyperactive children. The authors assert that Brunner et al misinterpreted the purpose of the study, miscalculated the prevalence of the effects, and ignored the toxicologic implications of the Feingold literature. (10 ref).

837. Weiss, Bernard et al. (1980). **Behavioral responses to artificial food colors.** *Science,* 207(4438), 1487–1489.
Assessed sensitivity to artificial colors in 15 male and 7 female 2.5–7 yr olds. Each S's problem behaviors had been reported as improved when given a diet free of artificial colors and flavors for the 3 mo before the study, but none had been diagnosed as hyperkinetic or had any clinically significant medical or psychiatric disorders. In the present double-blind study, where each S served as his or her own control, a diet excluding artificial colors and flavors, 14 fruits, 3 vegetables, certain spices and extracts, and 2 food preservatives was prescribed for 11 wks. Parental reports were used as data for assessing behavioral effects of the diet, although home visits by a behavioral specialist were also scheduled. At specified times on each of the 77 days in the study, S consumed a soft drink containing a blend of 7 artificial colors or placebo. One S that responded mildly to the challenge and one that responded dramatically were detected. The latter, a 34-mo-old female, also showed a significant increase in aversive behaviors. The need to include behavior as a criterion in future hazard evaluations of food additives is recommended.

838. Williams, J. Ivan & Cram, Douglas M. (1978). **Diet in the management of hyperkinesis: A review of the tests of Feingold's hypotheses.** *Canadian Psychiatric Association Journal,* 23(4), 241–248.
A series of clinical studies of the Feingold diet for treatment of hyperactivity have produced mixed results. More recently, there have been 4 sets of experimental studies that have resulted in rigorous tests of the original diet (elimination of salicylates and artificial flavors and colors) and a modified

diet with salicylates included but artificial additives excluded. None of the studies give unqualified support for the hypothesized diet effects, and there are reports that refute the thesis. Some findings suggest that some hyperactive children (10–25%), particularly younger ones, respond favorably to a diet free of artificial additives. The lack of conclusive evidence dictates that additional research needs to be conducted. (French summary) (26 ref).

Animal Research

839. Augustine, George J. & Levitan, Herbert. (1980). **Neurotransmitter release from a vertebrate neuromuscular synapse affected by a food dye.** *Science,* 207(4438), 1489–1490.
In view of reports showing behavioral effects of food additives, the present study examined the effects of the widely used food dye erythrosine (Erythrosin B; Red No. 3) on neuromuscular junctions and on spontaneous quantal release of acetylcholine in frogs (*Rana pipiens*). In concentrations of 10 μM or more, the dye produced an irreversible, dose-dependent increase in neurotransmitter release from presynaptic nerve terminals, as measured by spontaneous miniature end-plate potentials (MEPPs) recorded from muscle fibers. This increase did not depend on the presence of calcium ions in the bathing medium (the concentration of calcium in presynaptic nerve terminals is thought to affect the frequency of MEPPs). Results suggest that although erythrosine might be a useful pharmacological tool for studying transmitter release processes, its use as a food additive should be reexamined.

840. Barcus, Robert A. (1979). **Food additives and hyperactivity in dogs: An animal model of the hyperactive child syndrome.** *Dissertation Abstracts International,* 39(10-B), 5054.

841. Bogomolny, Alice. (1985). **Effects of Erythrosin B (FD&C Red #3) on developing rats.** *Dissertation Abstracts International,* 45(8-B), 2708–2709.

842. Dillon, Kathleen M. (1976). **Some historical, physiological, and psychological correlates of sodium chloride consumption.** *Dissertation Abstracts International,* 37(1-B), 488.

843. Galloway, W. D.; Olvey, K. M. & Brown, N. T. (1986). **Behavioral effects of erythrosine following light exposure.** *Neurobehavioral Toxicology & Teratology,* 8(5), 493–497.
Conducted 3 studies to examine the effects of erythrosine on the activity level of homozygous HRS/J hairless mice in a figure-8 maze. Results of the 1st study show that activity in a dark maze was not influenced by intraperitoneal doses as high as 1.25 mg/kg. In 2 additional studies, Ss were subjected to combinations of dye and preexposure to blue or blue and green light. Light exposure consistently produced increased activity levels. However, there was little evidence of a dye-light interaction effect.

844. Gold, Richard M. et al. (1979). **Non-effect of Massachusetts cement kiln dust upon the food intake, body weight, or activity of female rats.** *Pharmacology, Biochemistry & Behavior,* 10(1), 1–3.
The addition of Georgia cement kiln dust to the diet of cattle or weanling male rats has been reported to increase body weight and feed efficiency. The present study attempted to replicate these effects by adding kiln dust to the Purina laboratory chow of adult female CD rats. Massachusetts cement kiln dust caused no significant change in food intake, weight gain, or activity. The kiln dust effect appears to depend on (a) ingredients peculiar to Georgia kiln dust, (b) age (juveniles vs adults), (c) sex, and/or (d) deficiencies of the control diet. (7 ref).

845. Kantor, Mark A. (1982). **Effects of vitamin B-6 adequate or deficient diets, supplemented with food dyes, on locomotor activity, neurotransmitters, and cytochrome P-450 of male rats.** *Dissertation Abstracts International,* 43(4-B), 1046–1047.

846. Levitan, Herbert et al. (1984). **Brain uptake of a food dye, erythrosin B, prevented by plasma protein binding.** *Brain Research,* 322(1), 131–134.
In 8 experiments, [^{14}C] erythrosin B (EB) was administered into the circulation of mature male Osborne-Mendel rats, and the radioactivity was measured in brain regions several times thereafter. EB did not enter the brain from the blood but penetrated the blood-brain barrier if infused into the carotid circulation in the absence of blood protein. Results suggest that behavioral disorders caused by food colors may be due to sensitive individuals' altered plasma protein binding capacity, which can vary with age and disease. (43 ref).

847. Mailman, Richard B. et al. (1980). **Erythrosine (Red No. 3) and its nonspecific biochemical actions: What relation to behavioral changes?** *Science,* 207(4430), 535–537.
Biochemical studies have shown that the ability of erythrosine to inhibit dopamine uptake into brain synaptosomal preparations is dependent on the concentration of tissue present in the assay mixture. Thus, the present results from 16 Sprague-Dawley rats, which show that erythrosine inhibits dopamine uptake (possibly an explanation of the Feingold hypothesis of childhood hyperactivity), may simply be an artifact that results from nonspecific interactions with brain membranes. In addition, although erythrosine given parenterally (50 mg/kg) did not alter locomotor activity of control or 6-hydroxydopamine-treated Ss, erythrosine (50–300 mg/kg) attenuated the effect of punishment in a "conflict" paradigm. (11 ref).

848. Ohara, Ikuo & Naim, Michael. (1977). **Effects of monosodium glutamate on eating and drinking behavior in rats.** *Physiology & Behavior,* 19(5), 627–634.
In a study with male CD Charles River rats given preference tests in free choice situations, low or high protein casein diets containing up to 3% monosodium glutamate (MSG) were selected indifferently compared to plain casein diet in 7-day trials. The acceptability of diets containing 7% MSG, particularly those of low protein level, was significantly reduced. Except for Day 1, the proportional intake (MSG flavored diet intake/total diet intake) of the 9% protein/7% MSG diet was consistently lower than 18% protein/7% MSG diet. In brief exposure tests (10 min), solutions of MSG (0.02–8%) were preferred over deionized water. The acceptance of solutions containing higher concentrations of MSG was significantly reduced. The total volume intake of both choices (MSG flavored water and water) was significantly increased in tests using solutions containing 3–8% MSG. In long-term tests (1–14 days), solutions containing 0.05–1% MSG were preferred over water. The acceptance of a solution containing 5% MSG was significantly reduced. In a series of 2-choice preference tests using solutions, MSG was preferred over sodium acetate and over sodium glutamate but was less preferred than monosodium aspartate. Results are explained in terms of sensory quality. (34 ref).

849. Ohara, Ikuo; Tanaka, Yoshiharu & Otsuka, Shinichiro. (1979). **Discrimination of monosodium glutamate and sodium chloride solutions by rats.** *Physiology & Behavior,* 22(5), 877–882.
Data from 4 experiments with 305 weanling male Sprague-Dawley rats indicate that Ss might recognize monosodium glutamate (MSG) solution as a favorable substance, differently from sodium chloride solution. Ss' preferences for MSG were not entirely due to the Na+ and, hence, a weak salty taste. (16 ref).

FOOD ADDITIVES

850. Reisen, C. A. & Rothblat, L. A. (1986). **Effect of certified artificial food coloring on learning and activity level in rats.** *Neurobehavioral Toxicology & Teratology,* 8(3), 317–320.
Chronic oral administration of a formula consisting of 7 certified artificial food dyes, given in 0, 2.0, and 5.0 mg/kg doses, failed to produce changes in measures of physical or motor development in Long-Evans hooded rat pups. Two learning tasks, one given during development and the other at maturity, also revealed no differences among groups. In addition, 2 activity-level measures, time-sampled observations and the open field task, were taken on 5 occasions. These measures also failed to demonstrate any effects of food coloring. Although food dyes may have toxic effects at higher dose levels or under unusual dietary or environmental conditions, results suggest that orally ingested low doses do not reliably elicit behavioral changes.

851. Reisen, Carol A. (1984). **The effect of certified artificial food coloring on learning and activity level in rats.** *Dissertation Abstracts International,* 44(9-B), 2926.

852. Viveiros, Donna M. & Tondat, Lynn M. (1978). **Effects of sodium nitrite on DRL performance in the rat.** *Pharmacology, Biochemistry & Behavior,* 8(2), 125–127.
15 Sprague-Dawley rats were administered sodium nitrite (0.10 or 0.15% solutions) in their drinking water from the age of 45 days to the end of the study. Six controls received only tap water. At 80 days of age, Ss were trained to barpress for food pellets on a continuous reinforcement schedule. After reaching criterion performance Ss were switched to a DRL-20 schedule for 6 days to test for response inhibition, which was measured as a ratio of responses to reinforcements. Results indicate no significant differences between groups for response inhibition. All groups showed significant increases in learning as reflected by a decrease in ratios and an increase in total reinforcements over days. However, sodium-nitrite Ss compared to controls, obtained significantly fewer reinforcements over sessions and a greater number of no-responding periods (time-outs). The possibility that sodium nitrite produced an increase in responding to distractible (non-task-related) cues is discussed. (15 ref).

GASES

853. Laties, Victor G. & Merigan, William H. (1979). **Behavioral effects of carbon monoxide on animals and man.** *Annual Review of Pharmacology & Toxicology,* 19, 357–392.
Reviews literature in this area through July 1978 (chiefly experimental laboratory studies), where research has proliferated during the 1970's. Animal studies have covered many behaviors, but have dealt with only a few species and have not examined thoroughly all the important questions (such as the effects of prenatal exposure to CO). These studies consistently show a decreasing response rate due to CO in both conditioned and unconditioned Ss. Studies of human performance have dealt with the effects of CO on visual and auditory functions, on motor behavior (coordination, tracking, and driving), on time discrimination, and on vigilance (detection of small environmental changes). Results are not definitive; contradictory findings are reported by different investigators and even by the same investigators at different times. A few tentative generalizations seem warranted: (a) Interactions exist between CO effects and characteristics of the behavior studied. (b) The effects of short-term low-level exposure are marginal. (c) The dose-effect and time-effect relationships may not be monotonic. Future experiments should emphasize parametric studies of those variables that appear to be most crucial to the behavioral toxicity of CO. (120 ref).

854. Svenson, Ola & Fischhoff, Baruch. (1985). **Levels of environmental decisions.** *Journal of Environmental Psychology,* 5(1), 55–67.
Uses the language of decision theory to model the perspectives of 2 parties in the management of an environmental hazard (i.e., radon releases into homes from granite rock and shale and bricks made of light-weight concrete). The parties involved are (a) individuals whose homes are polluted by radon by-products that thereby pose an uncertain health hazard and (b) the public authorities concerned about those individuals' welfare. Decision trees from each perspective are presented. The analysis provides a means of anticipating ways in which the perceptions and decisions of these parties are intertwined, as well as how they can come into conflict. It also suggests ways in which these difficulties might be ameliorated by altering the respective decison problems. The heuristic value of modeling decision problems in other contexts is discussed, with consideration of the substantive issues arising with acid rain and seatbelt use. (34 ref).

Human Research

855. Ahlström, Richard; Berglund, Birgitta; Berglund, Ulf; Lindvall, Thomas et al. (1986). **Impaired odor perception in tank cleaners.** *Scandinavian Journal of Work, Environment & Health,* 12(6), 574–581.
Studied the olfactory perception of 20 male tank cleaners (aged 26–62 yrs) exposed to petroleum products while cleaning oil tanks. Two reference groups (controls)—each matched with the tank cleaners with respect to sex, age, and smoking habits—were recruited from oil company officers and security guards. The results suggest that Ss had higher absolute odor thresholds for n-butanol and oil vapor than did controls. Ss displayed an odor deficit called "odor intensity recruitment," which seems to be associated with occupational exposure to oil vapor.

856. Benignus, Vernon A.; Muller, Keith E.; Barton, Curtis N. & Prah, James D. (1987). **Effect of low level carbon monoxide on compensatory tracking and event monitoring.** *Neurotoxicology & Teratology,* 9(3), 227–234.
Replicated experiments by V. R. Putz et al (1976, 1979) concerning the effect of carbon monoxide (CO) exposure on compensatory tracking and monitoring in healthy young men. Task and procedural variables were reproduced as closely as practical. 24 19–31 yr old males who had not smoked in 5 yrs were exposed to either room air or 100 ppm CO. Mean carboxyhemoglobin (COHb) levels in the high CO exposure groups were 5.1% for Putz et al (1976, 70 ppm exposure) and 8.24% for the present study (100 ppm exposure). Findings show that in both studies elevated COHb produced a significant increase over time in log mean absolute deviation scores (tracking error) with respect to control groups. The magnitude of the effect was smaller in the present study. In contrast to Putz et al (1976), no significant effect of COHb in monitoring behavior was found.

857. Benignus, Vernon A.; Otto, David A.; Prah, James D. & Benignus, Gayla. (1977). **Lack of effects of carbon monoxide on human vigilance.** *Perceptual & Motor Skills,* 45(3, Pt 1), 1007–1014.
Previous publications on the effects of low levels of carbon monoxide (CO) on human vigilance performance have found conflicting results. This article presents a critical review of the literature and the results of a study employing 52 male Ss performing a numeric monitoring task. CO levels were 0, 100, and 200 ppm which produced mean carboxyhemoglobin levels 0.01, 4.61 and 12.62%, respectively. No CO-exposure levels produced any effect on vigilance performance. The power of the statistical test for CO effects was shown to be quite high, even for fairly trivial possible decrements of performance. (20 ref).

858. Berglund, Birgitta & Lindvall, Thomas. (1983). **Sensory reactions to "sick buildings."** *Reports from the Department of Psychology, U. Stockholm,* 60, 29 p.
Discusses a type of "sick building," in which the occupants show reactions and symptoms similar to those known to be caused by formaldehyde but in which the concentrations of formaldehyde are well below known reaction thresholds. Occupants complain of poor indoor air quality and suffer subtle medical symptoms that may be related to the indoor air, although the specific perceptual mechanisms are largely unknown. In the stimulus-response model of sensory evaluation, the symptoms generated by sick buildings easily fit into the sensory part of the model. The sick building syndrome is best understood by assuming that the sensory systems perform a pattern-recognition analysis. (95 ref).

859. Biersner, R. J.; Hall, D. A. & Linaweaver, P. G. (1976). **Associations between psychological factors and pulmonary toxicity during intermittent oxygen breathing at 2 ATA.** *Aviation, Space, & Environmental Medicine,* 47, 173–176.
Tests of digit span, short-term memory for easy and difficult word associations, simple and complex psychomotor performance, and mood questionnaires were administered over a 15-hr period to 4 experienced divers who breathed intermittent oxygen at 2 atmospheres absolute and to a 5th control diver who breathed only normoxic oxygen. Short-term memory for difficult word associations and self-reported moods of Activity, Depression, Fatigue, and Happiness correlated significantly with a criterion of oxygen toxicity (development of a 10% reduction in vital capacity). However, some of this impairment appeared, from the performance of the control S, to be related to the absence of adequate sleep and rest. Other tests were not affected.

860. Bolter, John F.; Stanczak, Daniel E. & Long, Charles J. (1983). **Neuropsychological consequences of acute, high-level gasoline inhalation.** *Clinical Neuropsychology,* 5(1), 4–7.
Presents WAIS, MMPI, Wechsler Memory Scale, and Halstead-Reitan Neuropsychological Test Battery results for 2 men (aged 28 and 32 yrs) who were exposed to gasoline fumes during an industrial accident. At a 2-yr follow-up, both Ss were left with residual left-hemispheric deficits; and at 3 yrs, 1 S developed severe emotional disturbances. Cases are discussed in terms of the dose-related neurotoxic effects of leaded gasoline inhalation, possible biochemical explanations for the observed lateralized neuropsychological deficits, and interaction of emotional and neurological factors in recovery of function. (9 ref).

861. Bryer, Jeffrey B.; Heck, Edward T. & Reams, Steven H. (1988). **Neuropsychological sequelae of carbon monoxide toxicity at eleven-year follow-up.** *Clinical Neuropsychologist,* 2(3), 221–227.
Presents a case study of a 38-yr-old man who experienced accidental carbon monoxide (CO) poisoning and who developed neurological sequelae that led to his psychiatric hospitalization 4 yrs later. Skull x-rays, EEG, brain scan, and computerized tomography (CT) scan were all within normal limits at the time of hospitalization, but the S demonstrated moderate intellectual impairment, including marked visual/spatial deficits, as well as other neuropsychological difficulties. A follow-up evaluation 11 yrs after the poisoning indicated moderate improvement; however, the visual/spatial deficits were relatively unimproved.

862. Bunnell, David E. & Horvath, Steven M. (1988). **Interactive effects of physical work and carbon monoxide on cognitive task performance.** *Aviation, Space, & Environmental Medicine,* 59(12), 1133–1138.
The simple and interactive effects of carbon monoxide (CO) exposure and prior physical work on cognitive performance were evaluated in 18 Ss (aged 18–29 yrs). Three levels of carboxyhemoglobin (HbCO) and 3 workloads were crossed. Following administration of CO, Ss exercised or rested for 50 min, then performed 5 cognitive tasks. HbCO levels were assessed. Performance on the 2nd of 2 sequentially presented interference tasks (using identical stimuli but with instructions reversed) was impaired with increasing HbCO level, suggesting a reduced ability to adapt to a new response set. An interaction between HbCO level and exercise level was seen for visual search performance: in rest conditions, performance was improved with increasing HbCO level; however, performance was impaired with increasing HbCO levels following 60% work.

863. Campion, John & Latto, Richard. (1985). **Apperceptive agnosia due to carbon monoxide poisoning: An interpretation based on critical band masking from disseminated lesions.** European Brain and Behaviour Society Workshop: The effect of hypoxia on brain and behaviour (1984, Rotterdam, Netherlands). *Behavioural Brain Research,* 15(3), 227–240.
Apperceptive visual agnosia is usually held to be a specific deficit in apperception—a hypothetical postsensory stage in visual processing. The present authors describe a male patient diagnosed as having a classical apperceptive agnosia resulting from carbon monoxide poisoning. Controlled behavioral testing confirmed the apparent agnosia but revealed that he could be trained to make a number of visual discriminations that had not been apparent from routine clinical examination and that he suffered a number of subtle sensory impairments that also had not been apparent. Evoked potential recordings to grating patterns showed a complex pattern of brain responses involving interactions between spatial frequency, orientation, and hemisphere. Data suggest that the agnosia was caused by sensory impairments rather than a deficit in apperception. It is proposed that the impairments were caused by loss of certain spatial frequency and orientation information; data from normal Ss whose visual fields were artificially masked support an interpretation based on object contour masking by a multifocal field defect caused by disseminated lesions. Implications for theories of visual agnosia and vision based on the concept of processing channels are discussed. (22 ref).

864. Chapel, James L. & Husain, Arshad. (1978). **The neuropsychiatric aspects of carbon monoxide poisoning.** *Psychiatric Opinion,* 15(3), 33–37.
Describes the neuropsychiatric picture of a family of 4 who were poisoned by carbon monoxide from a faulty muffler. Two of the surviving three appear to have overcome most of the major complications but still have tinnitus and "forgetfulness." The most seriously affected member, a 13-yr-old girl, is still seriously handicapped by a frontal (limbic) syndrome and a temporal lobe seizure disorder with associated interictal psychosis. (8 ref).

865. Christensen, C. L. et al. (1977). **Effects of three kinds of hypoxias on vigilance performance.** *Aviation, Space, & Environmental Medicine,* 48, 491–496.
Five men and 5 women performed a visual vigilance task under 4 atmospheric conditions while measures of heart rate, blood pressure, and ventilation were obtained. Physiological and subjective responses showed no changes attributable to the atmospheric conditions simulated in a chamber. A significant decline in vigilance performance (signals detected) was obtained for the low oxygen (17%) condition when compared with the control condition. However, performance under carbon monoxide (114 ppm) and carbon monoxide plus low oxygen did not differ from control. (31 ref).

866. Crystal, H. A.; Schaumburg, H. H.; Grober, E.; Fuld, P. A. et al. (1988). **Cognitive impairment and sensory loss associated with chronic low-level ethylene oxide exposure.** *Neurology,* 38(4), 567–569.
A 29-yr-old female college graduate worked for 10 yrs adjacent to an ethylene oxide (EtO) chemical sterilizer. When the sterilizer was closed, levels of EtO in the air around the

sterilizer were 4.2 ppm (Occupational Safety and Health Administration maximum level, 1 ppm). Seven years after beginning work with EtO, the S experienced impaired memory, increased irritability, clumsiness, and falling. Three years later exposure ceased, and symptoms markedly improved over the next few months but did not disappear entirely. Neurologic and neuropsychological exams 1 yr after exposure ceased demonstrated emotional lability, impaired concentration, cognitive slowing, impaired recent and remote memory, and impaired thermal and vibratory sense in distal limbs. The S's pattern of relatively preserved learning and profound forgetting distinguished her from most other Ss with memory disorders. No other causes for the condition were identified.

867. Dalen, Knut. (1986). **Nevropsykologiske følgjer av karbonmonoksydforgifting. / Delayed neuropsychological sequelae in carbon monoxide intoxication.** *Tidsskrift for Norsk Psykologforening,* 23(4), 215–220.
Reviews the 1983–1984 literature on neuropsychological sequelae in carbon monoxide intoxication (COI) and presents the case of a 62-yr-old man who was neuropsychologically examined as part of a vocational compensation suit 16 yrs after having severe COI and developing several neuropsychological symptoms. (English abstract).

868. Estrin, William J.; Cavalieri, Stuart A.; Wald, Peter; Becker, Charles E. et al. (1987). **Evidence of neurologic dysfunction related to long-term ethylene oxide exposure.** *Archives of Neurology,* 44(12), 1283–1286.
Examined neurological function in 8 female hospital workers chronically exposed to low-dose ethylene oxide and in 8 matched controls. The exposed group produced lower scores on measures of cognition, memory, reaction time, attention, and coordination. There was a dose–response relationship between years of exposure and decreasing preformance on the Continuous Performance Test and the slowing of sural nerve conduction velocity.

869. Frederiksen, Lee W. & Martin, John E. (1979). **Carbon monoxide and smoking behavior.** *Addictive Behaviors,* 4(1), 21–30.
Reviews the health risks of carbon monoxide (CO) and its relationship to smoking behavior. Special emphasis is placed on behavioral determinants of carbon monoxide uptake. The role of CO in measurement and modification of smoking risk is also discussed. (41 ref).

870. Gliner, Jeffrey A.; Horvath, Steven M. & Mihevic, Patricia M. (1983). **Carbon monoxide and human performance in a single and dual task methodology.** *Aviation, Space, & Environmental Medicine,* 54(8), 714–717.
Studied whether CO exposure would limit the ability to time share 2 concurrent tasks in an experiment in which 15 Ss (aged 20–32 yrs) underwent 2 2.5 hr exposures to either filtered air or 100 ppm CO. Ss performed 2 tasks singly and in combination. The central task was a compensatory tracking task with 3 levels of difficulty; the peripheral task was a signal detection task with 3 probabilities of signal occurrence. When CO levels reached 5% (during the last 30 min of exposure), performance on the peripheral signal detection task was altered. This was demonstrated by a 6% decline in signals detected correctly. This decline was found when the signal detection task was performed alone. Results suggest that exposure to CO decreased arousal and interacted with fatigue to produce decreases in performance. (13 ref).

871. Grattan, Lynn; Eslinger, Paul J. & Faust, David. (1988). **Case report: Reversible neuropsychological impairment after severe carbon monoxide poisoning in a child.** *Developmental Neuropsychology,* 4(1), 37–46.
Neurobehavioral examination at 2 wks postonset of a 10-yr-old girl who suffered severe CO intoxication revealed specific impairments in functions associated with the frontal and parietal areas. Follow-up examinations throughout the next 4 wks revealed recovery of all functions to estimated premorbid levels. Recovery was maintained at follow-up. This recovery pattern was different from recovery observed in adults.

872. Groll-Knapp, E. et al. (1982). **Moderate carbon monoxide exposure during sleep: Neuro- and psychophysiological effects in young and elderly people.** *Neurobehavioral Toxicology & Teratology,* 4(6), 709–716.
To assess age-related effects of carbon monoxide on brainwave activity and sleep, auditory EPs were measured during sleep in 10 20–25 yr olds and 10 55–72 yr olds under counterbalanced control and exposure conditions. Memory performance and subjective feeling were assessed before and after sleep. In young Ss there was a significant increase in deep sleep and a decrease in REM sleep during CO exposure, whereas in elderly Ss similar but nonsignificant changes occurred. Some CO-related changes in auditory EPs within different sleep stages, namely shorter latencies in elderly Ss and higher amplitudes in young Ss, approached significance. CO exposure tended to cause impaired memory consolidation and depressed mood in young Ss; no such effects were observed in elderly Ss. (29 ref).

873. Harbin, Thomas J.; Benignus, Vernon A.; Muller, Keith E. & Barton, Curtis N. (1988). **The effects of low-level carbon monoxide exposure upon evoked cortical potentials in young and elderly men.** *Neurotoxicology & Teratology,* 10(2), 93–100.
Investigated the effects of a 5% carboxyhemoglobin level upon 2 indices of neurophysiological function, reaction time (RT), and the late positive component of the visual evoked potential in 33 young males (aged 18–28 yrs) and 22 elderly males (aged 60–86 yrs). Results indicate no effects of carbon monoxide (CO) on any of the neurophysiological indices and greater absorption of CO by young than by elderly men. Findings indicate that acute, low-level CO exposure is probably not neurotoxic in normal, healthy men.

874. Jaeckle, Richard S. & Nasrallah, Henry A. (1985). **Major depression and carbon monoxide-induced parkinsonism: Diagnosis, computerized axial tomography, and response to L-dopa.** *Journal of Nervous & Mental Disease,* 173(8), 503–508.
Reports a case of major depressive disorder complicated by CO-induced Parkinson's syndrome in a 40-yr-old male. Computerized axial tomography (CAT) revealed bilateral globus pallidus necrosis. Clinical, CAT, and neuropathological findings in other cases of CO encephalopathy with and without parkinsonism are reviewed. There was no clinical response to a tricyclic antidepressant, but both the mood and movement disorders responded fully to levodopa. The implications of these findings with regard to the central neurochemical pathophysiology in this S and in major depressive disorder in general are discussed. (34 ref).

875. Jefferson, James W. (1976). **Subtle neuropsychiatric sequelae of carbon monoxide intoxication: Two case reports.** *American Journal of Psychiatry,* 133(8), 961–964.
Describes 2 male patients, 23 and 35 yrs old, who developed subtle but troublesome emotional and cognitive problems following carbon monoxide poisoning. The value of sequential neuropsychological testing and judicious psychiatric counseling in such cases is stressed.

876. Johnson, F. Reed & Luken, Ralph A. (1987). **Radon risk information and voluntary protection: Evidence from a natural experiment.** *Risk Analysis,* 7(1), 97–107.

Surveyed 221 householders in Maine to determine the efficacy of a program designed to provide them with information concerning health risks from indoor radon. All households had received information through the program. Results suggest that the risk information approach failed as indicated by evocation of perceived risk that understated objective risk and the lack of a statistically significant relationship between mitigating behavior and objective risk.

877. Kohler, G.-K. & Petzold, J. (1974). **Clinical and electroencephalographic course of a psychosis following poisoning with cesspool gases.** *Nervenarzt,* 45(11), 607-612.
Reports a case of toxic psychosis over a period of 18 mo. Abnormal EEG rhythms correlated with episodic exacerbations of psychopathological symptoms. (22 ref).

878. Laursen, Peter & Netterstrøm, Bo. (1982). **Psychological functions of urban busdrivers exposed to exhaust gases: A cross sectional study of urban busdrivers in Denmark.** *Scandinavian Journal of Psychology,* 23(4), 283-290.
A cross-sectional study using questionnaires and psychological tests was conducted on 171 urban busdrivers from the 3 largest cities in Denmark (Copenhagen, Aarhus, and Odense). 47 commuter train drivers, assumed to be exposed to air pollutants no more than the average citizen, were studied as controls. The air of the busdrivers' breathing zone was analyzed for toxic agents. The hygienic effect in the winter season was 0.63 and in the summer season 0.36. The year mean hygienic effect was 0.42. Neurasthenic complaints such as difficulties in concentration, verbal retrieval, and tiredness were significantly more frequent among the busdrivers, particularly in Copenhagen. On psychological tests of verbal and spatial learning, retrieval and memory, psychomotor functions, visual perception, and vigilance, the Copenhagen busdrivers compared to controls showed significant dysfunctions only of verbal learning and long-term memory. Busdrivers from the 2 smaller cities did not differ significantly from controls. It is suggested that the subjective complaints are due to psychosocial stressors in the busdrivers' condition of work, whereas the few differences in psychological test results may indicate a subclinical effect caused by the presence of neurotoxic agents in the working environment. (48 ref).

879. Lindvall, Thomas & Stevensson, Leif T. (1974). **Equal unpleasantness matching of malodorous substances in the community.** *Journal of Applied Psychology,* 59(3), 264-269.
Five odorants, produced through combustion procedures of animal manure, were matched with hydrogen sulfide with regard to unpleasantness by 30 female 20-47 yr olds. Power functions described the unpleasantness matchings for 5 combustion toilets tested. The exponents of the equal sensation functions indicated a relative invariance of the various combustion procedures on the exponent. Different combustion procedures resulted in different levels of odor unpleasantness, but these differences were small from a practical point of view. Results demonstrate the practical applicability of psychophysical methods in environmental health research. (18 ref).

880. Luria, S. M. (1977). **Visual masking and carbon monoxide toxicity.** *Perceptual & Motor Skills,* 44(1), 47-53.
Measured thresholds for letters with and without a masking stimulus (presented either to the same eye as the letters or to the other eye) before and after exposure of 6 smokers and 3 nonsmokers to 500 ppm CO in air for 1 hr. Identification of the unmasked letters was not degraded by CO but a number of thresholds of the masked letters were significantly affected among the smokers. The effects of the CO on binocular and interocular masking were similar. These results suggest that the first effects of CO toxicity are neither on the receptors nor central but are on the transmission lines in between and that smokers are more susceptible than nonsmokers to short-term increases in the level of CO. The masking phenomenon, however, does not appear to be an unusually sensitive measure of CO toxicity. (18 ref).

881. Mihevic, Patricia M.; Gliner, Jeffrey A. & Horvath, Steven M. (1981). **Perception of effort and respiratory sensitivity during exposure to ozone.** *Ergonomics,* 24(5), 365-374.
Investigated (1) the effects of exposure to the air pollutant ozone during exercise on perception of effort and (2) perceptual sensitivity to respiratory responses during this exposure. 14 male university students were exposed to various ozone concentrations during both resting and bicycle ergometer exercises. It is concluded that perceptual responses to exercise and respiratory stimuli during ozone exposure reflected the decrements in pulmonary function observed with the exposure. (29 ref).

882. Min, Sung Kil. (1986). **A brain syndrome associated with delayed neuropsychiatric sequelae following acute carbon monoxide intoxication.** *Acta Psychiatrica Scandinavica,* 73(1), 80-86.
Summarizes clinical data on 86 34-82 yr olds with delayed neuropsychiatric sequelae following acute carbon monoxide intoxication. Possible etiological factors in the development of the brain syndrome were age, duration of unconsciousness on acute intoxication, and previous physical illness. The onset was relatively sudden after the apparent clear period that ranged from 2 to 40 days. The most frequent symptoms were apathy, dull facial expressions, amnesia and disorientation, hypokinesia, mutism, irritable distractibility, incontinence, gait disturbance, and abnormal neurological signs and reflexes. EEG was abnormal in 33 of the 57 Ss assessed. Of 27 Ss who were given a computed tomographic brain scan, 15 Ss were abnormal. The prognosis was relatively good in a follow-up study of 56 Ss. Only age was related to a better prognosis. (18 ref).

883. Ohlin, P.; Lundh, B. & Westling, H. (1976). **Carbon monoxide blood levels and reported cessation of smoking.** *Psychopharmacology,* 49(3), 263-265.
Carboxyhemoglobin (COHb) levels were estimated in patients attending an anti-smoking clinic. A surprisingly large number of patients who reported "no smoking" had abnormally high COHb levels. Because this discrepancy may be due to the patients not reporting their smoking habits correctly, this phenomenon is seen as further evidence that smoking should be regarded as a form of drug addiction in some persons. Results of stop-smoking cures should be evaluated by other means than the patient's own reports.

884. Otto, D. A.; Benignus, Vernon A. & Prah, James D. (1979). **Carbon monoxide and human time discrimination: Failure to replicate Beard-Wertheim experiments.** *Aviation, Space, & Environmental Medicine,* 50, 40-43.
R. R. Beard and G. A. Wertheim (1967) described a dose-related deficit in human time perception during low level CO exposure. Two other laboratories were unable to replicate this finding, although methodological differences could explain the failures. This study more precisely repeated the original experiment, but failed again to obtain any CO-related deficit. The bulk of evidence, therefore, does not indicate any adverse effect of low level CO exposure on time perception in healthy young adults. (23 ref).

885. Perez, Edgardo L. & Silverman, Marvin. (1981). **Case report: CO_2 intoxication.** *Psychiatric Journal of the University of Ottawa,* 6(4), 226-228.
Discusses the case of a 31-yr-old male employee in a dry ice factory who suffered from industrial CO_2 poisoning. Following an accident, he developed a seizure disorder and had impaired visual-motor coordination and memory. The most significant etiological factor for the seizures was hypoxic encephalopathy secondary to exposure to a high concentration of CO_2. (12 ref).

GASES

886. Prelipceanu, D. (1985). **Sindrom psihoorganic alcoolic cronic acutizat heterotoxic. / Acute heterotoxic, chronic alcoholic psychoorganic syndrome.** *Neurologie, Psihiatrie, Neurochirurgie,* 30(1), 65–69.
Describes a case of chronic alcoholic psychoorganic syndrome that presented problems of differential diagnosis (Korsakoff-like syndrome, true Korsakoff's syndrome, idiopathic dementia, or brain tumor). When the etiological circumstances leading to the development of the clinical picture were determined, it was concluded that a partial, Alzheimer-like condition with dementia was caused by accidental carbon monoxide poisoning of a patient previously intoxicated with alcohol. (English & Russian abstracts).

887. Putz, Vernon R. (1979). **The effects of carbon monoxide on dual-task performance.** *Human Factors,* 21(1), 13–24.
30 18–26 yr old nonsmokers were exposed for 4 hrs to 1 of 3 concentrations of carbon monoxide (CO)—5 ppm, 35 ppm, and 70 ppm—to produce blood levels of either 1, 3, or 5% carboxyhemoglobin (COHb) after the 3rd hr of exposure. Performance was assessed by a tracking task paired with a peripheral monitoring task, each possessing 2 levels of difficulty. Results indicate that visual-manual tracking was significantly impaired by about 30% during the 4th hr of exposure to 70 ppm of CO (when 5% COHb was reached) as compared to performance at 5 and 35 ppm. The impairment occurred only during the high frequency tracking condition. Ss' response times to the peripheral light-intensity changes also increased during the 3rd and 4th hrs. Findings suggest that an assessment of the effects of low-level CO on human performance should include an analysis of the demand characteristics of the tasks and data on concentration and exposure duration. (27 ref).

888. Roche, S. et al. (1981). **Sustained visual attention and carbon monoxide: Elimination of adaptation effects.** *Human Factors,* 23(2), 175–184.
18 Ss (aged 20–30 yrs) performed a 1-hr visual vigilance task, once during a control condition (filtered air) and once during an experimental condition (CO). The carboxyhemoglobin (COHb) level was elevated to 5% utilizing a bolus maintenance technique, which raised the COHb level rapidly so that there would be no possibility of an adaptation occurring prior to vigilance testing. Physiological measurements included heart rate, blood pressure, and ventilation. Neither vigilance performance nor the physiological variables was statistically affected by the 5% COHb level. Ss identified a significantly higher percentage of signals with the high frequency of signal presentation as compared to the low frequency under both filtered air and the 5% COHb level. Signal detection improved in 12 Ss during minutes 0–15, while 10 Ss showed improvement during minutes 31–45 with an elevated COHb level. The subjective questionnaire indicated that CO significantly decreased Ss' confidence concerning their performance on the vigilance task and caused significant irritation of the eyes and throat. (25 ref).

889. Rummo, Nicholas & Sarlanis, Kiriako. (1974). **The effect of carbon monoxide on several measures of vigilance in a simulated driving task.** *Journal of Safety Research,* 6(3), 126-130.
In a 2-hr vigilance task in a driving simulator, Ss under low blood levels of carbon monoxide (CO) were significantly slower in responding to lead car speed changes and nonsmokers made significantly fewer steering wheel corrections. There was no decrement under CO in responding to a dashboard warning light or in maintenance of lane position.

890. Salvatore, Santo. (1974). **Performance decrement caused by mild carbon monoxide levels on two visual functions.** *Journal of Safety Research,* 6(3), 131–141.
Used 6 20–27 yr old volunteers to determine the effects of mild levels of carbon monoxide (CO) on the time necessary to detect static and dynamic visual targets. In the static phase, S adapted for 1 min to an illumination of 17 ft-L and detected low-contrast targets when the ambient illumination dropped to .02 ft-L. In the dynamic phase, the illumination was constant at 6 ft-L and S detected the targets moving into the visual field. There was a significant decrement in target detection time due to CO for the dynamic task, indicating some constriction of the visual field. The CO-related decrement for the static task was not statistically significant.

891. Sandman, Peter M.; Weinstein, Neil D. & Klotz, M. L. (1987). **Public response to the risk from geological radon.** *Journal of Communication,* 37(3), 93–108.
Assessed the awareness and reactions of the public in New Jersey to naturally occurring radon using (1) questionnaire data from 141 residents who were potentially at risk who had already been reached by radon information and had made an initial response and (2) data from a 1986 statewide survey of 800 residents. Three areas of public reactions were evaluated: emotional response, perception of radon as a threat, and relevant behaviors. Although the most common response to the radon issues was apathy, predictors of monitoring, perceived problem seriousness, and emotional distress were identified.

892. Smith, W. Lynn. (1986). **The thirteenth nerve: Sieben mit einem Streich.** *International Journal of Clinical Neuropsychology,* 8(1), 41–42.
Describes an industrial accident in which 7 workers suffered carbon monoxide poisoning and were later treated with hyperbaric oxygen. Ss showed signs of anxiety and depression, somatic displacement, and posttraumatic reaction. Complaints of headache, fatigue, and personality changes of irritability and impulsiveness persisted. The roles of emotional and organic factors in these impairments are discussed.

893. Strahilevitz, Meir; Strahilevitz, Aharona & Miller, John E. (1979). **Air pollutants and the admission rate of psychiatric patients.** *American Journal of Psychiatry,* 136(2), 205–207.
Studied the correlation between mean daily levels of several air pollutants and the number of emergency room visits and inpatient admissions to a psychiatric hospital in St. Louis during the summer and fall of 1972. Nitrogen dioxide and carbon monoxide showed a positive correlation with emergency room visits by all patients, while nitrogen monoxide showed a negative correlation with inpatient admissions during working days. (3 ref).

894. Svensson, Leif T. (1977). **A symmetric and an asymmetric model for the equal-sensation function in olfaction.** *Perception & Psychophysics,* 21(6), 535–544.
Data from 3 intramodel matching experiments in olfaction were analyzed with regard to a symmetric and an asymmetric model for the equal-sensation function. The asymmetric model is discussed in relation to the symmetric model. In all, 11 equal-sensation functions were investigated in a total of 11 Ss, and of these functions 9 were with different pairs of odorants. The following odorants were investigated: hydrogen sulfide, pyridine, demethyl disulfide, and 5 odorants obtained by different combustion procedures of animal manure. It was found that the equal-sensation function can be written in asymmetric and symmetric forms; equations are derived in which φ_i and φ_k are stimuli expressed in multiples of respective absolute thresholds, λ and C are general constants invariant of experimental matching method and matched attribute (perceived unpleasantness or intensity). The constants λ and C are calculated for both group and individual data. The asymmetric form of the equal-sensation function is interpreted in terms of relativity and the symmetric form in terms of measurement. (26 ref).

895. Treanor, J. J. (1977). **Cold weather aviation psychology: A case report.** *Aviation, Space, & Environmental Medicine,* 48, 377–379.
Presents a case study of gradually worsening apparent anxiety symptoms in an aircraft pilot that were fortuitously traced to carbon monoxide exposure from a faulty home heating unit.

896. Vicente, Peter J. (1980). **Neuropsychological assessment and management of carbon monoxide intoxication patient with consequent sleep apnea: A longitudinal case report.** *Clinical Neuropsychology,* 2(2), 91–94.
Demonstrates via standardized neuropsychological assessment procedures the longitudinal course of a carbon monoxide poisoning patient (34-yr-old female). Also described is the psychological management of S from the initial assessment through the delayed and subsequent development of sleep apnea and cataleptic seizures. (7 ref).

897. von Restorff, W. & Hebisch, S. (1988). **Dark adaptation of the eye during carbon monoxide exposure in smokers and nonsmokers.** *Aviation, Space, & Environmental Medicine,* 59(10), 928–931.
Dark adaptation time and light sensitivity of the dark adapted eye were measured in 10 young healthy smokers and nonsmokers (aged 19–23 yrs) during carbon monoxide (CO) exposure. Breathing 70 and 100 ppm CO in the inspired air after a prime dose of 5,000 ppm for 5 or 8 min resulted in an almost linear increase of carboxyhemoglobin (HbCO) saturation up to 19.1% HbCO in smokers as compared with 17.5% in nonsmokers. Dark adaptation time was longer and light sensitivity of the dark adapted eye was reduced in smokers as compared with nonsmokers at comparable levels of both inspired CO and HbCO. Data suggest that the cause for this may be the chronic poisoning with CO, stemming from cigarette smoking.

898. Wright, Geoffrey R. (1978). **Effects of carbon monoxide on human performance.** *Dissertation Abstracts International,* 39(3-B), 1224–1225.

899. Zeller, W. Patrick et al. (1984). **Accidental carbon monoxide poisoning.** *Clinical Pediatrics,* 23(12), 694–695.
Presents the case of a 58-yr-old female who brought her 2 4-yr-old grandchildren to the emergency room after the children had experienced accidental automobile carbon monoxide poisoning (CMP) and reviews the pathogenesis of CMP. It is suggested that other pediatric diseases (e.g., flulike syndrome, acute psychiatric illness) may mimic CMP, requiring a high index of suspicion from the emergency-room physician. Emergency room treatment and suggested criteria for hyperbaric oxygen use in pediatric patients are discussed. (15 ref).

Animal Research

900. Annau, Zoltan. (1987). **Complex maze performance during carbon monoxide exposure in rats.** First Joint International Union of Toxicology and Italian Society of Toxicology Symposium: Behavioral toxicology: New experimental approaches (1986, Bari, Italy). *Neurotoxicology & Teratology,* 9(2), 151–155.
Attempted to provide a model of human escape behavior from toxic gases using animals by building a complex maze with 8 "choice points" that resembled a human dwelling and yet closely approximated a rodent's natural habitat. Ss were 24 male Long-Evans hooded rats. After stable running times were established, different groups of 6 Ss were exposed to 2,000, 3,000, 3,500, and 4,000 ppm of carbon monoxide (CO) when placed in the maze. Results show that the effect of increasing CO concentrations was to increase maze running times as well as to decrease the number of animals reaching the goal. Carboxyhemoglobin concentrations reached asymptote sooner but were not at a markedly higher level at high CO concentrations. Behavior of the rats in this situation may be similar to human confusion and feelings of lethargy often reported by survivors of residential fires.

901. Ator, Nancy A. (1979). **Modulation of the behavioral effects of carbon monoxide by reinforcement contingencies.** *Dissertation Abstracts International,* 39(9-B), 4638.

902. Boja, J. W.; Nielsen, J. A.; Foldvary, E. & Truitt, Edward B. (1985). **Acute low-level formaldehyde behavioural and neurochemical toxicity in the rat.** Eighth Annual Meeting of the Canadian College of Neuropsychopharmacology: Perspectives in Canadian neuro-psychopharmacology (1985, London, Canada). *Progress in Neuro-Psychopharmacology & Biological Psychiatry,* 9(5–6), 671–674.
Determined the effects of low-level formaldehyde (HCHO) exposure on behavior and neurochemistry in male Sprague-Dawley rats. Ss were exposed to either air or HCHO vapor (5, 10, or 20 parts/million) for 3 hrs on 2 consecutive days, during which behavioral observations were made. Following the 2nd exposure session, the Ss' brains were analyzed for norepinephrine, dopamine, 5-hydroxytryptamine (5-HT), and their major metabolites. HCHO exposure resulted in decreased motor activity and neurochemical changes in dopamine and 5-HT neurons. Results suggest that low-level HCHO vapor exposure may affect the central nervous system (CNS). (6 ref).

903. Culver, Bruce & Norton, Stata. (1976). **Juvenile hyperactivity in rats after acute exposure to carbon monoxide.** *Experimental Neurology,* 50(1), 80-98.
It has been proposed that perinatal anoxia may be one cause of the syndrome of minimal brain dysfunction in children in which hyperactivity develops at an early age and diminishes or disappears with maturation of the brain during adolescence. Results of the present study, which show rapid onset and complete reversibility of hyperactivity in rats exposed to carbon monoxide as neonates, make this form of anoxic damage an interesting and useful model for further investigation. (41 ref).

904. Davis, Michael & Gendelman, Phillip M. (1977). **Plasticity of the acoustic startle response in the acutely decerebrate rat.** *Journal of Comparative & Physiological Psychology,* 91(3), 549–563.
In 4 experiments, plasticity of the acoustic startle reflex was measured in male albino Sprague-Dawley rats in which a complete transection between the forebrain and midbrain was made. During a period from 60 to 100 min after surgery, startle amplitude in the transected Ss was relatively stable and comparable with that of controls (anesthetized with halothane and placed in a stereotaxic instrument). During this period the transection did not alter the temporal recovery process (with intervals of 2, 4, 8, or 16 sec) or auditory prepulse inhibition (with intervals of 25, 50, 100, 500, or 1,000 msec) or the normal reduction in startle caused by high levels of background noise. The transection did prevent the normal increase in startle caused by moderate levels of background noise and eliminated within-session habituation. The effect on habituation was particularly noticeable since the curves of the transected and nontransected Ss actually crossed. Results are dicussed in terms of how the transection procedure can be used to evaluate various hypotheses about underlying mechanisms of startle plasticity. (50 ref).

905. Koëter, Herman B. & Rodier, Patricia M. (1986). **Behavioral effects in mice exposed to nitrous oxide or halothane: Prenatal vs postnatal exposure.** *Neurobehavioral Toxicology & Teratology,* 8(2), 189–194.
DUB/ICR mice exposed to 4 or 6 hrs of nitrous oxide or halothane differed from controls on a variety of tests conducted before weaning. Both treatment times and both agents were associated with delays in the appearance of developmen-

GASES

tal landmarks and delays in the appearance of righting reflexes and locomotion. The level of general activity just before weaning was significantly depressed in males exposed to N_2O postnatally. The distribution of activity scores was shifted significantly in both postnatal groups compared to controls. Data are compatible with human studies suggesting that inhalants at parturition have an effect on early behavior. The persistence of effects over the 1st 3 wks of life does not fit with the idea that the behavioral effects are mediated by continued presence of the drug.

906. Koob, George F.; Annau, Zoltan; Rubin, Robert J. & Montgomery, Mark R. (1974). **Effect of hypoxic hypoxia and carbon monoxide on food intake, water intake, and body weight in two strains of rats.** *Life Sciences,* 14(8), 1511-1520.
Exposed Long-Evans hooded and Sprague-Dawley albino male rats for 24 hrs to 3 different levels of hypoxic hypoxia and 3 different levels of carbon monoxide. Both rat strains showed a decrease in food and water intake and body weight gain that were directly related to the degree of hypoxia or carbon monoxide exposure. Results demonstrate the importance of considering nutritional alterations in biochemical studies of prolonged exposure to hypoxia or carbon monoxide. (19 ref).

907. Mactutus, Charles F. & Fechter, Laurence D. (1984). **Prenatal exposure to carbon monoxide: Learning and memory deficits.** *Science,* 223(4634), 409–411.
Two experiments studied the offspring of 34 female Long-Evans hooded rats exposed during pregnancy to average daily carbon monoxide (CO) concentrations of 150 parts/million and compared them to offspring of 34 Ss who were exposed only to air. Three male and 3 female pups from 16 randomly selected litters were evaluated in a 2-way avoidance task. Results demonstrate that chronic prenatal CO exposure may produce a functional deficit in the CNS in the absence of any overt toxicity. Multiple dependent measures and specific control groups confirmed that this deficit was independent of nonassociative or motivational alterations. Although no impairment was observed in avoidance acquisition, young adult Ss prenatally exposed to CO demonstrated impaired retention as indexed by reacquisition. It is noted that results resemble the often cited impairment in achievement test scores noted during early childhood in the children of women who were heavy smokers during pregnancy.

908. Merigan, William H. & McIntire, Roger W. (1976). **Effects of carbon monoxide on responding under a progressive ratio schedule in rats.** *Physiology & Behavior,* 16(4), 407–412.
Under a progressive ratio schedule the response requirement increases arithmetically with each reinforcement, and the session is terminated when responding ceases for 15 min. Four male Long-Evans rats, responding for food on this schedule, were exposed to 4 levels of carbon monoxide, ranging from 155 to 700 ppm, beginning 30 min before the test session and continuing throughout the session. Four additional, catheterized Ss were used for carboxy hemoglobin tests. The size of the last completed ratio and the local rate of responding decreased during exposure to the higher levels of carbon monoxide. Postreinforcement pause time was slightly increased for 3 of 4 Ss during exposure to the highest level of carbon monoxide. (19 ref).

909. Norton, Stata; Mullenix, Phyllis & Culver, Bruce. (1976). **Comparison of the structure of hyperactive behavior in rats after brain damage from X-irradiation, carbon monoxide and pallidal lesions.** *Brain Research,* 116(1), 49-67.
Nocturnal hyperactivity, as measured by photocell counts of locomotion in a residential maze, was produced in Charles River rats by 3 different kinds of brain damage, X-irradiation at gestational Day 14 or 15, exposure to carbon monoxide on the 5th day of postnatal life, or bilateral stereotaxic lesions of the globus pallidus in adult rats. These brain-damaged Ss and their controls were photographed during their 1st exploratory experience in a simple cage. Frequency of 15 motor acts, duration of each occurrence, and associations of pairs of acts were calculated. The 15 motor acts were divided into 3 clusters of acts: grooming, exploratory, and attention behaviors. Hyperactivity was associated with shortened durations and increases in frequency of exploratory acts, while grooming and attention behaviors tended to decrease in duration and frequency. Sequences of behavior acts were less structured in hyperactive Ss than in controls. No changes in behavior structure were found which were uniquely associated with one kind of brain damage. Hyperactivity appeared to be a continuum in that the intensity of effects produced on behavior as measured by the photographic technique correlated well with the amount of increase in photocell activity. (17 ref).

910. Plevova, J. & Frantik, E. (1974). **The influence of various saturation rates on motor performance of rats exposed to carbon monoxide.** *Activitas Nervosa Superior,* 16(2), 101-102.

911. Quimby, Kelvin L. et al. (1974). **Enduring learning deficits and cerebral synaptic malformation from exposure to 10 parts of halothane per million.** *Science,* 185(4151), 625-627.
Chronic exposure of Sprague-Dawley rats to halothane (10 ppm) during early life produced later deficits in learning a shock-motivated light-dark discrimination and a food-motivated maze pattern, correlated with enduring synaptic membrane malformation in cerebral cortex. Adult exposure had no effect. Halothane may provide a useful analytical tool for study of brain. The behavioral-ultrastructural techniques also suggest a standard for assessing the safety of trace toxicants with central nervous system effects.

912. Rodier, Patricia M. & Koëter, Herman B. (1986). **General activity from weaning to maturity in mice exposed to halothane or nitrous oxide.** *Neurobehavioral Toxicology & Teratology,* 8(2), 195–199.
Mice exposed to 6 hrs of 75% nitrous oxide (N_2O) or 0.5% halothane on the 14th day of gestation or to 4 hrs of 75% N_2O or 0.5% halothane on the 2nd day of life were tested for general activity at 3 ages. Just before weaning, all treated groups appeared hypoactive, and there was a significant effect in the postnatal N_2O group. Both postnatal groups had deviant distributions of scores, compared to sham-exposed controls. The main effect of treatment was greater in young adulthood, when the prenatal halothane group differed from controls. This group and the postnatal groups had excess numbers of low-scoring Ss. At 6 mo, the main effect of treatment was no longer significant, but the unusual distribution of scores was still present in the postnatal halothane group. Early activity measures were significantly related to later scores. Within treatment groups, controls and postnatal N_2O Ss were the most consistent over time.

913. Schrot, J. & Thomas, J. R. (1986). **Multiple schedule performance changes during carbon monoxide exposure.** *Neurobehavioral Toxicology & Teratology,* 8(3), 225–230.
Studied behavioral effects of carbon monoxide (CO) in 4 male hooded rats during 90-min exposures to concentrations ranging from 250 to 850 ppm. Ss performed on a multiple FR/differential-reinforcement-of-low-rates (DRL) schedule of food reinforcement. Periodically, Ss were individually exposed to either air or CO for 30-min periods prior to as well as during 60-min test sessions. Concentrations of 650 ppm or higher produced response rate reductions. The decreased response rates were due primarily to abrupt cessation of responding during CO exposures. Response patterning in both FR and DRL components remained intact until responding ceased. The accuracy of responding in the DRL component was not systematically affected by CO exposure.

914. Schrot, J.; Thomas, J. R. & Robertson, R. F. (1984). **Temporal changes in repeated acquisition behavior after carbon monoxide exposure.** *Neurobehavioral Toxicology & Teratology,* 6(1), 23–28.

Behavioral effects of carbon monoxide were studied in 8 male Sprague-Dawley rats following 90-min exposures to concentrations ranging from 500 to 1,200 ppm. Ss performed on a repeated acquisition of behavioral chains procedure in which food reinforcement depended on the correct completion of a 4-member response sequence on 3 separate response levers. Concentrations of 850 and 1,200 ppm produced increased pausing between responses throughout the test sessions. Accuracy of responding as measured by total error and timeout responses was not affected by carbon monoxide exposure. (16 ref).

915. Smith, Marcia D.; Merigan, William H. & McIntire, Roger W. (1976). **Effects of carbon monoxide on fixed-consecutive-number performance in rats.** *Pharmacology, Biochemistry & Behavior,* 5(3), 257–262.

Four male Long-Evans rats were trained under a fixed-consecutive-number (FCN) schedule to make sequences of 20 or more consecutive responses on 1 lever followed by a single response on a 2nd lever. When performance was stable, they were exposed to 200, 400, and 600 ppm carbon monoxide (CO) for either 30 or 60 min before and during a 45-min session. Decreases in response rate at CO levels as low as 200 ppm were due to both decreased local response rate and extended pauses. A lowered percentage of reinforcement, due to decreases in response sequence length, was also found at CO levels as low as 200 ppm. This decreased sequence length may reflect effects of CO on response rate, or a disruption of discriminative aspects of FCN schedule performance.

916. Smith, Robert F. & Goldman, Larry. (1983). **Behavioral effects of prenatal exposure to ethylene dibromide.** *Neurobehavioral Toxicology & Teratology,* 5(5), 579–585.

48 pregnant female Long-Evans hooded rats were exposed to 0, 0.43, 6.67, or 66.67 ppm ethylene dibromide via inhalation for 4 hrs/day 3 days/wk from Day 3 to 20 gestation. 66.67 ppm produced an increase in defecation during exposure, decreased gestational weight gain, and enhanced rotorod performance and T-maze brightness discrimination acquisition in the offspring. Similar changes were noted in the dams and offspring exposed to 6.67 ppm, but the magnitude of the effects was reduced. No effects of exposure to 0.43 ppm were detected, nor were litter size, litter composition, nest building, pup retrieval, DRL-20 acquisition, straight-alley running speed, or passive avoidance affected by exposure to any dose. It is suggested that the behavioral effects of the medium and high doses may be secondary to stress reactions in the dams to exposure to these doses. (26 ref).

917. Stupfel, Maurice; Halberg, Franz; Mordelet-Dambrine, Madeleine & Magnier, Monique. (1977). **Perspectives in chronobiology of air pollution.** *Chronobiologia,* 4(4), 333–351.

In 18 experiments, groups of 28–41 male or female Sprague Dawley rats kept on a 12 hr/12 hr light–dark cycle inhaled 5 different concentrations of carbon monoxide at each of the 2 test times, 12 hrs apart. A decrease in flow of CO_2 resulting from CO inhalation was greater in the active dark (D) than in the resting light (L) span. Experimental hypoxic mortality of male and female Ss also showed circadian variations greater in the D than in the L span. (56 ref).

918. Vogel, Richard A. (1976). **Effects of carbon monoxide, hypoxic hypoxia, and drugs on animal models of complex learned behavior.** *Dissertation Abstracts International,* 37(5-B), 2565.

Section II. Citations to Recently Published Journal Articles

This section includes the most recent citations from the journal literature on the psychological, behavioral, and sociocultural aspects of environmental toxins, retrieved from the PsycALERT database and arranged alphabetically by author. When abstracting and full indexing are completed, the records will appear in *Psychological Abstracts* and the PsycINFO database.

919. Adams, Perrie M.; Hanlon, Roger T. & Forsythe, John W. (1988). **Toxic exposure to ethylene dibromide and mercuric chloride: Effects on laboratory-reared octopuses.** *Neurotoxicology & Teratology,* 10(6), 519–523.

920. Akaike, M.; Tanaka, K.; Goto, M. & Sakaguchi, T. (1988). **Impaired Biel and radial arm maze learning in rats with methylnitrosourea-induced microcephaly.** *Neurotoxicology & Teratology,* 10(4), 327–332.

921. Bellinger, David; Leviton, Alan; Waternaux, Christine; Needleman, Herbert et al. (1988). **Low-level lead exposure, social class, and infant development.** *Neurotoxicology & Teratology,* 10(6), 497–503.

922. Bertazzi, Pier-Alberto. (1989). **Industrial disasters and epidemiology: A review of recent experiences.** *Scandinavian Journal of Work, Environment & Health,* 15(2), 85–100.

923. Braun, Claude M.; Daigneault, Sylvie & Gilbert, Brigitte. (1989). **Color discrimination testing reveals early printshop solvent neurotoxicity better than a neuropsychological test battery.** *Archives of Clinical Neuropsychology,* 4(1), 1–13.

924. Brody, Julia G. (1988). **Responses to collective risk: Appraisal and coping among workers exposed to occupational health hazards.** *American Journal of Community Psychology,* 16(5), 645–663.

925. Bushnell, Philip J. (1988). **Behavioral effects of acute p-xylene inhalation in rats: Autoshaping, motor activity, and reversal learning.** *Neurotoxicology & Teratology,* 10(6), 569–577.

926. Bushnell, Philip J. (1988). **Effects of delay, intertrial interval, delay behavior and trimethyltin on spatial delayed response in rats.** *Neurotoxicology & Teratology,* 10(3), 237–244.

927. Champagne, Francine & Kirouac, Gilles. (1989). **The effects of formaldehyde on voluntary ethanol consumption in the laboratory rat: A comparison of two methods of determination of a single test solution.** *Journal of General Psychology,* 116(1), 91–101.

928. Connor, Donald J.; Jope, Richard S. & Harrell, Lindy E. (1988). **Chronic, oral aluminum administration to rats: Cognition and cholinergic parameters.** *Pharmacology, Biochemistry & Behavior,* 31(2), 467–474.

929. DeLuca, John; Burright, Richard G. & Donovick, Peter J. (1989). **Genotypic influences on lead-induced hyperactivity in mice.** *Behavior Genetics,* 19(2), 171–181.

930. Eccles, Christine U. (1988). **EEG correlates of neurotoxicity.** Satellite Symposium to the Second World Congress of Neuroscience: Biological markers of neurotoxicity (1987, Szeged, Hungary). *Neurotoxicology & Teratology,* 10(5), 423–428.

931. Farage-Elawar, Miranda. (1988). **Toxicity of aldicarb in young chicks.** *Neurotoxicology & Teratology,* 10(6), 549–554.

932. Gordon, Christopher J. & Watkinson, William P. (1988). **Behavioral and autonomic thermoregulation in the rat following chlordimeform administration.** *Neurotoxicology & Teratology,* 10(3), 215–219.

933. Gunderson, Virginia M.; Grant-Webster, Kimberly S.; Burbacher, Thomas M. & Mottet, N. Karle. (1988). **Visual recognition memory deficits in methylmercury-exposed *Macaca fascicularis* infants.** *Neurotoxicology & Teratology,* 10(4), 373–379.

934. Hagstadius, Stefan; Ørbæk, Palle; Risberg, Jarl & Lindgren, May. (1989). **Regional cerebral blood flow at the time of diagnosis of chronic toxic encephalopathy induced by organic-solvent exposure and after the cessation of exposure.** *Scandinavian Journal of Work, Environment & Health,* 15(2), 130–135.

935. Hänninen, Helena. (1988). **The psychological performance profile in occupational intoxications.** Satellite Symposium to the Second World Congress of Neuroscience: Biological markers of neurotoxicity (1987, Szeged, Hungary). *Neurotoxicology & Teratology,* 10(5), 485–488.

936. Horowitz, Jordan & Stefanko, Michael. (1989). **Toxic waste: Behavioral effects of an environmental stressor.** *Behavioral Medicine,* 15(1), 23–28.

937. Korpela, Marja. (1989). **Inhibition of synaptosome membrane-bound integral enzymes by organic solvents.** *Scandinavian Journal of Work, Environment & Health,* 15(1), 64–68.

938. Kulig, Beverly M. (1988). **The neurobehavioral effects of chronic styrene exposure in the rat.** *Neurotoxicology & Teratology,* 10(6), 511–517.

939. Lehotzky, Kornelia; Szeberenyi, Judit M.; Ungvary, G. & Kiss, Anna. (1988). **Behavioral effects of prenatal methoxy-ethyl-mercury chloride exposure in rat pups.** Satellite Symposium to the Second World Congress of Neuroscience: Biological markers of neurotoxicity (1987, Szeged, Hungary). *Neurotoxicology & Teratology,* 10(5), 471–474.

940. Levin, Edward D. & Bowman, Robert E. (1988). **Long-term effects of chronic postnatal lead exposure on delayed spatial alternation in monkeys.** *Neurotoxicology & Teratology,* 10(6), 505–510.

941. Lilienthal, Hellmuth; Lenaerts, Claudia; Winneke, Gerhard & Hennekes, Raimund. (1988). **Alteration of the visual evoked potential and the electroretinogram in lead-treated monkeys.** Satellite Symposium to the Second World Congress of Neuroscience: Biological markers of neurotoxicity (1987, Szeged, Hungary). *Neurotoxicology & Teratology,* 10(5), 417–422.

942. Lyngbye, Troels; Hansen, Ole N. & Grandjean, Philippe. (1988). **Neurological deficits in children: Medical risk factors and lead exposure.** *Neurotoxicology & Teratology,* 10(6), 531–537.

CURRENT CITATIONS

943. Mattsson, J. L. & Albee, R. R. (1988). **Sensory evoked potentials in neurotoxicology.** Satellite Symposium to the Second World Congress of Neuroscience: Biological markers of neurotoxicity (1987, Szeged, Hungary). *Neurotoxicology & Teratology,* 10(5), 435–443.

944. McDonald, Brian E.; Costa, Lucio G. & Murphy, Sheldon D. (1988). **Spatial memory impairment and central muscarinic receptor loss following prolonged treatment with organophosphates.** *Toxicology Letters,* 40, 47–56.

945. Mikkelsen, Sigurd; Jørgensen, Merete; Browne, Ellen & Gyldensted, Carsten. (1988). **Mixed solvent exposure and organic brain damage: A study of painters.** *Acta Neurologica Scandinavica,* 78(Suppl 118), 143 p.

946. Newland, M. Christopher; Ng, Wendy W.; Baggs, Raymond B.; Gentry, G. David et al. (1986). **Operant behavior in transition reflects neonatal exposure to cadmium.** *Teratology,* 34, 231–241.

947. Norton, Stata & Kimler, Bruce F. (1988). **Comparison of functional and morphological deficits in the rat after gestational exposure to ionizing radiation.** *Neurotoxicology & Teratology,* 10(4), 363–371.

948. O'Flynn, R. R. (1988). **Do organic solvents "cause" dementia?** *International Journal of Geriatric Psychiatry,* 3(1), 5–15.

949. Piikivi, Leena. (1989). **Health effects of low level, long-term exposure to mercury (Hg°) vapour.** *Acta Universitatis Ouluensis: Series D Medica,* 183, 1–98.

950. Piikivi, Leena & Hänninen, Helena. (1989). **Subjective symptoms and psychological performance of chlorine-alkali workers.** *Scandinavian Journal of Work, Environment & Health,* 15(1), 69–74.

951. Pilisuk, Marc & Acredolo, Curt. (1988). **Fear of technological hazards: One concern or many?** *Social Behaviour,* 3(1), 17–24.

952. Poul, Jean-Michel. (1988). **Effects of perinatal ivermectin exposure on behavioral development of rats.** *Neurotoxicology & Teratology,* 10(3), 267–272.

953. Sandmark, Björn; Broms, Inger; Löfgren, Lennart & Ohlson, Carl-Göran. (1989). **Olfactory function in painters exposed to organic solvents.** *Scandinavian Journal of Work, Environment & Health,* 15(1), 60–63.

954. Singer, Raymond & Scott, Nancy E. (1987). **Progression of neuropsychological deficits following toluene diisocyanate exposure.** *Archives of Clinical Neuropsychology,* 2(2), 135–144.

955. Singh, Jaya; Dwivedi, Kamal & Saxena, Vinod B. (1988). **Psychological performance and subjective symptoms of welders in an automobile workshop.** *Journal of Personality & Clinical Studies,* 4(2), 179–182.

956. Thompson, Christopher; Dent, J. & Saxby, P. (1988). **Effects of thallium poisoning on intellectual function.** *British Journal of Psychiatry,* 153, 396–399.

957. Tupper, Charles R. (1989). **Chemical hazards in aeromedical aircraft.** *Aviation, Space, & Environmental Medicine,* 60(1), 73–75.

958. Vyner, Henry M. (1988). **The psychological dimensions of health care for patients exposed to radiation and the other invisible environmental contaminants.** Special Issue: Social policy for pollution-related diseases. *Social Science & Medicine,* 27(10), 1097–1103.

959. Wada, Hiromi; Hosokawa, Toshiyuki & Saito, Kazuo. (1988). **Repeated toluene exposure and changes of response latency in shock avoidance learning.** *Neurotoxicology & Teratology,* 10(4), 387–391.

960. Webb, Dianne B. (1989). **PBB: An environmental contaminant in Michigan.** *Journal of Community Psychology,* 17(1), 30–46.

961. Wigg, N. R.; Vimpani, G. V.; McMichael, A. J.; Baghurst, P. A. et al. (1988). **Port Pirie Cohort Study: Childhood blood lead and neuropsychological development at age two years.** *Journal of Epidemiology & Community Health,* 42(3), 213–219.

962. Willers, Stefan; Schütz, Andrejs; Attewell, Robyn & Skerfving, Staffan. (1988). **Relation between lead and cadmium in blood and the involuntary smoking of children.** *Scandinavian Journal of Work, Environment & Health,* 14(6), 385–389.

Section III. Subject Index

This is a subject index to entries in Section I. Subject terms in this index are taken from the *Thesaurus of Psychological Index Terms,* (Fifth Edition, 1988). *See* references are used to refer to preferred forms of entry, or from conceptually broader terms to narrower ones. *See also* references alert the reader to more specific terms. Each document is indexed with the most specific terms that are appropriate for that document's content.

Academic Achievement [See Also Reading Achievement] 194, 261, 493, 584, 594, 816, 831
Academic Achievement Prediction 603
Academic Environment [See Classroom Environment]
Accident Prevention 32, 49, 72, 124, 190
Accident Proneness 515
Accidents [See Also Home Accidents, Industrial Accidents, Transportation Accidents] 16, 98, 114
Acetylcholine 292, 605, 685, 839
Acetylcholinesterase 274, 283, 326, 607, 633
Achievement [See Academic Achievement, Reading Achievement]
Achievement Measures [See Stanford Achievement Test]
Acids [See Also Adenosine, Ascorbic Acid, Gamma Aminobutyric Acid, Glutamic Acid, Methionine] 298, 696
Acoustic Reflex 181, 904
Acoustic Stimuli [See Auditory Stimulation]
Acquired Immune Deficiency Syndrome 192
Active Avoidance [See Avoidance Conditioning]
Activist Movements 128, 154, 200
Activity Level 188, 226, 294, 300, 308, 322, 414, 419, 495, 608, 615, 617, 631, 639, 645, 646, 652, 658, 659, 669, 676, 704, 709, 731, 746, 757, 769, 774, 779, 827, 834, 843, 845, 850, 851, 905, 912
Acute Psychosis [See Acute Schizophrenia]
Acute Schizophrenia 351
Adaptation [See Also Environmental Adaptation] 888
Adaptation (Dark) [See Dark Adaptation]
Adaptation (Environmental) [See Environmental Adaptation]
Addiction [See Alcoholism]
Adenosine 691
Adjudication 64
Adjunctive Behavior [See Also Polydipsia] 642
Adjustment [See Also Related Terms] 177
Administrators [See Management Personnel]
Admission (Psychiatric Hospital) [See Psychiatric Hospital Admission]
Adolescents 93, 94, 208, 532, 534, 589, 816, 822, 829, 832

Adrenal Cortex Hormones [See Corticosterone]
Adrenal Medulla Hormones [See Norepinephrine]
Adrenergic Blocking Drugs [See Hydroxydopamine (6-), Phenoxybenzamine]
Adrenergic Drugs [See Amphetamine, Dextroamphetamine]
Adrenergic Nerves 429
Adrenolytic Drugs [See Chlorpromazine]
Adult Attitudes 160
Adults [See Also Aged, Middle Aged, Young Adults] 131
Aerospace Personnel [See Aircraft Pilots]
Aesthetics 130
Aetiology [See Etiology]
Affective Disorders [See Affective Disturbances]
Affective Disturbances [See Also Mania, Manic Depression] 445, 558, 578
Age Differences 173, 423, 542, 543, 560, 580, 589, 628, 652, 662, 690, 694, 741, 779, 810, 872, 873, 912
Aged 24
Agencies (Groups) [See Organizations]
Aggressive Behavior [See Also Animal Aggressive Behavior, Animal Predatory Behavior, Attack Behavior] 141, 183, 539, 826
Aging (Physiological) [See Physiological Aging]
Agnosia 863
Agonistic Behavior [See Aggressive Behavior]
Agricultural Workers 133, 248, 253
AIDS [See Acquired Immune Deficiency Syndrome]
Aircraft 113, 121
Aircraft Pilots 98
Airplanes [See Aircraft]
Akinesia [See Apraxia]
Albino Rats [See Rats]
Alcohol Abuse [See Alcoholism]
Alcoholic Hallucinosis [See Korsakoffs Psychosis]
Alcoholic Psychosis [See Korsakoffs Psychosis]
Alcoholism [See Also Korsakoffs Psychosis] 332, 369
Alcohols [See Also Ethanol, Methanol] 344, 387, 426
Alienation 90, 169, 170
Alkaloids [See Apomorphine, Atropine, Caffeine, Cocaine, Morphine, Nicotine, Physostigmine, Scopolamine]

Allergic Disorders [See Also Food Allergies] 42
Alphabets [See Letters (Alphabet)]
Alzheimers Disease 70, 76, 102, 108, 117, 118, 123, 164, 179, 180, 189, 207, 214, 216, 331, 337, 391, 545, 577, 776, 780
Amentia [See Mental Retardation]
Amines [See Also Amphetamine, Atropine, Catecholamines, Chlordiazepoxide, Chlorpromazine, Cocaine, Dextroamphetamine, Dopamine, Methylphenidate, Norepinephrine, Phenoxybenzamine, Physostigmine, Scopolamine, Serotonin] 779
Amino Acids [See Gamma Aminobutyric Acid, Glutamic Acid, Methionine]
Amphetamine 647, 701, 742, 761, 779
Amphetamine (d-) [See Dextroamphetamine]
Amphetamine (dl-) [See Amphetamine]
Amphetamine Sulfate [See Amphetamine]
Amphibia [See Also Frogs, Salamanders] 228
Amplitude (Response) [See Response Amplitude]
Amygdaloid Body 294
Anabolites [See Metabolites]
Analgesia 619
Analgesic Drugs [See Atropine, Morphine, Scopolamine]
Analysis [See Also Related Terms] 791
Ancestors [See Parents]
Anesthetic Drugs [See Also Cocaine, Hexobarbital, Pentobarbital] 362, 399, 415, 905, 911, 912, 916
Anger 141
Angst [See Anxiety]
Anguish [See Distress]
Animal Aggressive Behavior [See Also Animal Predatory Behavior, Attack Behavior] 272, 330, 611, 628, 646, 673, 744, 767
Animal Behavior [See Animal Ethology]
Animal Biological Rhythms [See Also Animal Circadian Rhythms] 689
Animal Breeding 228, 229, 297, 651
Animal Circadian Rhythms 329, 917
Animal Communication 237
Animal Courtship Behavior 272
Animal Defensive Behavior [See Also Animal Escape Behavior] 230
Animal Development [See Also Related Terms] 223, 312, 409, 420, 610, 616, 629, 643, 646, 650, 651, 666, 669, 681, 684, 706, 733, 736, 772, 785, 841, 905, 912

SUBJECT INDEX

Animal Dominance 662
Animal Drinking Behavior 236, 429, 654, 682, 718, 759, 848, 849, 906
Animal Emotionality 274, 316, 666
Animal Environments 221, 234, 237, 271, 770
Animal Escape Behavior 611, 653, 900
Animal Ethology [See Also Animal Aggressive Behavior, Animal Biological Rhythms, Animal Circadian Rhythms, Animal Communication, Animal Courtship Behavior, Animal Defensive Behavior, Animal Dominance, Animal Drinking Behavior, Animal Escape Behavior, Animal Exploratory Behavior, Animal Feeding Behavior, Animal Foraging Behavior, Animal Maternal Behavior, Animal Mating Behavior, Animal Open Field Behavior, Animal Play, Animal Predatory Behavior, Animal Sex Differences, Animal Sexual Behavior, Animal Social Behavior, Attack Behavior, Nest Building] 61, 63, 239, 263, 764, 768
Animal Exploratory Behavior 265, 645, 763
Animal Feeding Behavior 221, 224, 317, 429, 682, 718, 848, 906
Animal Foraging Behavior 279
Animal Instinctive Behavior 313
Animal Locomotion 408, 413, 608, 639, 652, 659, 757, 905
Animal Maternal Behavior 313, 314, 616, 618, 916
Animal Mating Behavior 232, 286, 297, 328, 641
Animal Motivation 266, 312, 718
Animal Open Field Behavior 267, 274, 279, 294, 300, 320, 407, 419, 625, 626, 641, 653, 654, 666, 688, 705, 734, 743, 763, 767, 779
Animal Parental Behavior [See Animal Maternal Behavior]
Animal Play 677
Animal Predatory Behavior 279, 281
Animal Sex Differences 272, 681, 917
Animal Sexual Behavior [See Also Animal Courtship Behavior, Animal Mating Behavior] 421, 422, 649
Animal Social Behavior [See Also Animal Aggressive Behavior, Animal Communication, Animal Courtship Behavior, Animal Dominance, Animal Maternal Behavior, Animal Mating Behavior, Animal Predatory Behavior, Attack Behavior] 236, 309, 629, 637, 649, 650, 651, 662, 675, 676, 677, 689, 770
Animal Strain Differences 627, 738
Animals [See Also Related Terms] 235, 853
Anoxia 865, 903, 906, 917, 918
Antabuse [See Disulfiram]
Antibiotics 58
Anticholinergic Drugs [See Cholinergic Blocking Drugs]
Anticholinesterase Drugs [See Cholinesterase Inhibitors]

Anticonvulsive Drugs [See Also Pentobarbital, Phenobarbital] 412
Antidepressant Drugs [See Also Methylphenidate] 316
Antiemetic Drugs [See Chlorpromazine, Sulpiride]
Antiepileptic Drugs [See Anticonvulsive Drugs]
Antihypertensive Drugs [See Chlorpromazine, Phenoxybenzamine]
Antipathy [See Aversion]
Antisocial Behavior [See Crime, Homicide, Recidivism]
Antispasmodic Drugs [See Atropine]
Anxiety 42, 166, 253, 255, 402, 479, 892, 895
Anxiety Neurosis [See Panic Disorder, Posttraumatic Stress Disorder]
Anxiousness [See Anxiety]
Aphasia [See Agnosia]
Apnea 896
Apomorphine 636, 711, 735
Apomorphine Hydrochloride [See Apomorphine]
Appalachia 536
Apparatus 448
Appetite 760, 842
Appetite Depressing Drugs [See Amphetamine, Dextroamphetamine]
Appetite Disorders 710
Applied Psychology [See Environmental Psychology]
Apprehension [See Anxiety]
Apraxia 270
Architecture 858
Arrhythmias (Heart) [See Bradycardia]
Arteries (Anatomy) [See Carotid Arteries]
Arthropoda [See Beetles, Crabs, Crustacea, Diptera, Insects]
Arts [See Architecture, Literature]
Ascorbic Acid 588
Asia [See India, Japan]
Asphyxia [See Anoxia]
Assessment [See Measurement]
Associations (Groups) [See Organizations]
Associations (Word) [See Word Associations]
At Risk Populations 73, 74, 114, 149, 476, 494, 583
Ataxia 262, 372
Atmospheric Conditions 7, 39, 80, 88, 100, 109, 112, 176, 186, 198, 204, 211
Atropine 306
Attack Behavior 274, 276
Attempted Suicide 77, 259
Attention [See Also Monitoring, Vigilance] 495, 501, 807, 827
Attention Span 282, 389
Attitude Change 125, 172, 175, 206, 218
Attitude Measurement 35, 154
Attitude Similarity 185
Attitudes [See Also Related Terms] 45, 93, 96, 132, 140, 161, 169, 174, 218, 513

Attraction (Interpersonal) [See Interpersonal Attraction]
Audiogenic Seizures 606
Audition [See Auditory Perception]
Auditory Discrimination 717, 719
Auditory Evoked Potentials 431, 432, 717, 719, 872
Auditory Perception [See Also Auditory Discrimination, Loudness Perception] 319, 468
Auditory Stimulation [See Also White Noise] 55, 85, 182, 293
Auditory Thresholds 425, 427, 432
Australia 52, 96, 484
Authoritarianism 130
Autism [See Early Infantile Autism]
Autistic Children 567, 581
Automobiles 49, 81, 82, 83, 84, 85, 182, 206
Autonomic Nervous System [See Also Adrenergic Nerves, Cholinergic Nerves] 281
Autonomic Nervous System Disorders 369
Autoshaping 681
Aversion 688
Aversion Conditioning 231, 308, 320, 393, 638, 738
Aversive Stimulation 703
Aviation 895
Aviators [See Aircraft Pilots]
Avoidance 763
Avoidance Conditioning 233, 238, 283, 285, 294, 299, 301, 302, 305, 437, 604, 606, 614, 623, 631, 634, 635, 641, 642, 657, 671, 679, 686, 687, 688, 705, 734, 741, 746, 767, 769, 907
Awareness [See Attention, Monitoring, Vigilance]
Axons 262

Babies [See Infants]
Baboons 918
Background (Family) [See Family Background]
Barbiturates [See Hexobarbital, Pentobarbital, Phenobarbital]
Barometric Pressure [See Atmospheric Conditions]
Basal Ganglia [See Also Amygdaloid Body] 728, 739
Basal Metabolism 223
Bayes Theorem [See Statistical Probability]
Beetles 329
Behavior Analysis [See Behavioral Assessment]
Behavior Change 847
Behavior Disorders [See Also Alcoholism, Attempted Suicide, Crime, Homicide, Korsakoffs Psychosis, Recidivism] 8, 97, 440, 452, 466, 474, 481, 533, 534, 569, 800, 801, 815
Behavior Modification 127, 496, 525
Behavior Problems 42, 168, 529, 534, 535, 552, 553, 582, 593, 802, 814, 826, 829, 836, 837

SUBJECT INDEX

Behavior [See Also Related Terms] 12, 109, 112, 220, 430, 548, 568, 585, 599, 605, 756, 777
Behavioral Assessment 40
Beliefs (Nonreligious) [See Attitudes]
Bender Gestalt Test 464
Benzedrine [See Amphetamine]
Benzodiazepines [See Also Chlordiazepoxide, Diazepam] 619
Bibliography 65, 790
Biochemistry [See Also Neurochemistry] 51, 380, 464, 519, 564, 609, 777, 847
Biological Clocks (Animal) [See Animal Biological Rhythms]
Biological Rhythms [See Animal Biological Rhythms, Animal Circadian Rhythms]
Bipolar Depression [See Manic Depression]
Birds [See Also Chickens, Ducks, Pigeons, Quails, Sea Gulls] 271, 276, 279, 280, 285, 297
Birth Weight 136
Bitterness [See Taste Perception]
Blacks 462, 488, 490, 555, 590
Blood [See Also Blood Plasma] 504, 508, 561, 563, 573, 598, 599, 706
Blood Cells [See Also Erythrocytes] 225
Blood Flow 89, 338, 370, 376, 379
Blood Plasma 253, 299, 846
Blood Pressure Disorders [See Hypertension]
Blood Proteins [See Also Hemoglobin] 846
Blood Vessels [See Carotid Arteries]
Blue Collar Workers 75, 187, 215, 337, 352, 355, 375, 528, 596
Body Fluids [See Blood, Blood Plasma, Cerebrospinal Fluid]
Body Size [See Body Weight]
Body Weight [See Also Birth Weight] 419, 647, 675, 679, 686, 693, 710, 735, 767, 844, 906, 916
Borderline Mental Retardation 532
Borderline Mentally Retarded [See Slow Learners]
Boys [See Human Males]
Bradycardia 293
Brain [See Also Amygdaloid Body, Basal Ganglia, Cerebellum, Cerebral Cortex, Geniculate Bodies (Thalamus), Hippocampus, Hypothalamo Hypophyseal System, Hypothalamus, Limbic System, Mesencephalon, Motor Cortex, Reticular Formation, Superior Colliculus, Visual Cortex] 227, 379, 459, 664, 691, 706, 716, 727, 846
Brain Ablation [See Brain Lesions]
Brain Damage 520, 864
Brain Damaged 349
Brain Disorders [See Also Alzheimers Disease, Brain Damage, Korsakoffs Psychosis, Microcephaly, Minimal Brain Disorders, Organic Brain Syndromes, Parkinsons Disease, Toxic Encephalopathies, Toxic Psychoses] 456
Brain Injuries [See Brain Damage]

Brain Lesions 286, 298, 765, 909
Brain Metabolism [See Neurochemistry]
Brain Self Stimulation 438
Brain Stem [See Reticular Formation]
Brain Stimulation [See Brain Self Stimulation, Chemical Brain Stimulation]
Breast Feeding 122, 251
Breathing [See Respiration]
Breeding (Animal) [See Animal Breeding]
Brightness Perception 785
Bromides 89, 193
Budgets [See Costs and Cost Analysis]
Burnout [See Occupational Stress]
Business 133
Business and Industrial Personnel [See Also Blue Collar Workers, Management Personnel, White Collar Workers] 58, 69, 127, 147, 201, 212, 241, 335, 342, 343, 345, 356, 365, 370, 376, 379, 385, 386, 466, 502, 516, 570, 572, 586, 855
Businessmen [See Business and Industrial Personnel]
Buying [See Consumer Behavior]

Caffeine 378
Calcium [See Also Calcium Ions] 522, 581, 664, 739, 759, 760
Calcium Ions 406
Cancers [See Neoplasms]
Carbohydrates [See Also Sugars] 816
Carbon Monoxide 853, 856, 857, 862, 865, 867, 869, 870, 873, 880, 883, 884, 887, 888, 889, 890, 898, 899, 900, 901, 903, 906, 907, 908, 909, 910, 913, 914, 915, 917, 918
Carbon Monoxide Poisoning 853, 861, 863, 864, 871, 872, 874, 875, 882, 886, 892, 895, 896, 897, 898
Carboxyhemoglobinemia [See Carbon Monoxide Poisoning]
Carcinogens 25, 72, 876
Carcinomas [See Neoplasms]
Cardiac Rate [See Heart Rate]
Cardiovascular Disorders [See Bradycardia, Hypertension]
Cardiovascular System [See Also Carotid Arteries] 78
Careers [See Occupations]
Carotid Arteries 846
Carp [See Goldfish]
Case History [See Patient History]
Case Law 460
Case Report 89, 193, 197, 217, 248, 348, 485, 512, 521, 821, 875, 877, 885, 895, 896
Catabolites [See Metabolites]
Cataplexy 896
Catecholamines [See Also Dopamine, Norepinephrine] 242, 457, 670, 684, 845
Categorizing [See Classification (Cognitive Process)]
Cathode Ray Tubes [See Video Display Units]
Cats 269, 295, 634, 635

Caucasians [See Whites]
Cells (Biology) [See Axons, Blood Cells, Dendrites, Epithelial Cells, Erythrocytes, Neurons, Sensory Neurons, Sperm]
Central Nervous System [See Also Amygdaloid Body, Basal Ganglia, Brain, Cerebellum, Cerebral Cortex, Geniculate Bodies (Thalamus), Hippocampus, Hypothalamo Hypophyseal System, Hypothalamus, Limbic System, Mesencephalon, Motor Cortex, Reticular Formation, Spinal Cord, Superior Colliculus, Visual Cortex] 75, 295, 296, 367, 411, 643, 776
Central Nervous System Disorders [See Also Alzheimers Disease, Ataxia, Brain Damage, Brain Disorders, Korsakoffs Psychosis, Microcephaly, Minimal Brain Disorders, Organic Brain Syndromes, Parkinsons Disease, Toxic Psychoses] 348, 374, 481, 598, 626, 907
Cerebellar Cortex [See Cerebellum]
Cerebellar Nuclei [See Cerebellum]
Cerebellopontile Angle [See Cerebellum]
Cerebellum 473, 707
Cerebral Cortex [See Also Amygdaloid Body, Basal Ganglia, Hippocampus, Limbic System, Motor Cortex, Visual Cortex] 338, 342, 362, 370, 685, 728, 773, 911
Cerebral Lesions [See Brain Lesions]
Cerebrospinal Fluid 359
Chance (Fortune) [See Statistical Probability]
Change (Social) [See Social Change]
Character Disorders [See Personality Disorders]
Chemical Brain Stimulation 436, 634, 635, 686
Chemical Elements [See Also Calcium, Calcium Ions, Cobalt, Copper, Iron, Lead (Metal), Lithium, Magnesium, Mercury (Metal), Metallic Elements, Nitrogen, Oxygen, Phosphorus, Sodium, Sodium Ions, Zinc] 34, 37, 38, 51, 201, 365, 379, 386, 519, 537, 564, 570, 581, 588, 598, 634, 721, 806, 881
Chemistry [See Biochemistry, Neurochemistry]
Chemoreceptors 237
Chemotherapy [See Drug Therapy]
Chickens 262, 678, 743
Child Care Workers 513
Child Guidance Clinics 497
Child Psychiatric Clinics [See Child Guidance Clinics]
Childhood Development [See Also Early Childhood Development] 439, 472, 489, 517, 554, 556, 568, 732
Childhood Play Behavior 526
Childhood Psychosis [See Early Infantile Autism]
Childrearing Practices [See Also Weaning] 513
Children [See Also Infants, Neonates, Preschool Age Children, School Age

SUBJECT INDEX

Children] 32, 139, 142, 467, 474, 477, 478, 501, 506, 513, 523, 540, 547, 548, 550, 556, 557, 565, 573, 574, 612, 648, 790, 800, 802, 812, 820, 825, 835, 836
Chlordiazepoxide 287, 288
Chlorpromazine 775
Choice Behavior 161
Cholinergic Blocking Drugs [See Also Atropine, Nicotine, Scopolamine] 778
Cholinergic Drugs [See Also Physostigmine] 310, 753
Cholinergic Nerves 604, 607
Cholinesterase 253, 262, 281, 299, 300
Cholinesterase Inhibitors [See Also Physostigmine] 320, 322
Cholinolytic Drugs [See Cholinergic Blocking Drugs]
Cholinomimetic Drugs [See Acetylcholine, Physostigmine]
Choroid [See Eye (Anatomy)]
Chronic Schizophrenia [See Schizophrenia]
Cigarette Smoking [See Tobacco Smoking]
Circadian Rhythms (Animal) [See Animal Circadian Rhythms]
Cities [See Urban Environments]
Classical Conditioning [See Also Conditioned Responses, Conditioned Suppression] 293, 703
Classification (Cognitive Process) 79, 587
Classroom Behavior 8, 529, 535, 539, 549, 551, 553, 602, 804, 814
Classroom Environment 159, 194
Climate (Meteorological) [See Atmospheric Conditions]
Clinical Judgment (Med Diagnosis) [See Medical Diagnosis]
Clinical Judgment (Psychodiagnosis) [See Psychodiagnosis]
Clinics [See Child Guidance Clinics]
CNS Affecting Drugs [See Amphetamine, Caffeine, Chlorpromazine, Dextroamphetamine, Methylphenidate, Pentylenetetrazol, Scopolamine]
CNS Depressant Drugs [See Chlorpromazine, Scopolamine]
CNS Stimulating Drugs [See Amphetamine, Caffeine, Dextroamphetamine, Methylphenidate, Pentylenetetrazol]
Cobalt 623
Cocaine 192, 627
Cognition 583
Cognitive Ability [See Also Reading Ability, Spatial Ability, Verbal Ability] 1, 18, 59, 71, 97, 104, 331, 381, 493, 508, 511, 520, 522, 554, 561, 562, 563, 597, 862, 866, 871
Cognitive Complexity 154
Cognitive Development [See Also Intellectual Development, Language Development, Perceptual Development] 208, 246, 470, 480, 490, 548, 580, 700, 702
Cognitive Dissonance 172
Cognitive Functioning [See Cognitive Ability]

Cognitive Processes [See Also Choice Behavior, Classification (Cognitive Process), Concept Formation, Decision Making, Imagination, Problem Solving] 121, 188, 255, 335, 355, 551, 574, 601, 868
Cognitive Style [See Cognitive Complexity]
Cognitive Techniques 358
Coitus (Animal) [See Animal Mating Behavior]
College Teachers 75
Commerce [See Business]
Communication Disorders [See Hearing Disorders, Language Disorders, Speech Disorders]
Communication [See Also Related Terms] 23
Communications Media [See Mass Media]
Community Attitudes 35, 73, 86, 105, 106, 107, 120, 170, 200, 891
Community Mental Health 110, 200
Community Services 139
Comparative Psychology 690, 853
Complexity (Cognitive) [See Cognitive Complexity]
Computer Applications [See Also Computer Assisted Diagnosis, Computer Assisted Instruction, Computer Assisted Testing, Computer Simulation] 1, 44, 75, 171
Computer Assisted Diagnosis 874
Computer Assisted Instruction 103
Computer Assisted Testing 143
Computer Peripheral Devices [See Video Display Units]
Computer Simulation 50
Computers [See Microcomputers]
Concept Formation 79
Concept Learning [See Concept Formation]
Concept Validity [See Construct Validity]
Conceptualization [See Concept Formation]
Conditioned Inhibition [See Conditioned Suppression]
Conditioned Reflex [See Conditioned Responses]
Conditioned Responses [See Also Conditioned Suppression] 266, 315
Conditioned Suppression 722
Conditioning [See Autoshaping, Aversion Conditioning, Avoidance Conditioning, Classical Conditioning, Conditioned Responses, Conditioned Suppression, Escape Conditioning, Operant Conditioning]
Conditioning (Avoidance) [See Avoidance Conditioning]
Conditioning (Classical) [See Classical Conditioning]
Conditioning (Escape) [See Escape Conditioning]
Conditioning (Operant) [See Operant Conditioning]

Conditioning (Verbal) [See Verbal Learning]
Conference Proceedings [See Professional Meetings and Symposia] 25
Congenital Disorders 10, 499
Consciousness Disturbances [See Delirium, Sleep Disorders]
Consciousness States [See Also Attention, Monitoring, Vigilance, Wakefulness] 390
Conservation (Ecological Behavior) 30, 128
Conservatism 130
Construct Validity 475
Consumer Attitudes 72, 162, 247
Consumer Behavior 72, 131, 161
Consumer Protection 32, 247
Consumer Research 162
Contingent Negative Variation 559
Continuous Reinforcement [See Reinforcement Schedules]
Contour [See Form and Shape Perception]
Contribution (Professional) [See Professional Criticism]
Convulsions [See Also Audiogenic Seizures] 266, 292, 348, 362, 395, 412, 499, 627, 743, 750, 885
Coordination (Motor) [See Motor Coordination]
Coordination (Perceptual Motor) [See Perceptual Motor Coordination]
Coping Behavior 107, 122, 131
Copper 558, 581, 603, 689, 716, 725, 775
Copulation (Animal) [See Animal Mating Behavior]
Corpus Striatum [See Basal Ganglia]
Cortex (Cerebral) [See Cerebral Cortex]
Cortex (Motor) [See Motor Cortex]
Cortex (Visual) [See Visual Cortex]
Cortical Evoked Potentials [See Also Contingent Negative Variation] 559, 560, 595, 781, 873
Corticosteroids [See Corticosterone]
Corticosterone 294
Cost Effectiveness [See Costs and Cost Analysis]
Costs and Cost Analysis 35, 156
Counseling (Group) [See Group Counseling]
Courts [See Adjudication]
Courtship (Animal) [See Animal Courtship Behavior]
Crabs 778
Craving [See Appetite]
Creative Writing [See Literature]
Crime [See Also Homicide] 39
Crippled [See Physically Handicapped]
Crises 211
Crisis (Reactions to) [See Stress Reactions]
Critical Flicker Fusion Threshold 375, 392, 448, 449, 674
Criticism (Professional) [See Professional Criticism]
Cross Cultural Differences 96, 259
CRT [See Video Display Units]

106

SUBJECT INDEX

Crustacea [See Also Crabs] 221, 224, 225, 232
Cuban Americans [See Hispanics]
Cues 129, 231
Cultural Differences [See Cross Cultural Differences]
Curriculum [See Reading Education, Science Education, Social Studies Education, Spelling]
Cutaneous Sense [See Also Vibrotactile Thresholds] 866
Cyclic Adenosine Monophosphate 685, 691
Czechoslovakia 71

Daily Biological Rhythms (Animal) [See Animal Circadian Rhythms]
Dark Adaptation 448, 449, 897
DDT (Insecticide) 313
Death and Dying 211, 917
Death Rate [See Mortality Rate]
Decarboxylases 728
Decerebration 904
Decision Making [See Also Choice Behavior] 30
Decoding [See Human Information Storage]
Defecation 916
Defense Mechanisms [See Denial]
Defensive Behavior (Animal) [See Animal Defensive Behavior]
Deja Vu [See Consciousness States]
Delayed Development 462, 490, 573
Delirium 388
Dementia 95, 498
Dementia Praecox [See Schizophrenia]
Demographic Characteristics 162, 168, 219, 590
Dendrites 707, 708
Denial 122
Denmark 878
Dental Treatment 446, 455, 512
Depression (Emotion) 134, 255, 527, 874, 892
Deprivation [See Food Deprivation]
Design (Experimental) [See Experimental Design]
Design (Man Machine Systems) [See Man Machine Systems Design]
Desires [See Motivation]
Detection (Signal) [See Signal Detection (Perception)]
Development [See Also Related Terms] 459
Developmental Age Groups [See Adolescents, Adults, Aged, Children, Infants, Middle Aged, Neonates, Preschool Age Children, School Age Children, Young Adults]
Developmental Differences [See Age Differences]
Developmental Disabilities 488, 555, 567
Developmental Stages [See Also Embryo, Fetus, Prenatal Developmental Stages] 646
Devices (Experimental) [See Apparatus]

Dexamphetamine [See Dextroamphetamine]
Dexedrine [See Dextroamphetamine]
Dextroamphetamine 263, 433, 657, 681, 735, 784, 918
Diagnosis [See Also Computer Assisted Diagnosis, Differential Diagnosis, Electroencephalography, Electroretinography, Medical Diagnosis, Psychodiagnosis, Urinalysis] 9, 119, 148, 464, 587, 896
Diazepam 354, 390, 402
Dieldrin 264, 276, 277, 295, 323, 324, 325
Diencephalon [See Geniculate Bodies (Thalamus), Hypothalamo Hypophyseal System, Hypothalamus]
Diets 9, 474, 503, 616, 630, 721, 724, 787, 791, 793, 794, 795, 796, 800, 801, 803, 804, 805, 806, 811, 813, 814, 815, 816, 817, 820, 821, 823, 824, 826, 830, 831, 838, 842, 844, 845, 848
Differential Diagnosis 95, 192, 332, 337, 349, 391, 886
Differential Limen [See Thresholds]
Differential Reinforcement 414, 606, 657, 713, 852, 913
Digestive System [See Gastrointestinal System, Mouth (Anatomy), Teeth (Anatomy)]
Diptera 223
Disasters [See Also Natural Disasters] 15, 16, 115, 819
Discrimination Learning [See Also Drug Discrimination, Reversal Shift Learning] 238, 282, 283, 403, 617, 659, 700, 701, 704, 749, 767, 784, 916
Discriminative Learning [See Discrimination Learning]
Diseases [See Disorders]
Dislike [See Aversion]
Disorders [See Also Related Terms] 25, 43, 58, 64, 98, 142, 349, 569, 892
Displays [See Visual Displays]
Disruptive Behavior [See Behavior Problems]
Dissonance (Cognitive) [See Cognitive Dissonance]
Distress 101, 157
Disulfiram 731
Diuretics [See Also Caffeine] 690
Dogs 840
Dominance (Animal) [See Animal Dominance]
Domination [See Authoritarianism]
Dopamine 99, 267, 270, 324, 404, 636, 709, 731, 847
Dopamine Agonists [See Also Amphetamine, Apomorphine, Morphine] 774
Dopamine Metabolites 222
Doxepin [See Antidepressant Drugs]
Drinking Behavior [See Animal Drinking Behavior, Water Intake]
Drinking Behavior (Animal) [See Animal Drinking Behavior]
Drive [See Motivation]
Drivers 206, 878
Driving Behavior 889, 898

Drug Abuse [See Inhalant Abuse]
Drug Administration Methods 308, 315, 396, 427, 640, 690
Drug Adverse Reactions [See Side Effects (Drug)]
Drug Discrimination 434, 711, 742
Drug Dissociation [See State Dependent Learning]
Drug Dosages 268, 281, 282, 315, 396, 405, 407, 657, 668, 676, 688, 709, 742, 771, 828, 897, 901, 916
Drug Effects [See Drugs] 248, 253, 255, 262, 264, 265, 266, 267, 269, 272, 274, 276, 278, 285, 290, 291, 292, 295, 297, 299, 305, 306, 307, 311, 312, 313, 314, 316, 317, 319, 323, 324, 325, 329, 366, 410, 441, 458, 599, 624, 637, 640, 641, 647, 648, 653, 655, 664, 666, 668, 673, 674, 678, 679, 680, 681, 688, 690, 691, 694, 703, 734, 735, 743, 745, 747, 748, 751, 753, 755, 761, 763, 771, 773, 775, 778, 781, 783, 833, 837, 839, 852, 853, 869, 880, 889, 901, 903, 906, 908, 910, 915, 918
Drug Interactions 289, 344, 355, 419, 426, 731
Drug Potentiation [See Drug Interactions] 748
Drug Sensitivity 329
Drug Synergism [See Drug Interactions]
Drug Therapy 482, 500, 579, 806, 822
Drug Tolerance 283, 407, 422, 433
Drug Usage [See Tobacco Smoking]
Drug Withdrawal 883
Drug Withdrawal Effects [See Drug Withdrawal]
Drugs [See Also Related Terms] 10, 316, 366, 389, 403, 430, 671, 710, 756
Ducks 324
Dying [See Death and Dying]
Dysmetria [See Ataxia]

Ear (Anatomy) [See Middle Ear, Vestibular Apparatus]
Ear Disorders 342, 423
Ear Ossicles [See Middle Ear]
Early Childhood [See Preschool Age Children]
Early Childhood Development [See Also Infant Development] 136, 484, 491
Early Experience 580, 630, 637, 648, 718, 733, 758
Early Infantile Autism 462
Eating [See Also Diets] 794, 810
Eating Disorders [See Appetite Disorders]
Eating Patterns [See Eating]
Echinodermata 406
Ecological Factors [See Also Pollution] 10, 49, 51, 228
Ecology 96, 153, 271
Educable Mentally Retarded 483, 532, 536, 603
Educational Personnel [See College Teachers]

SUBJECT INDEX

EEG (Electrophysiology) [See Electroencephalography]
Effort [See Energy Expenditure]
Electrical Activity [See Also Auditory Evoked Potentials, Cortical Evoked Potentials, Evoked Potentials, Somatosensory Evoked Potentials, Visual Evoked Potentials] 300, 492, 596, 753
Electrical Stimulation [See Electroconvulsive Shock]
Electroconvulsive Shock 627
Electroencephalography 5, 81, 82, 83, 84, 85, 241, 392, 625, 626, 634, 877
Electrolytes [See Also Calcium Ions, Sodium Ions, Zinc] 151
Electrophysiology [See Also Auditory Evoked Potentials, Cortical Evoked Potentials, Electrical Activity, Electroencephalography, Electroretinography, Evoked Potentials, Somatosensory Evoked Potentials, Visual Evoked Potentials] 29, 36, 41, 202
Electroretinography 278, 404
Elementary School Students 50, 173, 518, 529, 535, 539, 549, 553, 804, 814, 831
Elimination (Excretion) [See Excretion]
Embryo 229, 743
Emergency Services 899
Emetic Drugs [See Apomorphine, Disulfiram]
Emotional Adjustment [See Also Coping Behavior] 104, 157, 188
Emotional Control [See Coping Behavior]
Emotional Maladjustment [See Emotional Adjustment]
Emotional Responses 184, 199, 891
Emotional States [See Also Alienation, Anxiety, Depression (Emotion), Distress, Fear, Optimism, Panic, Pessimism] 344, 357, 527, 596, 859
Emotionally Disturbed [See Also Autistic Children] 531, 533, 860
Emotions [See Also Related Terms] 15, 583
Empirical Methods [See Also Experimental Methods] 236, 239
Employee Attitudes 167, 212
Employee Benefits [See Workmens Compensation Insurance]
Employee Characteristics [See Employee Attitudes]
Employee Health Insurance [See Workmens Compensation Insurance]
Employees [See Personnel]
Encephalography [See Electroencephalography]
Encephalopathies [See Toxic Encephalopathies]
Encoding [See Human Information Storage]
Endocrine Glands [See Hypothalamo Hypophyseal System]
Endocrine System [See Hypothalamo Hypophyseal System]
Energy Expenditure 268, 862, 881
England 133, 213

Environment [See Also Animal Environments, Classroom Environment, Home Environment, Rural Environments, Social Environments, Urban Environments, Working Conditions] 46, 47, 54, 120, 136, 173, 494, 498, 526
Environmental Adaptation 84, 111
Environmental Attitudes 6, 65, 73, 74, 94, 103, 105, 106, 125, 128, 129, 130, 131, 133, 146, 156, 165, 166, 175, 177, 194, 203, 204, 206, 250, 891
Environmental Effects [See Also Atmospheric Conditions, Heat Effects, Noise Effects, Seasonal Variations, Temperature Effects, Underwater Effects] 20, 22, 34, 40, 51, 67, 81, 82, 83, 84, 85, 88, 97, 110, 142, 150, 158, 159, 182, 185, 186, 194, 211, 223, 224, 280, 858, 879, 898
Environmental Psychology 19, 47, 52, 67, 854
Environmental Stress 6, 25, 115, 134, 139, 157, 689
Enzyme Inhibitors [See Cholinesterase Inhibitors]
Enzymes [See Also Acetylcholinesterase, Cholinesterase, Decarboxylases, Hydroxylases, Phosphatases] 380
Epidemiology 4, 34, 148, 201, 210, 376, 386, 448, 449, 475
Epilepsy [See Experimental Epilepsy]
Epileptic Seizures [See Experimental Epilepsy]
Epithelial Cells 225
Epithelium [See Skin (Anatomy)]
Equipment [See Apparatus]
Ergonomics [See Human Factors Engineering]
Erythrocytes 299, 497, 625
Escape [See Avoidance]
Escape Behavior (Animal) [See Animal Escape Behavior]
Escape Conditioning 300, 305, 746
Eserine [See Physostigmine]
Esterases [See Acetylcholinesterase, Cholinesterase]
Estimation [See Time Estimation]
Estrogens 456
Ethanol 274, 340, 357, 378, 401, 403, 415, 416, 417, 419, 721, 723, 724
Ethics [See Personal Values, Social Values]
Ethnic Differences [See Racial and Ethnic Differences]
Ethnic Groups [See Hispanics]
Ethology (Animal) [See Animal Ethology]
Ethyl Alcohol [See Ethanol]
Etiology 42, 70, 76, 91, 99, 102, 108, 117, 118, 123, 148, 164, 179, 180, 189, 196, 207, 214, 216, 244, 332, 442, 443, 444, 452, 479, 482, 483, 498, 519, 533, 552, 565, 761, 799, 800, 824
Europe [See Czechoslovakia, Finland, Ireland, Italy, Spain]
Eustachian Tube [See Middle Ear]
Evaluation 12

Evoked Potentials [See Also Auditory Evoked Potentials, Cortical Evoked Potentials, Somatosensory Evoked Potentials, Visual Evoked Potentials] 3, 171, 295
Excretion [See Also Defecation] 223
Exercise 881
Exhaustion [See Fatigue]
Experiences (Events) [See Early Experience, Life Experiences]
Experiences (Life) [See Life Experiences]
Experimental Apparatus [See Apparatus]
Experimental Design [See Also Followup Studies, Repeated Measures] 4, 13, 32, 556, 801
Experimental Epilepsy 412, 750
Experimental Methods 3, 5, 7, 17, 29, 32, 41, 44, 53, 220, 239, 320, 566, 659, 661, 749, 764, 798
Experimental Replication 154, 817, 884
Experimentation [See Also Related Terms] 2, 11, 32, 37, 69, 439, 795, 835
Exploratory Behavior [See Animal Exploratory Behavior]
Extinction (Learning) 631, 766
Eye (Anatomy) [See Also Retina] 778
Eye Disorders [See Nystagmus]
Eye Movements [See Also Nystagmus] 373, 502

Factor Analysis 465
Factory Environments [See Working Conditions]
Family Background [See Also Family Socioeconomic Level] 168, 565
Family Life [See Family Relations]
Family Members [See Also Fathers, Housewives, Mothers, Parents, Siblings, Twins] 193
Family Relations [See Also Childrearing Practices, Mother Child Relations, Parent Child Relations, Parental Attitudes] 126, 168, 200, 478, 575
Family Socioeconomic Level 590
Family Structure 168
Family [See Also Related Terms] 101
Fantasy [See Imagination]
Farmers [See Agricultural Workers]
Fathers 261
Fatigue 449
Fear [See Also Panic] 247, 294
Feeding Behavior (Animal) [See Animal Feeding Behavior]
Feeding Practices [See Breast Feeding, Weaning]
Feelings [See Emotions]
Felonies [See Crime]
Femininity 130
Fenfluramine 436
Fetus 727
Fiction [See Literature]
Fighting [See Aggressive Behavior]
Finland 37
Firearms [See Weapons]

SUBJECT INDEX

Fishes [See Also Goldfish] 268, 309, 672, 689
Fixed Interval Reinforcement 284, 416, 714, 786, 901
Fixed Ratio Reinforcement 414, 417, 632, 901, 913
Flicker Fusion Frequency [See Critical Flicker Fusion Threshold]
Flies [See Diptera]
Fluid Intake [See Also Water Intake] 723
Followup Studies 361, 528, 560
Food 824
Food Additives 10, 66, 205, 787, 788, 789, 790, 791, 792, 793, 794, 795, 797, 798, 799, 800, 802, 803, 804, 805, 806, 810, 811, 812, 813, 814, 815, 817, 820, 821, 822, 823, 824, 825, 826, 827, 828, 829, 830, 831, 832, 833, 834, 835, 836, 837, 838, 839, 840, 841, 842, 843, 844, 845, 846, 847, 848, 849, 850, 851, 852
Food Allergies 205, 787, 794, 815, 822, 824
Food Deprivation 297, 317, 642, 652, 747, 779
Food Intake [See Also Diets, Eating] 208, 268, 273, 638, 639, 640, 642, 696, 747, 760, 844
Food Preferences 842, 848
Foraging (Animal) [See Animal Foraging Behavior]
Forensic Psychology 64
Form and Shape Perception 785
Form Perception [See Form and Shape Perception]
Fowl [See Birds]
Frequency (Response) [See Response Frequency]
Frogs 264, 270, 839
Frontal Lobe [See Motor Cortex]

Games [See Simulation Games]
Gamma Aminobutyric Acid 789
Ganglia [See Basal Ganglia]
Ganglion Blocking Drugs [See Nicotine]
Gastrointestinal System 696
Gender Differences [See Human Sex Differences]
Genetics [See Also Related Terms] 123, 228, 906
Geniculate Bodies (Thalamus) 293, 633
Geographic Regions [See Geography]
Geography 22
Gerbils 305, 307
Gestation [See Pregnancy]
Glands [See Hypothalamo Hypophyseal System]
Glutamic Acid 728, 730
Goldfish 234
Government Agencies 2, 69
Government Personnel [See Military Personnel]
Government Policy Making [See Also Laws, Legislative Processes] 11, 20, 25, 347

Gradepoint Average [See Academic Achievement]
Great Britain [See Also England] 585
Group Counseling 830
Group Dynamics [See Intergroup Dynamics]
Group Psychotherapy [See Therapeutic Community]
Groups (Organizations) [See Organizations]
Growth [See Development]
Guanosine 685
Guinea Pigs 775
Gulls [See Sea Gulls]
Gustatory Perception [See Taste Perception]

Habits [See Tobacco Smoking]
Habituation 274
Hair 440, 530, 533, 535, 537, 564, 569, 581, 593
Hallucinosis [See Korsakoffs Psychosis]
Halstead Reitan Test Battery [See Neuropsychological Assessment]
Handicapped [See Autistic Children, Brain Damaged, Educable Mentally Retarded, Emotionally Disturbed, Institutionalized Mentally Retarded, Physically Handicapped, Slow Learners]
Haptic Perception [See Cutaneous Sense]
Hawaii 583
Hazards 32, 73, 177, 854, 891
Headache [See Also Migraine Headache] 349
Health [See Also Community Mental Health, Mental Health] 19, 24, 25, 67, 73, 98, 109, 156, 158, 195, 334, 343, 389, 869
Health Attitudes 250, 876
Health Care Professionals [See Medical Personnel]
Health Insurance [See Workmens Compensation Insurance]
Health Locus of Control [See Health Attitudes]
Hearing Disorders 126, 428, 461
Heart Disorders [See Bradycardia]
Heart Rate 293, 898
Heart Rate Affecting Drugs [See Caffeine]
Heartbeat [See Heart Rate]
Heat Effects 232
Help Seeking Behavior 77
Helplessness (Learned) [See Learned Helplessness]
Hemoglobin 625, 883
Heredity [See Genetics]
Hexobarbital 311, 748
High Risk Populations [See At Risk Populations]
High School Students 103, 125, 831
Hippocampus 604, 606, 607, 619, 620, 626, 720, 765
Hispanics 590
Home Accidents 168

Home Environment 43, 106, 509, 513, 542, 543, 565, 876
Homicide 151
Hormones [See Corticosterone, Estrogens, Norepinephrine, Parathyroid Hormone]
Hospital Admission [See Psychiatric Hospital Admission]
Hospital Programs [See Therapeutic Community]
Hospital Staff [See Medical Personnel]
Hospitalization [See Psychiatric Hospital Admission]
Hospitals 439
Housewives 161, 162
Human Development [See Also Related Terms] 20, 458
Human Factors Engineering 21, 33, 49
Human Females [See Housewives, Mothers]
Human Information Processes [See Cognitive Processes]
Human Information Storage 79
Human Males [See Also Fathers] 248
Human Sex Differences 120, 168, 173
Hydroxydopamine (6-) 294
Hydroxylases 845
Hydroxytryptamine (5-) [See Serotonin]
Hygiene [See Health]
Hyoscine [See Scopolamine]
Hyoscyamine (dl-) [See Atropine]
Hyperactivity [See Hyperkinesis]
Hyperkinesis 9, 66, 159, 205, 261, 482, 487, 524, 542, 544, 629, 648, 734, 754, 755, 788, 789, 790, 791, 792, 793, 794, 795, 796, 797, 798, 799, 802, 803, 805, 810, 811, 812, 813, 817, 820, 821, 822, 823, 824, 825, 826, 832, 833, 835, 836, 838, 840, 903, 909
Hypertension 503
Hypnotic Drugs [See Apomorphine, Hexobarbital, Pentobarbital, Phenobarbital]
Hypoglycemia 815
Hypothalamo Hypophyseal System 321
Hypothalamus [See Also Hypothalamo Hypophyseal System] 286
Hypothermia 292, 397
Hypoxia [See Anoxia]
Hysteria [See Mass Hysteria]

Ideation [See Imagination]
Illness (Physical) [See Disorders]
Illumination [See Also Scotopic Stimulation] 159, 843, 890, 911
Imagination 129
Imitation (Learning) 183
Immunologic Disorders [See Acquired Immune Deficiency Syndrome, Allergic Disorders, Food Allergies]
Incidental Learning [See Latent Learning]
India 138, 259
Individual Problem Solving [See Problem Solving]
Industrial Accidents 68, 200, 212, 382, 385, 892

SUBJECT INDEX

Industrial Personnel [See Business and Industrial Personnel]
Industrial Safety [See Occupational Safety]
Industrialization 24, 46
Industry [See Business]
Infancy [See Infants]
Infant Development [See Also Neonatal Development] 251, 471
Infants [See Also Neonates] 137, 251, 469, 471, 480, 543, 544, 590
Infants (Animal) 275, 301, 302, 423, 604, 605, 607, 613, 615, 616, 617, 621, 625, 629, 643, 658, 665, 666, 671, 676, 677, 683, 706, 707, 708, 713, 714, 726, 728, 734, 757, 766, 850, 912, 916
Infections [See Infectious Disorders]
Infectious Disorders [See Also Acquired Immune Deficiency Syndrome, Parasitic Disorders] 225
Infirmaries [See Hospitals]
Influences (Social) [See Social Influences]
Information (Messages) [See Messages]
Information Processes (Human) [See Cognitive Processes]
Information Storage (Human) [See Human Information Storage]
Information [See Also Related Terms] 23, 79, 876
Inhalant Abuse 372, 408
Injections [See Intraperitoneal Injections]
Injuries [See Also Self Inflicted Wounds] 49, 64
Inner City [See Urban Environments]
Insanity [See Mental Disorders, Psychosis]
Insecticides [See Also DDT (Insecticide), Dieldrin, Parathion] 66, 241, 243, 244, 245, 247, 248, 250, 251, 253, 256, 257, 259, 260, 262, 263, 265, 266, 267, 268, 269, 270, 272, 273, 274, 275, 279, 282, 283, 284, 285, 287, 288, 289, 290, 292, 296, 297, 299, 300, 302, 303, 304, 305, 306, 307, 308, 309, 310, 311, 312, 314, 315, 316, 317, 318, 320, 321, 322, 327, 328, 329, 330
Insects [See Also Beetles, Diptera, Wasps] 272, 290
Institutionalized Mentally Retarded 834
Instruction (Computer Assisted) [See Computer Assisted Instruction]
Instrumental Conditioning [See Operant Conditioning]
Instrumental Learning [See Operant Conditioning]
Insurance [See Workmens Compensation Insurance]
Intellectual Development [See Also Language Development] 506, 538, 574
Intellectual Functioning [See Cognitive Ability]
Intelligence 261, 389, 445, 468, 487, 506, 507, 511, 520, 524, 543, 553, 582, 584, 585, 594, 596, 816
Intelligence Measures 465

Intelligence Quotient 454, 509, 510, 522, 538, 557, 569, 807
Intensity (Stimulus) [See Stimulus Intensity]
Interaction (Interpersonal) [See Interpersonal Interaction]
Intergroup Dynamics 146
Intermittent Reinforcement [See Reinforcement Schedules]
Internal External Locus of Control 128, 166, 209
Interpersonal Attraction 185
Interpersonal Interaction [See Also Interpersonal Attraction, Participation] 77
Interresponse Time 752
Intersensory Processes 87, 468
Interval Reinforcement [See Fixed Interval Reinforcement, Variable Interval Reinforcement]
Intoxication [See Toxic Disorders]
Intra Aural Muscle Reflex [See Acoustic Reflex]
Intracranial Self Stimulation [See Brain Self Stimulation]
Intraperitoneal Injections 640, 690
Invertebrates [See Beetles, Crabs, Crustacea, Diptera, Echinodermata, Insects, Worms]
Investigation [See Experimentation]
Involvement 153, 154
Ions [See Electrolytes]
Ireland 497
Iron 716, 725, 775
Irradiation [See Radiation]
Italy 476
Item Content (Test) 128

Japan 130
Jobs [See Occupations]
Journalists 178
Judgment 68, 74
Junior High School Students 173, 831
Juvenile Court [See Adjudication]

Kindergarten Students 518
Knowledge Level 73, 74, 206
Korsakoffs Psychosis 886

L Dopa [See Levodopa]
Labor Unions 62
Laborers (Construct and Indust) [See Blue Collar Workers]
Laborers (Farm) [See Agricultural Workers]
Lactation 251, 718, 781
Language [See Also Vocabulary] 485, 601
Language Arts Education [See Reading Education, Spelling]
Language Development 542
Language Disorders 501, 540
Language Handicaps [See Language Disorders]
Latent Learning 712
Latinos [See Hispanics]

Law Enforcement [See Adjudication]
Laws 32, 162, 213
Lead (Metal) 66, 92, 246, 339, 454, 463, 471, 482, 483, 501, 505, 506, 508, 511, 522, 534, 537, 542, 561, 562, 573, 581, 591, 599, 606, 617, 619, 624, 628, 629, 637, 638, 640, 644, 645, 646, 647, 649, 651, 654, 663, 664, 668, 670, 684, 694, 697, 706, 717, 718, 719, 723, 725, 731, 733, 734, 739, 740, 742, 747, 751, 753, 759, 760, 766, 770, 784, 786
Lead Poisoning 439, 443, 445, 451, 453, 456, 457, 459, 461, 462, 463, 464, 466, 467, 468, 469, 470, 472, 474, 475, 477, 478, 479, 480, 481, 482, 484, 486, 487, 488, 489, 490, 491, 492, 493, 494, 495, 496, 497, 499, 502, 506, 507, 509, 510, 513, 514, 517, 520, 523, 524, 525, 526, 528, 531, 532, 534, 536, 540, 541, 543, 544, 546, 547, 548, 549, 550, 551, 552, 553, 554, 555, 556, 557, 559, 560, 562, 563, 565, 568, 574, 575, 576, 578, 579, 580, 582, 584, 585, 588, 590, 594, 595, 598, 600, 601, 602, 604, 605, 607, 612, 613, 614, 615, 616, 620, 621, 622, 625, 626, 627, 630, 632, 633, 639, 640, 643, 648, 650, 652, 653, 662, 663, 665, 666, 667, 668, 673, 677, 684, 693, 694, 698, 699, 700, 701, 702, 704, 707, 708, 709, 711, 712, 713, 714, 716, 720, 722, 732, 735, 737, 738, 741, 747, 750, 752, 754, 755, 756, 758, 761, 762, 769, 774, 779, 785
Learned Helplessness 277, 611
Learning Ability 1, 624, 737
Learning Disabilities 42, 453, 474, 477, 481, 530, 564, 567, 573, 603, 788, 789, 792, 803, 806, 811, 835
Learning Disorders [See Also Learning Disabilities] 8, 552, 569, 591, 813
Learning Rate 414, 914
Learning [See Also Related Terms] 645, 697, 726, 766, 827, 878, 907, 918
Legal Liability (Professional) [See Professional Liability]
Legal Processes [See Adjudication, Legislative Processes]
Legal Psychology [See Forensic Psychology]
Legislative Processes 156
Lesions [See Brain Lesions]
Letters (Alphabet) 518, 880
Levodopa 701
Librium [See Chlordiazepoxide]
Life Change [See Life Experiences]
Life Experiences 110
Life Satisfaction 90
Light [See Illumination]
Limbic System [See Also Amygdaloid Body, Hippocampus, Medial Forebrain Bundle] 70, 76, 102, 108, 117, 118, 164, 179, 180, 189, 207, 214, 216, 473
Limen [See Thresholds]
Lipids 773
Listening [See Auditory Perception]
Literature 440
Literature Review 69, 97, 109, 112, 114, 180, 195, 205, 237, 245, 336, 347,

SUBJECT INDEX

350, 383, 444, 453, 459, 475, 506, 507, 540, 556, 569, 584, 606, 788, 791, 793, 794, 800, 838, 853, 867
Lithium 217, 643, 691
Local Anesthetics [See Cocaine]
Locus of Control [See Internal External Locus of Control]
Loudness Perception 87
Luminance Threshold [See Brightness Perception, Visual Thresholds]
Lung Disorders 476
Luria Nebraska Tests [See Neuropsychological Assessment]

Magnesium 581, 603, 759
Maladjustment (Emotional) [See Emotional Adjustment]
Male Animals 286, 422
Males (Human) [See Human Males]
Malignant Neoplasms [See Neoplasms]
Malnutrition [See Nutritional Deficiencies]
Malpractice [See Professional Liability]
Mammals [See Also Baboons, Cats, Dogs, Gerbils, Guinea Pigs, Mice, Monkeys, Rabbits, Rats, Sheep] 296
Mammillary Bodies (Hypothalamic) [See Hypothalamus]
Man Machine Systems Design 49
Management Personnel 138
Management [See Also Related Terms] 48
Mania 217
Manic Depression 690
Manic Depressive Psychosis [See Manic Depression]
Manufacturing [See Business]
Marketing 190
Masculinity 130
Masking [See Visual Masking]
Mass Hysteria 43, 163
Mass Media 178, 211
Maternal Behavior (Animal) [See Animal Maternal Behavior]
Maternal Behavior (Human) [See Mother Child Relations]
Mating Behavior (Animal) [See Animal Mating Behavior]
Maturation [See Human Development]
Maze Learning 400, 606, 667, 668, 712, 720, 741, 758, 765, 785, 900, 911
Measurement [See Also Related Terms] 1, 28, 60, 61, 63, 75
Medial Forebrain Bundle 286
Medical Diagnosis [See Also Electroencephalography, Electroretinography, Urinalysis] 36, 145, 603
Medical History [See Patient History]
Medical Patients 527
Medical Personnel 571, 597, 868
Medical Sciences [See Epidemiology, Neurology, Neuropathology, Neuropsychiatry, Psychopathology]
Medical Treatment (General) 896
Medication [See Drug Therapy]
Membranes [See Also Nasal Mucosa] 225

Memory [See Also Short Term Memory, Spatial Memory] 137, 287, 288, 291, 331, 355, 358, 360, 370, 384, 385, 487, 697, 698, 699, 807, 808, 878, 898
Memory Disorders 345, 398, 589
Men [See Human Males]
Mental Deficiency [See Mental Retardation]
Mental Disorders [See Also Related Terms] 34, 55, 58, 98, 142, 148, 186, 191, 201, 240, 335, 377, 386, 460, 466, 501, 504, 512, 515, 569, 572, 864, 867, 875
Mental Health [See Also Community Mental Health] 389, 809
Mental Illness [See Mental Disorders]
Mental Retardation [See Also Borderline Mental Retardation, Microcephaly] 439, 537, 547, 552, 569
Mentally Retarded [See Educable Mentally Retarded, Institutionalized Mentally Retarded]
Mercury (Metal) 66, 500, 504, 512, 586, 597, 641, 655, 659, 661, 669, 674, 678, 679, 682, 688, 692, 729, 743, 744, 745, 749, 764, 771, 772
Mercury Poisoning 257, 441, 442, 445, 446, 448, 449, 450, 455, 458, 512, 514, 516, 521, 527, 531, 538, 546, 571, 583, 586, 587, 592, 596, 597, 622, 636, 657, 658, 660, 674, 678, 679, 680, 681, 682, 683, 687, 695, 703, 710, 715, 728, 730, 746, 781, 782, 783
Mesencephalon [See Also Superior Colliculus] 222, 753
Messages 190
Metabolism [See Also Basal Metabolism, Metabolites, Protein Metabolism] 227, 436
Metabolism Disorders 789
Metabolites [See Also Dopamine Metabolites] 264, 457, 745
Metallic Elements [See Also Calcium, Calcium Ions, Cobalt, Copper, Iron, Lead (Metal), Lithium, Magnesium, Mercury (Metal), Sodium, Sodium Ions, Zinc] 66, 70, 76, 102, 108, 117, 118, 123, 150, 164, 179, 180, 189, 207, 214, 216, 242, 246, 440, 444, 447, 452, 473, 501, 503, 522, 529, 530, 532, 533, 535, 539, 546, 567, 569, 577, 589, 591, 595, 603, 608, 610, 618, 622, 631, 672, 675, 676, 686, 690, 691, 705, 716, 724, 725, 726, 748, 757, 763, 767, 773, 775, 776, 780, 816
Methanol 406
Methionine 380
Methodology [See Also Related Terms] 6, 12, 13, 31, 198, 298, 450, 556, 584
Methyl Alcohol [See Methanol]
Methylatropine [See Atropine]
Methylphenidate 735, 753
Metrazole [See Pentylenetetrazol]
Mice 266, 278, 457, 627, 628, 637, 645, 647, 648, 679, 680, 681, 718, 735, 738, 745, 754, 755, 763
Microcephaly 573
Microcomputers 18, 95, 220

Midbrain [See Mesencephalon]
Middle Aged 248
Middle Ear 566
Migraine Headache 830
Mildly Mentally Retarded [See Educable Mentally Retarded]
Military Personnel [See Also Navy Personnel] 895
Military Veterans 145, 240, 243, 252, 254, 261
Minimal Brain Disorders 648, 755, 761, 765
Minor Tranquilizers [See Chlordiazepoxide]
Misbehavior [See Behavior Problems]
Misconduct [See Behavior Problems]
Misdemeanors [See Crime]
Modeling [See Simulation]
Modeling Behavior [See Imitation (Learning)]
Models 14, 17, 235
Money 35
Monitoring [See Also Vigilance] 828, 856, 887
Monkeys 227, 239, 241, 275, 291, 319, 325, 412, 629, 630, 674, 682, 697, 771
Monoamines (Brain) [See Catecholamines]
Moods [See Emotional States]
Morphine 751
Mortality [See Death and Dying]
Mortality Rate 249, 353
Mother Child Relations 543
Mothers 122, 479, 543
Motion Perception 890
Motivation [See Also Animal Motivation] 199
Motor Coordination 645
Motor Cortex 708
Motor Development [See Also Psychomotor Development] 246, 301, 469, 486, 517, 591, 618, 729, 754, 850
Motor Disorders [See Nervous System Disorders]
Motor Evoked Potentials [See Somatosensory Evoked Potentials]
Motor Performance 226, 435, 680, 910
Motor Processes [See Also Activity Level, Animal Locomotion, Exercise, Motor Coordination, Motor Performance, Motor Skills, Swimming] 264, 265, 267, 269, 272, 299, 303, 316, 406, 410, 419, 480, 542, 574, 594, 613, 631, 647, 648, 654, 664, 666, 670, 673, 683, 684, 693, 735, 747, 805, 844
Motor Skills 355, 508
Motor Vehicles [See Automobiles]
Mouth (Anatomy) 526
Movement Disorders [See Also Apraxia, Ataxia, Cataplexy, Myoclonia, Paralysis, Tremor] 729
Movement Perception [See Motion Perception]
Multiple Births [See Twins]
Multivariate Analysis [See Factor Analysis]
Murder [See Homicide]

SUBJECT INDEX

Muscarinic Drugs [See Cholinergic Drugs]
Muscle Contractions 316
Muscle Relaxation Therapy [See Relaxation Therapy]
Muscle Relaxing Drugs [See Diazepam]
Muscles 269
Muscular Disorders [See Cataplexy, Myoclonia]
Musculoskeletal Disorders [See Cataplexy, Myoclonia]
Musculoskeletal System [See Muscles]
Myelin Sheath 262
Myoclonia 348

Narcosis 334
Narcotic Drugs [See Apomorphine, Atropine, Morphine]
Nasal Mucosa 70, 76, 102, 108, 117, 118, 164, 179, 180, 189, 207, 214, 216
Natural Disasters 177
Navy Personnel 98, 353
Negroes [See Blacks] 468, 487, 524, 526, 561, 562, 563, 601
Nembutal [See Pentobarbital]
Neonatal Development 135, 242, 670, 677, 684, 903
Neonates 136, 314, 499
Neonates (Animal) [See Infants (Animal)]
Neoplasms 91, 476
Nerve Cells [See Neurons]
Nerve Endings [See Chemoreceptors, Neural Receptors, Photoreceptors, Synapses]
Nerve Tissues [See Myelin Sheath]
Nerves (Adrenergic) [See Adrenergic Nerves]
Nerves (Cholinergic) [See Cholinergic Nerves]
Nerves (Peripheral) [See Peripheral Nerves]
Nervous Breakdown [See Mental Disorders]
Nervous System [See Also Adrenergic Nerves, Amygdaloid Body, Autonomic Nervous System, Axons, Basal Ganglia, Brain, Central Nervous System, Cerebellum, Cerebral Cortex, Chemoreceptors, Cholinergic Nerves, Dendrites, Geniculate Bodies (Thalamus), Hippocampus, Hypothalamo Hypophyseal System, Hypothalamus, Limbic System, Mesencephalon, Motor Cortex, Myelin Sheath, Neural Receptors, Neurons, Peripheral Nerves, Photoreceptors, Reticular Formation, Sensory Neurons, Spinal Cord, Superior Colliculus, Synapses, Visual Cortex] 78
Nervous System Disorders [See Also Alzheimers Disease, Ataxia, Autonomic Nervous System Disorders, Brain Damage, Brain Disorders, Cataplexy, Central Nervous System Disorders, Convulsions, Hyperkinesis, Korsakoffs Psychosis, Microcephaly, Minimal Brain Disorders, Movement Disorders, Organic Brain Syndromes, Paralysis, Parkinsons Disease, Sclerosis (Nervous System), Toxic Psychoses] 36, 53, 197, 242, 260, 269, 332, 333, 334, 335, 336, 352, 367, 383, 386, 442, 443, 444, 445, 501, 515, 550, 587, 594, 730, 868, 875
Nest Building 313
Neural Development 559, 618, 626, 692, 707, 708, 772
Neural Pathways [See Limbic System, Medial Forebrain Bundle, Reticular Formation]
Neural Receptors [See Also Chemoreceptors, Photoreceptors] 613, 633, 709
Neural Regeneration [See Neural Development]
Neurasthenic Neurosis 144
Neurochemistry [See Also Receptor Binding] 97, 222, 264, 292, 299, 316, 324, 418, 430, 436, 456, 633, 647, 658, 660, 664, 665, 684, 685, 693, 705, 725, 728, 731, 740, 743, 745, 756, 762, 775, 779, 782, 783, 845, 902
Neuroinfections [See Infectious Disorders, Nervous System Disorders]
Neuroleptic Drugs [See Chlorpromazine, Sulpiride]
Neurological Disorders [See Nervous System Disorders]
Neurology 60, 63, 148
Neuromuscular Disorders [See Cataplexy, Paralysis, Parkinsons Disease]
Neurons [See Also Axons, Dendrites, Sensory Neurons] 635, 776
Neuropathology 2, 3, 4, 18, 29, 41, 44, 53, 59, 70, 75, 76, 102, 108, 117, 118, 123, 164, 171, 179, 180, 189, 193, 207, 214, 216, 683
Neuropathy [See Nervous System Disorders]
Neurophysiology [See Also Receptor Binding] 395
Neuropsychiatry 599, 882
Neuropsychological Assessment [See Also Wechsler Memory Scale] 18, 56, 59, 64, 69, 95, 116, 145, 147, 187, 188, 337, 347, 349, 350, 367, 368, 377, 528, 551, 576
Neuropsychology 26, 27, 339, 381, 463, 467, 485, 491, 514, 597, 598, 600, 860, 861, 867, 871, 896
Neurosciences [See Also Neurochemistry, Neurology, Neuropathology, Neurophysiology, Neuropsychiatry, Neuropsychology] 11
Neurosis [See Also Affective Disturbances, Neurasthenic Neurosis] 519
Neurosurgery [See Decerebration]
Neuroticism 809
Neurotoxins 5, 14, 17, 20, 26, 27, 36, 41, 54, 56, 57, 59, 60, 61, 63, 67, 69, 70, 76, 95, 97, 102, 104, 108, 117, 118, 123, 147, 164, 179, 180, 187, 188, 189, 197, 207, 214, 216, 222, 226, 235, 241, 242, 245, 249, 260, 286, 294, 298, 300, 301, 304, 321, 330, 336, 339, 342, 347, 350, 351, 360, 376, 383, 409, 418, 424, 425, 431, 432, 447, 456, 502, 528, 572, 596, 609, 622, 642, 656, 657, 658, 683, 685, 695, 710, 720, 736, 765, 769, 780, 868, 902
Neurotransmitters [See Also Acetylcholine, Catecholamines, Gamma Aminobutyric Acid, Glutamic Acid, Serotonin, Substance P] 762
Newborn Infants [See Neonates]
Nicotine 78, 753
Night Terrors [See Sleep Disorders]
Nitrogen 828
Noise (Sound) [See Auditory Stimulation]
Noise (Visual) [See Visual Stimulation]
Noise Effects 21, 35, 49, 86, 87, 113, 121, 181, 199
Nonmetallic Elements [See Nitrogen, Oxygen, Phosphorus]
Nonprojective Personality Measures [See Rotter Intern Extern Locus Cont Scal]
Nonverbal Ability [See Motor Skills, Spatial Ability]
Noradrenaline [See Norepinephrine]
Norepinephrine 267, 292, 324
North America [See United States]
Nortriptyline [See Antidepressant Drugs]
Nose [See Nasal Mucosa]
Novel Stimuli [See Stimulus Novelty]
Nuclear War 160
Nucleic Acids [See Adenosine, Cyclic Adenosine Monophosphate]
Nucleotides [See Cyclic Adenosine Monophosphate]
Nutrition 208, 440, 474, 567, 581, 759, 827
Nutritional Deficiencies [See Also Starvation] 22, 42, 609, 759, 760
Nystagmus 373, 374

Object Permanence 275
Occipital Lobe [See Visual Cortex]
Occupational Exposure 33, 56, 78, 98, 126, 147, 149, 150, 155, 181, 187, 195, 215, 249, 345, 346, 347, 356, 381, 384, 385, 514, 855, 866, 868
Occupational Safety 2, 37, 58, 62, 69, 127, 157, 197, 201, 212, 333, 334, 351, 353, 365, 368, 370, 379, 386, 391, 418, 466, 476, 572
Occupational Stress 90, 167, 382
Occupations [See Also Related Terms] 48
Oculomotor Response [See Eye Movements]
Odor Aversion Conditioning [See Aversion Conditioning]
Old Age [See Aged]
Olfactory Perception 7, 87, 204, 237, 381, 855, 879, 894
Olfactory Stimulation 7, 184
Oligophrenia [See Mental Retardation]
Ontogeny [See Development]
Open Field Behavior (Animal) [See Animal Open Field Behavior]

SUBJECT INDEX

Operant Conditioning [See Also Avoidance Conditioning, Conditioned Responses, Discrimination Learning, Escape Conditioning] 234, 273, 306, 307, 310, 327, 405, 414, 417, 433, 606, 612, 622, 629, 642, 673, 679, 695, 713, 722, 733, 746, 751, 752, 771, 773, 786, 908, 914
Ophthalmologic Examination [See Electroretinography]
Opiates [See Morphine]
Opinion (Public) [See Public Opinion]
Opinion Change [See Attitude Change]
Opinions [See Attitudes]
Optimism 152, 209
Optokinetic Nystagmus [See Nystagmus]
Organic Brain Syndromes [See Also Alzheimers Disease, Dementia, Korsakoffs Psychosis, Toxic Psychoses] 376, 882
Organic Therapies [See Also Drug Therapy, Vitamin Therapy] 796
Organizational Behavior 146
Organizations [See Also Government Agencies, Labor Unions] 146
Orthopedically Handicapped [See Physically Handicapped]
Overpopulation 94, 160
Oxygen 859
Oxygenation 329

Pain [See Headache, Migraine Headache]
Pain Perception [See Also Analgesia] 320, 769, 770
Paired Associate Learning 833
Palsy [See Paralysis]
Panic 163
Panic Disorder 346
Paralysis [See Also Parkinsons Disease] 262
Paralysis Agitans [See Parkinsons Disease]
Paramedical Sciences [See Pharmacology]
Parameters (Stimulus) [See Stimulus Parameters]
Parasitic Disorders 645
Parasympatholytic Drugs [See Cholinergic Blocking Drugs]
Parathion 255, 278, 281, 291, 319, 326
Parathyroid Hormone 631
Parent Child Relations [See Also Mother Child Relations, Parental Attitudes] 565
Parental Attitudes 72
Parental Influence [See Parent Child Relations]
Parents [See Also Fathers, Mothers] 72
Parkinsons Disease 99, 196, 227, 244, 248, 270, 498, 874
Parks (Recreational) [See Recreation Areas]
Partial Reinforcement [See Reinforcement Schedules]
Participation 176

Passive Avoidance [See Avoidance Conditioning]
Pathogenesis [See Etiology]
Pathology [See Neuropathology, Psychopathology]
Patient History 77
Patients [See Medical Patients, Psychiatric Patients]
Pattern Discrimination 704
Pavlovian Conditioning [See Classical Conditioning]
Pecking Order [See Animal Dominance]
Pedestrians 898
Pentobarbital 278, 434, 711, 779, 918
Pentylenetetrazol 295
Pentylenetetrazole [See Pentylenetetrazol]
Peptides [See Also Substance P] 359, 730
Perception [See Also Related Terms] 563
Perceptual Development 246, 469, 480, 486, 591
Perceptual Discrimination [See Also Auditory Discrimination, Pattern Discrimination, Visual Discrimination] 884
Perceptual Disturbances [See Also Agnosia] 445
Perceptual Motor Coordination 378
Perceptual Motor Development [See Motor Development, Perceptual Development]
Perceptual Motor Processes [See Also Perceptual Motor Coordination, Tracking, Visual Tracking] 18, 28, 53, 56, 71, 188, 255, 335, 392, 487, 516, 524, 542, 546, 561, 562, 671, 682, 808, 834, 859, 878, 887
Perceptual Stimulation [See Auditory Stimulation, Illumination, Olfactory Stimulation, Visual Stimulation, White Noise]
Performance [See Also Motor Performance] 88, 121, 184, 199, 356, 357, 365, 812, 859, 862, 865
Performance Tests 143, 350, 366, 598
Peripheral Nerves 29
Perseveration 765
Personal Adjustment [See Emotional Adjustment]
Personal Computers [See Microcomputers]
Personal Values 45, 153, 215
Personality Change 201, 804, 892
Personality Correlates 145, 150, 219
Personality Disorders 97
Personality Measures [See Bender Gestalt Test, Rorschach Test, Rotter Intern Extern Locus Cont Scal]
Personality Traits [See Authoritarianism, Conservatism, Femininity, Internal External Locus of Control, Masculinity, Neuroticism, Optimism, Pessimism, Tolerance]
Personnel [See Also Related Terms] 144, 389, 464, 898

Persuasive Communication 175, 247
Pessimism 209
Pesticides [See Insecticides]
Pharmacology 32
Pharmacotherapy [See Drug Therapy]
Phenobarbital 735
Phenothiazine Derivatives [See Chlorpromazine]
Phenoxybenzamine 289
Philippines 498
Phonetics 717
Phonology [See Phonetics]
Phosphatases 262
Phosphorus 256
Photic Threshold [See Illumination, Visual Thresholds]
Photoreceptors 778
Physical Development [See Also Motor Development, Neural Development, Prenatal Development, Psychomotor Development] 232, 268, 413, 608, 609, 617, 670, 679, 734, 754, 772, 773, 850
Physical Divisions (Geographic) [See Geography]
Physical Exercise [See Exercise]
Physical Geography [See Geography]
Physical Growth [See Physical Development]
Physical Illness [See Disorders]
Physical Trauma [See Injuries]
Physical Treatment Methods [See Decerebration, Dental Treatment]
Physically Handicapped 460
Physiological Aging 70, 76, 95, 102, 108, 117, 118, 164, 179, 180, 189, 207, 214, 216, 776
Physiological Correlates 208, 593, 768, 842
Physiological Psychology [See Neuropsychology]
Physiological Stress 223, 232, 880
Physiology [See Also Related Terms] 232, 239
Physostigmine 287, 288
Pica 496, 513, 525, 526, 565, 574, 759
Pictorial Stimuli 129
Pigeons 306, 695, 918
Pigments [See Also Hemoglobin] 756, 773
Pilots (Aircraft) [See Aircraft Pilots]
Pituitary Gland [See Hypothalamo Hypophyseal System]
Plasma (Blood) [See Blood Plasma]
Play [See Recreation]
Play (Animal) [See Animal Play]
Play Behavior (Childhood) [See Childhood Play Behavior]
Poisoning [See Toxic Disorders]
Poisons [See Also Neurotoxins] 8, 9, 40, 51, 52, 68, 71, 97, 99, 114, 119, 122, 127, 135, 136, 137, 191, 196, 200, 202, 212, 226, 230, 240, 252, 254, 258, 260, 261, 305, 342, 371, 394, 398
Policy Making [See Also Government Policy Making] 178
Policy Making (Government) [See Government Policy Making]

SUBJECT INDEX

Political Divisions (Geographic) [See Geography]
Pollution 6, 7, 19, 21, 23, 24, 30, 35, 38, 39, 42, 43, 45, 46, 48, 49, 50, 55, 57, 65, 71, 73, 74, 79, 80, 81, 82, 83, 84, 85, 86, 87, 88, 90, 93, 94, 96, 100, 103, 105, 106, 107, 109, 110, 111, 112, 113, 120, 121, 125, 128, 129, 130, 131, 132, 133, 134, 138, 139, 140, 141, 142, 146, 152, 153, 154, 156, 158, 160, 161, 162, 165, 166, 169, 170, 172, 173, 174, 175, 176, 177, 182, 183, 184, 185, 186, 194, 198, 199, 203, 204, 206, 209, 211, 213, 218, 219, 221, 223, 224, 228, 229, 232, 234, 237, 271, 280, 452, 511, 536, 878, 881, 893, 917
Polydipsia 643
Population [See Overpopulation]
Population Characteristics [See Demographic Characteristics]
Postnatal Period 263, 312, 321, 326, 458, 472, 669, 675, 680, 704, 719, 729, 741, 751, 768, 786
Posttraumatic Stress Disorder 149, 254, 382, 818
Posture 729
Potentiation (Drugs) [See Drug Interactions]
Power 169
Predatory Behavior (Animal) [See Animal Predatory Behavior]
Prediction [See Also Academic Achievement Prediction] 537
Predictive Validity 128, 465
Predisposition 335
Preferences [See Also Food Preferences] 401, 426, 710, 849
Pregnancy 313, 314, 419, 680, 727, 758, 781
Prenatal Development [See Also Embryo, Fetus, Prenatal Developmental Stages] 12, 13, 31, 135, 136, 137, 220, 238, 242, 246, 251, 263, 301, 321, 418, 419, 420, 458, 469, 470, 472, 484, 486, 491, 499, 548, 608, 610, 611, 613, 617, 618, 622, 625, 626, 636, 650, 655, 657, 658, 659, 660, 661, 663, 664, 669, 678, 680, 683, 692, 704, 719, 720, 731, 733, 734, 739, 744, 749, 764, 766, 772, 786, 907
Prenatal Developmental Stages [See Also Embryo, Fetus] 698
Preschool Age Children 124, 168, 188, 190, 208, 457, 480, 483, 488, 490, 496, 517, 524, 525, 526, 532, 542, 543, 544, 555, 559, 560, 561, 562, 563, 568, 590, 601, 798, 805, 816, 817, 822, 823, 827, 837, 899
Presenile Dementia [See Alzheimers Disease]
Prevention [See Also Related Terms] 139, 513
Primates (Nonhuman) [See Baboons, Monkeys]
Probability [See Statistical Probability]
Problem Solving 218
Process Schizophrenia [See Schizophrenia]

Professional Contribution [See Professional Criticism]
Professional Criticism 454, 802, 803, 806, 811, 825
Professional Criticism Reply 836
Professional Liability 64
Professional Meetings and Symposia 1, 2, 3, 4, 5, 12, 13, 14, 18, 28, 29, 31, 41, 44, 53, 54, 59, 69, 75, 95, 171, 220, 222, 263, 333, 336, 340, 342, 350, 369, 383, 559, 595, 613, 638, 669, 692, 772, 777, 863, 902
Professional Personnel [See Also Related Terms] 157
Professional Standards [See Professional Liability]
Professors [See College Teachers]
Prognosis 361, 364
Projective Personality Measures [See Bender Gestalt Test, Rorschach Test]
Projective Techniques [See Bender Gestalt Test, Rorschach Test]
Protein Metabolism 845
Proteins [See Also Blood Proteins, Hemoglobin] 848
Pseudopsychopathic Schizophrenia [See Schizophrenia]
Psychiatric Disorders [See Mental Disorders]
Psychiatric History [See Patient History]
Psychiatric Hospital Admission 893
Psychiatric Hospital Programs [See Therapeutic Community]
Psychiatric Hospitalization [See Psychiatric Hospital Admission]
Psychiatric Patients 588, 589, 690
Psychiatry [See Neuropsychiatry]
Psychoactive Drugs [See Drugs]
Psychodiagnosis 56, 211, 350, 377
Psychodynamics 503
Psychogenesis [See Cognitive Development, Intellectual Development, Language Development, Perceptual Development, Psychomotor Development]
Psychological Adjustment [See Emotional Adjustment]
Psychological Correlates [See Psychodynamics]
Psychological Reactance 38
Psychological Stress 157
Psychological Testing [See Psychometrics]
Psychologists 62
Psychology [See Comparative Psychology, Forensic Psychology, Neuropsychology]
Psychometrics 119, 542
Psychomotor Development 475
Psychomotor Processes [See Perceptual Motor Processes]
Psychoneurosis [See Neurosis]
Psychopathology 56, 583, 819, 877
Psychophysical Measurement 7, 41, 894
Psychophysiology 859
Psychosis [See Also Early Infantile Autism, Korsakoffs Psychosis, Schizophrenia, Toxic Psychoses] 519

Psychosocial Factors 126, 479, 494
Psychosocial Rehabilitation 818
Psychotherapy [See Therapeutic Community]
Psychotomimetic Drugs 380
Psychotropic Drugs [See Drugs]
Public Attitudes [See Public Opinion]
Public Opinion 169, 174, 178, 213, 250
Public Policy [See Government Policy Making]
Public Sector [See Government Agencies]
Puerto Rican Americans [See Hispanics]

Quails 281

Rabbits 725, 776
Racial and Ethnic Differences 590
Racial Differences [See Racial and Ethnic Differences]
Radiation 42, 238, 239, 641, 854, 891, 909
Rage [See Anger]
Rapport [See Interpersonal Attraction]
Rat Learning 231, 312, 608, 624, 693, 694, 761, 782, 783, 850, 851, 852, 915
Rating Scales 6
Ratio Reinforcement [See Fixed Ratio Reinforcement]
Rats 231, 233, 265, 267, 274, 283, 286, 292, 298, 299, 300, 301, 311, 312, 313, 314, 316, 317, 394, 410, 419, 430, 436, 447, 606, 612, 617, 624, 631, 641, 642, 644, 653, 654, 655, 656, 657, 658, 663, 664, 665, 666, 668, 670, 671, 673, 684, 686, 687, 688, 690, 691, 693, 694, 696, 703, 707, 710, 713, 716, 726, 727, 732, 733, 734, 746, 747, 748, 751, 752, 753, 756, 758, 759, 760, 761, 765, 766, 769, 773, 779, 781, 782, 783, 784, 785, 786, 841, 842, 844, 845, 847, 848, 849, 852, 901, 903, 904, 906, 908, 909, 910, 911, 915, 917
Reactance [See Psychological Reactance]
Reaction Time 182, 344, 355, 365, 375, 501, 551, 898
Reactive Schizophrenia [See Schizophrenia]
Readaptation [See Adaptation]
Reading Ability 208
Reading Achievement 468, 546, 582, 804
Reading Education 518
Rebuttal [See Professional Criticism Reply]
Receptor Binding 222, 326, 330, 429, 619, 636, 739, 846
Receptors (Neural) [See Neural Receptors]
Recidivism 478
Recognition (Learning) 137, 675
Recovery (Disorders) 394, 871
Recreation [See Also Childhood Play Behavior, Swimming] 100, 176
Recreation Areas 100, 176

SUBJECT INDEX

Red Nucleus [See Mesencephalon]
Reflexes [See Also Acoustic Reflex, Nystagmus, Startle Reflex] 28, 905
Rehabilitation [See Psychosocial Rehabilitation]
Rehabilitation (Psychosocial) [See Psychosocial Rehabilitation]
Reinforcement [See Also Differential Reinforcement, Fixed Interval Reinforcement, Fixed Ratio Reinforcement, Reinforcement Schedules, Variable Interval Reinforcement] 751
Reinforcement Schedules [See Also Fixed Interval Reinforcement, Fixed Ratio Reinforcement, Variable Interval Reinforcement] 433, 915
Reinnervation [See Neural Development]
Relaxation Therapy 830
Remembering [See Retention]
Repeated Measures 143
Replication (Experimental) [See Experimental Replication]
Reply (to Professional Criticism) [See Professional Criticism Reply]
Research [See Experimentation]
Research Design [See Experimental Design]
Research Methods [See Methodology]
Residential Care Institutions [See Hospitals]
Resonance [See Vibration]
Respiration 223, 410, 859, 881, 917
Respiration Stimulating Drugs [See Caffeine]
Respiratory Distress [See Apnea]
Respiratory System [See Nasal Mucosa]
Respiratory Tract Disorders [See Apnea, Lung Disorders]
Respondent Conditioning [See Classical Conditioning]
Response Amplitude 595
Response Frequency 405, 416, 612, 632, 659, 714, 749, 786, 901, 913
Response Lag [See Reaction Time]
Response Latency 395, 595, 659, 663, 749
Response Parameters [See Interresponse Time, Reaction Time, Response Amplitude, Response Frequency, Response Latency, Response Set]
Response Rate [See Response Frequency]
Response Set 129
Response Speed [See Reaction Time]
Response Time [See Reaction Time]
Responses [See Also Conditioned Responses, Conditioned Suppression, Emotional Responses] 644
Retardation (Mental) [See Mental Retardation]
Retention [See Also Recognition (Learning)] 323, 614, 623, 631, 635
Retention Measures [See Wechsler Memory Scale]
Reticular Formation 753
Retina 404, 633, 665
Reversal Shift Learning 325

Review (of Literature) [See Literature Review]
Rigidity (Muscles) [See Muscle Contractions]
Risk Populations [See At Risk Populations]
Risk Taking 68, 73, 250
Ritalin [See Methylphenidate]
Rodents [See Gerbils, Guinea Pigs, Mice, Rats]
Rorschach Test 84
Rotter Intern Extern Locus Cont Scal 128
RT (Response) [See Reaction Time]
Rural Environments 173, 536, 594

Saccadic Eye Movements [See Eye Movements]
Safety [See Also Occupational Safety] 258, 854
Safety Devices 215
Salamanders 230
Saltiness [See Taste Perception]
Sarcomas [See Neoplasms]
Satiation 317
Satisfaction [See Life Satisfaction]
Scandinavia [See Denmark]
Schedules (Reinforcement) [See Reinforcement Schedules]
Schizophrenia [See Also Acute Schizophrenia] 22
Schizophrenia (Residual Type) [See Schizophrenia]
Schizophreniform Disorder [See Acute Schizophrenia]
Scholastic Achievement [See Academic Achievement]
School Achievement [See Academic Achievement]
School Age Children 168, 208, 218, 246, 261, 468, 482, 483, 487, 490, 511, 520, 532, 533, 534, 536, 538, 543, 544, 551, 560, 564, 576, 585, 589, 591, 594, 602, 805, 815, 816, 821, 822, 823, 826, 829, 830, 832, 833
Schools 387
Science Education 50, 103, 125
Sciences [See Biochemistry, Comparative Psychology, Epidemiology, Forensic Psychology, Geography, Neurochemistry, Neurophysiology, Neuropsychiatry, Neuropsychology, Neurosciences]
Scientific Communication [See Professional Meetings and Symposia]
Scientific Methods [See Experimental Methods]
Scientists [See Also Related Terms] 90
Sclera [See Eye (Anatomy)]
Sclerosis (Nervous System) 498
Scopolamine 287, 665, 699, 701, 918
Scopolamine Hydrobromide [See Scopolamine]
Scores (Test) [See Test Scores]
Scotopic Stimulation 630, 674
Sea Gulls 229
Seasonal Variations 689

Secretion (Gland) [See Lactation]
Sedatives [See Atropine, Chlorpromazine, Hexobarbital, Pentobarbital, Phenobarbital, Scopolamine]
Seizures [See Convulsions]
Self Acceptance [See Self Perception]
Self Consciousness [See Self Perception]
Self Destructive Behavior [See Attempted Suicide, Self Inflicted Wounds, Suicide]
Self Inflicted Wounds 77
Self Perception 172
Self Report 145
Self Stimulation [See Also Brain Self Stimulation] 421, 644, 721
Senescence [See Aged]
Senior Citizens [See Aged]
Sensation [See Perception]
Sense Organ Disorders [See Ear Disorders, Nystagmus]
Sense Organs [See Eye (Anatomy), Middle Ear, Retina, Vestibular Apparatus]
Sensitivity (Drugs) [See Drug Sensitivity]
Sensorineural Hearing Loss [See Hearing Disorders]
Sensory Adaptation [See Dark Adaptation]
Sensory Motor Processes [See Perceptual Motor Processes]
Sensory Neurons [See Also Chemoreceptors, Photoreceptors] 41
Sentencing [See Adjudication]
Serotonin 267, 292, 316, 324, 330, 845
Servicemen [See Military Personnel]
Sex Differences (Animal) [See Animal Sex Differences]
Sex Differences (Human) [See Human Sex Differences]
Sex Hormones [See Estrogens]
Sexual Reproduction 155, 271, 280, 297, 318, 328
Shape Perception [See Form and Shape Perception]
Sheep 323
Shock 277
Shopping [See Consumer Behavior]
Short Term Memory 365, 375, 524, 586, 596, 737, 859
Siblings [See Also Twins] 520
Side Effects (Drug) [See Also Drug Sensitivity] 412, 500
Side Effects (Treatment) [See Side Effects (Drug)]
Signal Detection (Perception) 111, 319, 870, 888, 890
Signal Intensity [See Stimulus Intensity]
Simple Schizophrenia [See Schizophrenia]
Simulation [See Also Computer Simulation, Simulation Games] 54
Simulation Games 50
Simulators [See Simulation]
Skin (Anatomy) 230
Sleep 82, 311, 748, 872

SUBJECT INDEX

Sleep Disorders 202
Slow Learners 483, 532
Smell Perception [See Olfactory Perception]
Smoking (Tobacco) [See Tobacco Smoking]
Social Behavior [See Also Aggressive Behavior, Animal Social Behavior, Attack Behavior, Help Seeking Behavior, Interpersonal Attraction, Interpersonal Interaction, Involvement, Participation, Risk Taking] 45, 209
Social Change 46, 47, 209
Social Class 600
Social Environments [See Also Animal Environments, Classroom Environment, Home Environment, Rural Environments, Social Support Networks, Urban Environments, Working Conditions] 46, 47
Social Influences [See Also Power, Social Values] 105, 215, 585
Social Interaction [See Interpersonal Attraction, Interpersonal Interaction, Participation]
Social Learning [See Imitation (Learning)]
Social Movements [See Also Activist Movements] 146, 152, 153
Social Processes [See Industrialization]
Social Sciences [See Comparative Psychology, Neuropsychology]
Social Services [See Community Services]
Social Structure [See Social Class]
Social Studies Education 103, 125
Social Support Networks 115
Social Values 47
Society [See Socioeconomic Status]
Sociocultural Factors [See Also Cross Cultural Differences] 510
Socioeconomic Status [See Also Family Socioeconomic Level, Social Class] 507, 509, 510
Sodium [See Also Sodium Ions] 648
Sodium Ions 849
Sodium Pentobarbital [See Pentobarbital]
Solvent Abuse [See Inhalant Abuse]
Solvents 75, 332, 333, 334, 335, 336, 337, 338, 339, 340, 341, 343, 344, 346, 350, 352, 354, 355, 356, 357, 358, 359, 360, 362, 363, 364, 367, 368, 369, 370, 371, 372, 373, 374, 375, 376, 377, 378, 381, 383, 384, 385, 388, 390, 391, 392, 393, 395, 396, 397, 399, 400, 401, 402, 404, 405, 406, 407, 408, 409, 411, 413, 414, 415, 416, 417, 418, 419, 420, 421, 422, 423, 424, 425, 426, 427, 428, 429, 431, 432, 433, 434, 435, 437, 438, 866
Somatosensory Evoked Potentials 431, 492
Somesthetic Perception [See Also Cutaneous Sense, Pain Perception, Vibrotactile Thresholds] 881
Sorting (Cognition) [See Classification (Cognitive Process)]
Sound [See Auditory Stimulation]

Sourness [See Taste Perception]
South America 93
Southeast Asia [See Philippines]
Spain 818
Spanish Americans [See Hispanics]
Spatial Ability 697, 699, 737
Spatial Discrimination [See Spatial Perception]
Spatial Frequency 665
Spatial Memory 326
Spatial Perception [See Also Motion Perception] 325, 698
Special Education 8
Speech Disorders 540
Speed (Response) [See Reaction Time]
Spelling 546
Sperm 406
Spinal Cord 762
Spinal Fluid [See Cerebrospinal Fluid]
Spontaneous Alternation 625, 644
Sports [See Swimming]
Spouses [See Housewives]
Stanford Achievement Test 505
Stapedius Reflex [See Acoustic Reflex]
Starfish [See Echinodermata]
Startle Reflex 289, 669, 671, 904
Starvation 231
State Dependent Learning 399, 411
Statistical Analysis [See Factor Analysis, Statistical Probability]
Statistical Measurement [See Statistical Probability]
Statistical Probability 30
Statistical Validity [See Predictive Validity]
Status [See Socioeconomic Status]
Stereotaxic Techniques [See Chemical Brain Stimulation]
Stereotyped Behavior 636, 659, 734
Steroids [See Corticosterone]
Stimulation [See Auditory Stimulation, Aversive Stimulation, Olfactory Stimulation, Self Stimulation, Visual Stimulation]
Stimulus Change 901
Stimulus Control 433
Stimulus Deprivation [See Food Deprivation]
Stimulus Discrimination 291, 849, 918
Stimulus Intensity 887
Stimulus Novelty 233
Stimulus Parameters [See Also Spatial Frequency, Stimulus Intensity, Stimulus Novelty] 231
Strain Differences (Animal) [See Animal Strain Differences]
Stress [See Also Environmental Stress, Occupational Stress, Physiological Stress, Psychological Stress, Stress Reactions] 277, 610, 611, 694
Stress Reactions 6, 68, 110, 115, 157, 200, 211, 615, 721
Student Attitudes 173
Student Characteristics [See Student Attitudes]
Students [See Also Elementary School Students, High School Students, Junior High School Students, Kindergarten Students] 387
Studies (Followup) [See Followup Studies]
Subcortical Lesions [See Brain Lesions]
Substance P 619
Substantia Nigra [See Mesencephalon]
Subtests 465
Sugars 9, 823, 827, 831
Suicide 151, 249
Suicide (Attempted) [See Attempted Suicide]
Sulpiride 709
Superior Colliculus 633
Supervisors [See Management Personnel]
Suppression (Conditioned) [See Conditioned Suppression]
Surgery [See Decerebration]
Susceptibility (Disorders) 142, 534
Sweetness [See Taste Perception]
Swimming 232
Sympathomimetic Amines [See Amphetamine, Catecholamines, Dextroamphetamine, Dopamine, Norepinephrine]
Sympathomimetic Drugs [See Amphetamine, Catecholamines, Dextroamphetamine, Dopamine, Fenfluramine, Norepinephrine]
Symposia [See Professional Meetings and Symposia]
Symptoms [See Also Anoxia, Apnea, Appetite Disorders, Apraxia, Ataxia, Convulsions, Delirium, Fatigue, Headache, Hyperkinesis, Hypoglycemia, Hypothermia, Migraine Headache, Shock, Tremor] 145, 201, 254, 356, 357, 361, 384, 386, 550, 571, 572, 575, 682, 858, 895
Synapses 559, 762, 839, 911
Syndromes [See Also Acquired Immune Deficiency Syndrome, Alzheimers Disease, Korsakoffs Psychosis, Organic Brain Syndromes, Toxic Psychoses] 193, 473

Tactual Perception [See Vibrotactile Thresholds]
Taste Aversion Conditioning [See Aversion Conditioning]
Taste Discrimination [See Taste Perception]
Taste Perception 233, 237, 393, 503, 842, 848, 849
Teachers [See College Teachers]
Teaching [See Computer Assisted Instruction, Teaching Methods]
Teaching Methods [See Also Computer Assisted Instruction] 518
Technology 130
Teenagers [See Adolescents]
Teeth (Anatomy) 501, 585
Telencephalon [See Amygdaloid Body, Basal Ganglia, Cerebral Cortex, Hippocampus, Limbic System, Motor Cortex, Visual Cortex]

SUBJECT INDEX

Temperature Effects [See Also Heat Effects] 80, 656
Teratogens 486, 608, 659, 660, 661, 731, 744, 749, 764
Test Construction [See Also Item Content (Test), Test Validity] 126, 143, 187, 188
Test Interpretation 367
Test Scores [See Also Intelligence Quotient] 505
Test Validity 465
Testing [See Also Computer Assisted Testing, Item Content (Test), Repeated Measures, Test Interpretation, Test Validity] 896
Tests [See Measurement]
Tests (Intelligence) [See Intelligence Measures]
Thalamus [See Geniculate Bodies (Thalamus)]
Theory Verification 791
Therapeutic Community 16
Therapy [See Treatment]
Therapy (Drug) [See Drug Therapy]
Thorazine [See Chlorpromazine]
Thought Disturbances [See Memory Disorders, Perseveration]
Threat 170
Thresholds [See Also Auditory Thresholds, Critical Flicker Fusion Threshold, Dark Adaptation, Vibrotactile Thresholds, Visual Thresholds] 266, 784
Time [See Also Interresponse Time] 23
Time Estimation 437
Time Perception [See Also Time Estimation] 884
Tiredness [See Fatigue]
Tissues (Body) [See Membranes, Myelin Sheath, Nasal Mucosa, Skin (Anatomy)]
Tobacco (Drug) [See Nicotine]
Tobacco Smoking 139, 141, 194, 199, 869, 880, 883, 897
Tolerance 74, 184
Tolerance (Drug) [See Drug Tolerance]
Toxic Disorders [See Also Carbon Monoxide Poisoning, Lead Poisoning, Mercury Poisoning, Narcosis, Toxic Encephalopathies, Toxic Psychoses] 20, 27, 28, 32, 37, 64, 66, 67, 77, 92, 98, 101, 116, 119, 124, 144, 145, 148, 163, 167, 168, 190, 193, 197, 205, 231, 239, 240, 243, 252, 253, 258, 259, 262, 269, 270, 333, 339, 342, 348, 349, 352, 353, 355, 361, 364, 369, 372, 375, 387, 388, 394, 398, 473, 501, 515, 529, 532, 539, 545, 546, 570, 598, 807, 808, 809, 818, 819, 860, 864, 866, 867, 885, 899
Toxic Encephalopathies 210, 257, 331, 337, 338, 358, 371, 485, 520, 574, 579, 668, 693, 705, 725, 780
Toxic Psychoses 89, 192, 193, 256, 351, 541, 877
Toxicity 2, 3, 4, 5, 11, 12, 13, 17, 18, 25, 29, 31, 34, 42, 44, 53, 57, 58, 60, 61, 63, 106, 107, 115, 150, 157, 171, 201, 217, 220, 223, 225, 226, 230, 232, 233, 236, 246, 249, 263, 276, 284, 291, 302, 353, 365, 373, 379, 386, 409, 410, 412, 418, 424, 425, 428, 435, 459, 522, 558, 570, 629, 656, 672, 674, 727, 732, 739, 768, 772, 782, 853, 859, 880
Toxins [See Poisons]
Tracking [See Also Visual Tracking] 828
Traditionalism [See Conservatism]
Tranquilizing Drugs [See Chlordiazepoxide, Chlorpromazine, Diazepam]
Transportation 24
Transportation Accidents 49
Trauma (Physical) [See Injuries]
Treatment Facilities [See Child Guidance Clinics, Hospitals]
Treatment [See Also Related Terms] 77, 803, 806, 811
Tremor 270, 289
Tumors [See Neoplasms]
Twins 575
Tympanic Membrane [See Middle Ear]

Underwater Effects 859
United Kingdom [See Great Britain]
United States [See Also Appalachia, Hawaii] 93, 484
Urban Environments 21, 39, 100, 103, 173, 198, 487, 497, 508, 585, 878, 898
Urinalysis 457

Validity (Test) [See Test Validity]
Valium [See Diazepam]
Values [See Personal Values, Social Values]
Variable Interval Reinforcement 306
Vasoconstrictor Drugs [See Amphetamine, Norepinephrine, Serotonin]
Verbal Ability 520, 551
Verbal Conditioning [See Verbal Learning]
Verbal Learning [See Also Paired Associate Learning] 358, 834
Verdict Determination [See Adjudication]
Verification (of Theories) [See Theory Verification]
Vernier Acuity [See Visual Acuity]
Vertebrates [See Amphibia, Baboons, Birds, Cats, Chickens, Dogs, Ducks, Fishes, Frogs, Gerbils, Goldfish, Guinea Pigs, Mammals, Mice, Monkeys, Pigeons, Quails, Rabbits, Rats, Salamanders, Sea Gulls, Sheep]
Vestibular Apparatus 363
Vestibular Nystagmus [See Nystagmus]
Veterans (Military) [See Military Veterans]
Vibration 566
Vibrotactile Thresholds 352
Video Display Terminals [See Video Display Units]
Video Display Units 155, 195
Vigilance 340, 341, 354, 375, 378, 392, 596, 857, 865, 878, 888, 889
Viral Disorders [See Acquired Immune Deficiency Syndrome]

Vision [See Also Brightness Perception, Critical Flicker Fusion Threshold, Dark Adaptation, Visual Discrimination, Visual Field, Visual Perception, Visual Thresholds] 521
Vision Disorders 730
Visual Acuity 665
Visual Cortex 633, 665, 715
Visual Discrimination 323, 630, 653, 713, 749, 865, 911
Visual Displays [See Also Video Display Units] 124
Visual Evoked Potentials 395, 396, 397, 404, 431, 492, 625, 634, 655, 656, 663, 778, 783
Visual Field 715
Visual Masking 880
Visual Perception [See Also Brightness Perception, Critical Flicker Fusion Threshold, Dark Adaptation, Visual Acuity, Visual Discrimination, Visual Field, Visual Thresholds] 365, 468, 863, 878, 890, 897
Visual Search 344
Visual Stimulation [See Also Illumination, Scotopic Stimulation, Visual Displays] 85, 182, 449, 888
Visual Thresholds [See Also Critical Flicker Fusion Threshold] 715, 880
Visual Tracking 344, 856, 870, 887
Vitamin C [See Ascorbic Acid]
Vitamin Therapy 588, 806
Vitamins [See Also Ascorbic Acid] 815, 845
Vocabulary 518
Vocations [See Occupations]
Volunteer Civilian Personnel 146
Volunteer Personnel [See Volunteer Civilian Personnel]

Wakefulness 357
War [See Nuclear War]
Wasps 318
Water Intake 638, 640, 642
Weaning 668
Weapons 94
Weather [See Atmospheric Conditions]
Wechsler Memory Scale 345
Weight (Body) [See Body Weight]
Wellness [See Health]
White Collar Workers [See Also Management Personnel] 33
White Noise 83
White Rats [See Rats]
Whites 590
Within Subjects Design [See Repeated Measures]
Wives [See Housewives]
Word Associations 859
Words (Vocabulary) [See Vocabulary]
Work Environments [See Working Conditions]
Workers [See Personnel]
Working Conditions [See Also Occupational Safety] 33, 38, 43, 69, 78, 144, 149, 167, 195, 334, 343, 360, 366, 371, 389, 502, 515, 516, 570, 598, 878

SUBJECT INDEX

Working Memory [See Short Term Memory]
Workmens Compensation Insurance 460
Worms 303
Wounds [See Self Inflicted Wounds]
Writing (Creative) [See Literature]

Written Language [See Letters (Alphabet)]

Young Adults 890
Youth (Adolescents) [See Adolescents]

Youth (Adults) [See Young Adults]
Youth (Children) [See Children]

Zinc 522, 603

Section IV. Author Index

The Author Index contains references to all the records published in this bibliography. All authors whose works are cited are listed alphabetically by surname. This index is intended to be a name index only and not a person index. For example, a listing for "Barclay, A." will be listed separately from "Barclay, Allan," even though the names may refer to the same person; two listings for "Barclay, A." may refer to two different authors. As many as four authors are listed for each record; if there are more than four authors, the first author is listed, followed by "et al." Numbers cited refer to citation numbers in the bibliography.

Abou-Donia, Mohamed B., 262
Abrol, B. M., 566
Abueg, Francis R., 68
Abumrad, N. N., 705
Accardo, Pasquale, 462
Acredolo, Curt, 250, 951
Adams, J., 220
Adams, Jane, 263
Adams, Perrie M., 919
Adesso, Vincent J., 313, 314
Agnew, Jacqueline, 463
Agrawal, Ashok K., 330
Ahlström, Richard, 855
Akaike, M., 920
Åkerstedt, Torbjörn, 357
Akkermans, Louis M., 264
Albee, R. R., 943
Albee, Ralph R., 304
Albright, Michael E., 265
Alfano, Dennis P., 604, 605, 606, 607
Al-Hachim, Ghazi M., 266
Ali, M. M., 608
Ali, M. Mohamed et al, 609
Ali, S. Fatehyab, 267
Allen, Gary L., 1
Allen, James R., 630
Almirall Hernández, Pedro, 464
Anand, Mohini, 330
Anderson, Brenda J. et al, 610, 611
Anderson, Diane L., 101
Anderson, William J., 707, 708
Angell, Norman F., 612
Anger, W. Kent, 2, 69
Angiak, Robert, 667
Annau, Zoltan, 621, 655, 657, 658, 680, 900, 906
Ansari, Khurshed A., 70
Anshelm Olson, Birgitta, 357
Antti-Poika, Mari, 361, 364
Aragon, Polly, 785
Arezzo, Joseph C., 3, 54
Arlien-Søborg, P. et al, 338
Arlien-Søborg, Peter, 337
Armstrong, Eileen, 511
Árochová, Ol'ga, 71
Arredondo, J. M., 807
Arunachalam, S., 268
Atkinson, Elizabeth J., 687
Ator, Nancy A., 901
Attewell, Robyn, 962
Augustine, George J., 839
Avery, Carol E., 72

Baggs, Raymond B., 946
Baghurst, P. A., 961
Bailey, Kent G., 465
Baird, Brian N., 73, 74
Baker, Dorothy M., 721, 723
Baker, Edward L., 4, 215, 339, 466
Baker, Edward L. et al, 75
Baker, H., 76
Baker, Thomas, 269
Bakke, Hans K., 294
Balduini, Walter, 326
Balko, Stanley W., 666, 667
Ballowe, Tom, 533
Baloh, Robert, 467
Balster, Robert L., 416, 417, 434
Bancroft, John et al, 77
Bankovska, R., 78
Baraldi, Mario et al, 613
Barbeau, A. et al, 270
Barcus, Robert A., 840
Barker, M. L., 79
Barlow, Charles F., 439
Barrett, J., 614, 615, 616, 706
Barrett, Rowland P., 468
Barry, Timothy, 185

Barter, Marie J., 688
Barton, Curtis N., 856, 873
Bass, Rolf, 749
Baumann, Stephan, 171
Baumeister, Alan A., 617
Bautista, Samuel, 394
Bechard, Marc J., 271
Beck, Dave, 531
Becker, Charles E., 868
Beginn, U., 492
Bell, Paul A., 80
Bellinger, David, 470, 921
Bellinger, David C., 471, 472
Bellinger, David C. et al, 469
Beneš, V., 340, 341
Benignus, Gayla, 857
Benignus, Vernon A., 5, 856, 857, 873, 884
Benna, P., 82, 83, 84
Benson, D. Frank, 521
Ber, Abram, 787
Bercegeay, Mark S., 396
Bergamasco, B., 82, 83, 84, 85
Bergamasco, B. et al, 81
Berger, Philip A., 248
Bergholtz, L. M., 342
Berglund, Birgitta, 6, 7, 86, 87, 88, 855, 858
Berglund, Mats, 89
Berglund, Ulf, 86, 87, 88, 855
Berman, Mark S., 221
Berman, Robert F., 741
Bernuzzi, Viviane, 618
Berry, Paul, 814
Bertazzi, Pier-Alberto, 922
Besser, R., 473
Beuthin, Frederic C., 741, 742
Biela, Adam, 90
Bier, Mariana, 486
Biersner, R. J., 859
Biggs, James D., 272
Biondi, Massimo, 91
Bishry, Z., 168
Bjerke, Tore, 92
Blackburn, Archie B., 240
Blackshear, Pamela, 750
Bland, Jeffrey, 440
Bloom, A. S., 327
Bloom, Alan S., 273
Blouin, Arthur G., 474
Blouin, Jane H., 474
Bluhm, Louis H., 93
Blunden, Dale, 832
Bodis-Wollner, Ivan, 404
Bogat, G. Anne, 141
Bogomolny, Alice, 841
Bohl, J., 473
Boja, J. W., 902
Bolter, John F., 860
Bondy, Stephen C., 619
Bone, Craig M., 353
Bonithon-Kopp, C., 475
Bonithon-Kopp, Claire, 246
Boone, Lois, 544, 573
Booze, Rosemarie M., 620, 621
Bornhausen, M., 622
Bornschein, Robert L., 673
Bourg, Wendy J., 623
Bourgeois, Anthony E., 722
Bowman, Ann, 156
Bowman, R. E., 701
Bowman, Robert E., 630, 698, 699, 700, 714, 940
Boyes, Barry E., 729
Boyes, William K., 397
Brackbill, Yvonne, 8
Bracy, Odie L. et al, 274
Bradley, M., 649

Brady, Kathleen, 624
Braithwaite, V. A., 94
Branconnier, Roland J., 95
Bratton, Gerald R., 721
Braun, Claude M., 923
Brebner, J., 96
Breen, Timothy J., 435
Breidenbach, Steven T., 199
Brennan, Nancy E., 3
Brightwell, W. S., 418, 419
Brockhaus, Arthur, 704
Brody, Julia G., 924
Bromet, Evelyn J., 187
Broms, Inger, 953
Brown, D. R., 777
Brown, N. T., 843
Brown, W. J., 746
Browne, Ellen, 945
Brunner, Robert L., 802
Bryce-Smith, Derek, 97
Bryer, Jeffrey B., 861
Bælum,Jesper et al, 343
Buchanan, Stephen R., 9
Buckalew, L. W., 10
Buckholtz, Neil S., 11
Buckley, Robert, 803
Buelke-Sam, Judy, 31, 263
Buiatti, Eva et al, 476
Bull, R. J., 726
Bunnell, David E., 862
Burbacher, Thomas M., 275, 933
Burchfiel, James S., 241
Burdette, Linda J., 625, 626
Burg, J. R., 418
Burne, Thomas A., 769
Burr, Ralph G., 98
Burright, Richard G., 628, 646, 652, 662, 929
Burright, Richard G. et al, 627
Busbee, Everette L., 276
Bushnell, P. J., 398
Bushnell, Philip J., 393, 629, 630, 714, 925, 926
Butcher, Richard E., 12, 13, 669, 802
Butzirus, Sharyl M., 813

Cabetas, I., 807
Callahan, B. G., 777
Calne, D. B. et al, 99
Campbell, Joan M., 19
Campion, John, 863
Cañas, F., 819
Cann, Arnie, 206
Cantor, D. S., 208
Carlson, Jeffrey N., 277
Carlson, Shally L., 247
Carmichael, Neil F., 459
Carricaburu, Pierre, 278
Case, James C., 535
Catalano, Ralph, 110, 134
Cataldo, Michael F., 496, 525, 526
Caul, Jefferies, 462
Cavalieri, Stuart A., 868
Cawte, John, 242
Chaiklin, Harris, 477, 478, 479
Champagne, Francine, 927
Chandra, Om, 267
Chandra, S. V., 608
Chang, Louis W., 304
Chapel, James L., 864
Chapko, Michael K., 100
Chernick, Eleanor, 804
Cherry, Nicola et al, 344
Chimento, Barry E., 729
Chisolm, J. Julian, 457
Chouinard, Guy, 351
Christensen, C. L. et al, 865
Christian, W., 348

Chung, Eunyong, 404
Churkin, E. A., 256
Clark, Donald E., 623, 722, 723
Coggeshall, Ellen, 434
Coggeshall, Ellen M., 435
Cohen, Gerald, 222
Cohen, Randye E., 101
Colburn, Theodore R., 53
Coleman, Timothy L., 193
Colotla, Victor A., 394
Colowick, S. P., 705
Colvin, Bruce A., 279
Commissaris, Randall L. et al, 631
Congdon, William C., 412
Conners, C. Keith, 805
Connor, Donald J., 928
Conrad, Mary K., 480
Cook, Art, 768
Cook, Fay L., 178
Cook, Jeanne J., 478
Cook, Larry L., 322
Cook, Michelle P., 761
Coombes, Shannon, 233
Cooper, Gary P., 673
Copeland, R. L., 438
Correa Cruz, Manuel, 223
Corwin, June, 102
Cory-Slechta, Deborah A., 632
Cossairt, Ace, 530, 591
Costa, L. G., 633, 665
Costa, Lucio G., 320, 326, 944
Costikyan, Nancy S., 192
Cott, Allan, 806
Covacich, A. M., 83
Cowley, Deborah S., 346
Cram, Douglas M., 838
Crapper, D. R., 634, 635, 686
Creel, Donnell J., 14
Crim, Karen O., 103
Cripe, Lloyd I., 104
Crofton, Kevin M., 315
Crossen, John R., 345
Croxton, Jack S., 378
Crystal, H. A., 866
Cullen, Mark R., 382, 578
Cullen, Susan M., 565
Cullinane, Marie M., 565
Culver, Bruce, 903, 909
Cuomo, Vincenzo et al, 636
Curtin, Thomas R., 178
Custer, Thomas W., 280
Cuthbertson, Beverley H., 15, 16
Cutkomp, Laurence K., 329
Cutler, M. G., 649, 650, 651
Cutler, Margaret G., 637
Cutter, Susan C., 105
Czech, Donald A., 638, 639, 640, 747

Dager, Stephen R., 346
Daigneault, Sylvie, 923
Dalen, Knut, 867
Dalton, A. J., 634, 635
D'Amato, Robert J., 196
David, Oliver J., 481, 483
David, Oliver J. et al, 482
Davies, Helen N., 545
Davis, J. Michael, 484
Davis, Kenneth L., 248
Davis, Michael, 904
Dawson, R. G., 706
Day, H. D., 641, 682
Dean, Karen F., 322
de Boni, U., 686
Dehaven, Diane L., 774
DeHaven, Diane L., 642, 643
Delin, P., 96
Delouise, Edward R., 590
del Ser, T., 807

AUTHOR INDEX

Del Ser Quijano, T., 808
DeLuca, John, 929
de Man, A. F., 166
Demers, Francois X., 504
de Mol, J., 485
Dent, J., 956
de Rossett, Sarah E., 644
Desor, Didier, 618
Dick, Robert B., 347
Dickinson, Julie, 409, 423, 424, 425, 428
Dieringer, Therese, 273
Dietrich, Kim N., 486
Díez Manrique, J. F. et al, 809
Dillon, Kathleen M., 842
Dodrill, Carl B., 104
Dolinsky, Z. S. et al, 645
Dolinsky, Zelig S., 646
Domer, Floyd R., 647, 648
Donald, J. M., 649, 650, 651
Donohoe, Tim, 768
Donovick, Peter J., 628, 646, 652, 662, 929
Dooley, David, 110, 134
Doraz, Walter E., 831
Dorndorf, W., 348
Dortch, Annie L., 788
Dragan, Yvonne, 435
Drayton, Mary A., 576
Drew, Colleen, 762
Drew, Kelly L., 400
Driscoll, Janis W., 653, 654
Driver, Crystal J., 281
DuCharme, Larry L., 412
Duffy, Frank H., 241
Dunlap, W. P., 143
Dunner, David L., 346
Duva, Nicholas A., 487
Dvorzniak, Mark, 404
Dwivedi, Kamal, 56, 384, 955
Dyer, Robert S., 17, 396, 397, 655, 656
Dyer, Robert S. et al, 395

Ebert, John, 211
Eccles, Christine U., 655, 657, 658, 930
Eckerman, David A., 44, 54
Eckerman, David A. et al, 18
Edelstein, Michael R., 106, 107
Edinger, Jack, 465
Eisenbrandt, David L., 304
Elkington, Brian, 786
Elkins, John, 814
Elsner, Jürg, 659, 660, 661
Ely, Daniel, 198
Emmett, Edward A., 570
Engellenner, William J., 628, 662
Engen, Trygg, 88
Eriksson, H., 447
Ernhart, Claire B., 488, 489, 490, 491, 562, 563
Ernst, Karl, 211
Errera, John, 530, 531, 532, 533, 534, 535, 536, 537, 538, 539, 546, 591
Esiri, Margaret M., 108
Eskelinen, Leena, 349
Eslinger, Paul J., 871
Espasandin, P., 807
Estrin, William J., 868
Etuk, Ezekiel M., 810
Evans, G. W., 224
Evans, Gary W., 19, 109, 110, 111, 112, 134
Evans, H. L., 398
Evans, Hugh L., 441, 450, 695
Ewert, T., 492

Faed, James M., 582
Fairhurst, Stephen P., 234
Fantasia, Martha A., 721
Farage-Elawar, Miranda, 931
Farrell, Brian, 757
Farská, I., 690, 691
Faubert, Patricia, 638
Faust, David, 871
Fechter, Laurence D., 907
Feeney, Dennis M. et al, 663
Feeney, Ellen M., 423, 428
Fein, Greta G., 20, 136
Feingold, Benjamin F., 811
Feldman, Hobart T., 828

Feldman, Robert G., 442, 443, 444, 466
Ferguson, H. Bruce, 812
Ferguson, Sherry A., 702
Fergusson, D. M., 493, 494, 495
Fergusson, J. E., 493, 494, 495
Fiedler, Fred E., 113
Fiedler, Judith, 113
Field, Robert I., 331
Fifer, William E., 50
Finney, Jack W., 496
Fiori, Charles E., 498
Fischhoff, Baruch, 854
Fisher, Gerald H., 21
Fite, Kenneth, 669
Fitzgerald, Michael, 497
Flagler, Sally L., 114
Fleming, India C., 115
Flindt, Michael L., 385
Flynn, Eleanor R., 664
Foldvary, E., 902
Folio, Rhonda, 536
Forman, Samuel A., 353
Forness, Steven R., 791
Forsythe, John W., 919
Foster, Harold D., 22
Fox, D. A., 633, 665
Frager, Neal B., 111
Frank, Richard, 557
Frantík, E., 910
Frantík, E., 340, 341, 354, 390
Franzen, Michael D., 116
Frederiksen, Lee W., 869
Freimark, Steven J., 234
Frey, James, 185, 186
Friedhoff, Arnold J., 380
Fries, Cara R., 225
Fuld, P. A., 866
Furlan, P., 84
Fusco, Marc E., 80

Gabor, Silvia, 514
Gade, Anders, 399
Gál, E. M., 436
Galindo, Janine C., 281
Galloway, W. D., 843
Gallus, J. A., 289
Gamberale, Francesco, 350, 357
Garbe, Kurt, 720
Garruto, Ralph M., 498
Gartside, Peter S., 727
Gause, E. M., 282, 401, 402
Gause, Emily M., 403
Gaynor, Jeffrey J., 643
Gechman, Arthur S., 571
Gedney, B., 581
Geiger, Susan K., 557
Geist, Charles R., 400, 666, 667, 668
Geller, I., 282, 401, 402
Geller, Irving, 403
Gendelman, David S., 65
Gendelman, Phillip M., 904
Gentile, Christopher G., 293
Gentry, G. David, 946
Gerber, Gary J., 226
Getty, Louise, 126
Geyer, Mark A., 669
Ghafour, Siham Y., 499
Ghilardi, M. Felice, 404
Ghosh, T. K., 405, 438
Giardini, Valerio et al, 283
Gibbons, Barbara H., 406
Gibbons, I. R., 406
Gilbert, Avery N., 117
Gilbert, Brigitte, 923
Gilewsky, Michael J., 500
Gilka, Libuse, 789
Gillberg, Christopher, 501
Gillespie, David F., 45, 174
Gilli, M., 82, 83, 84, 85
Gittelman, Rachel, 820
Gittelman-Klein, Rachel, 821
Givens, David B., 23
Glenn, Allen D., 50
Gleser, Goldine, 467
Glickman, Linda A., 502
Gliner, Jeffrey A., 870, 881
Glowa, John R., 284
Gnelitsky, G. I., 58
Gold, Richard M., 696
Gold, Richard M. et al, 844
Goldberg, Alan M., 718, 754, 755

Goldbloom, D., 351
Golden, Charles J., 64, 116
Golden, Herbert M., 24
Goldman, Larry, 916
Goldsmith, Marshall, 784
Goldstein, M., 286
Goldstein, Robert, 626
Golter, Marianne, 670
Gordon, Christopher J., 932
Gordon, Cynthia M., 503
Gordon, Margaret T., 178
Goto, M., 920
Govoni, S., 739
Gowdy, John M., 504
Goyette, Charles H., 805
Grad, Gary, 483
Grandjean, Philippe, 942
Grant, Corbett V., 285
Grant, Kimberly S., 275
Grant-Webster, Kimberly S., 933
Grattan, Lynn, 871
Graves, Roger, 521
Green, Bonnie, 467
Green, Lois M., 249
Greenless, Robert M., 505
Gregory, Robert J., 506
Grober, E., 866
Groll-Knapp, E. et al, 872
Gross, Mortimer D., 813
Gunderson, Virginia M., 933
Guth, Lloyd, 118
Gutterman, Elane M., 157
Gyldensted, Carsten, 945

Hagen, U., 622
Häggblad, J., 447
Hagstadius, Stefan, 379, 934
Halberg, Franz, 329, 917
Hall, D. A., 859
Hall, Debra, 536
Hall, Wayne, 243
Halonen, J.-P., 352
Halonen, P., 352
Haluska, Marianne, 750
Hamlin, M. W., 508
Hammond, E. Cuyler, 25
Hanin, Israel, 753
Hanlon, Roger T., 919
Hänninen, Helena, 119, 445, 528, 935, 950
Hanse, S., 286
Hansen, Ole N., 942
Hanson, Mats, 446
Hantman, Elaine, 823
Harbin, Thomas J., 873
Hardison, Nancy M., 120
Härkönen, Hannu, 362
Harley, J. Preston, 466, 790
Harrell, Lindy E., 928
Harris, C. S., 121
Harry, Gaylia J., 671
Hartlage, Lawrence C., 26
Hartman, David E., 27
Hartmann, R. J., 401, 402
Hartmann, Roy J., 282, 402, 403
Hartwell, Stuart I., 672
Harvey, P. G., 507, 508
Hasan, Mahdi, 267
Hastings, Lloyd, 673
Hatcher, Sherry L., 122
Hawk, B. A. et al, 509
Hawk, Barbara A., 510
Hawkes, Glenn R., 250
Hayes, Margaret E., 478
Heard, G. S., 29
Hebben, Nancy, 521
Hebel, J. R., 511
Hebisch, S., 897
Heck, Edward T., 861
Heilbronn, E., 447
Heimstra, Norman W., 199
Heise, George A., 287, 288
Hellberg, Jan, 448, 449, 674
Hellström, Jonas, 674
Helmkamp, James C., 353
Henderson, Victor W., 123
Hendrickson, Edward C., 124
Hennekes, Raimund, 941
Henretig, Fred M., 579
Hensler, Gary L., 280
Hepburn, Mary A., 125

Hernberg, S., 528
Herr, D. W., 289
Herrera, Yolanda, 624
Hétu, Raymond, 126
Hetzler, Bruce E., 397
Hicks, Lou E., 517
Himnan, Donald J., 407
Hinman, Donald J., 408
Hobbes, Gary, 817
Hodel, Beat, 660
Hodge, David C., 177
Hodgson, Michael, 381
Hofferberth, B., 492
Hoffman, Jeanne S., 251
Hoiberg, Anne, 98
Hoium, Ellen, 639
Holborow, Patricia, 814
Holland, John P., 346
Hollingworth, Robert M., 290, 317
Holloway, William R., 675, 676, 677
Hong, J. S., 321
Hooisma, J., 57
Hopkins, B. L. et al, 127
Hopper, David L., 291
Horowitz, Jordan, 936
Horst, Richard L., 522
Horváth, M., 340, 341, 354, 390
Horvath, Steven M., 862, 870, 881
Horwood, L. J., 493, 494, 495
Hosokawa, Toshiyuki, 437, 959
Howard, Rosanne B., 565
Howd, Robert A., 409, 424, 425, 426, 427, 432
Howell, William E., 656
Hrdina, Pavel D., 292
Hudson, Jeffrey D., 287, 288
Huebner, Robert B., 128
Huel, G., 475
Huel, Guy, 246
Huggins, Hal A., 512
Hughes, J. A., 678
Hughes, John A., 679, 680, 681
Hughes, Pauline, 582
Hummel, Carl F., 80, 129
Hunt, Thomas J., 513
Hupp, E. W., 682
Hupp, Eugene W., 641
Husain, Arshad, 864
Hyytiäinen, Asko, 364

Ibarra Fernández de la Vega, Enrique, 464
Ibrahim, Hanem S., 499
Inouye, Minoru, 238, 683
Iregren, Anders, 355, 356, 357
Isaacson, Robert L., 694
Ishikawa, Terry T., 410
Ison, James R., 28
Istoc-Bobis, Mariana, 514
Iwata, Osamu, 131
Iwata, Osamu, 130, 132

Jacobs, Abraham H., 133
Jacobs, Jim, 532, 533, 538
Jacobs, Stephen V., 110, 111, 112, 134
Jacobson, Joseph L., 20, 136
Jacobson, Joseph L. et al, 135
Jacobson, Sandra W., 25
Jacobson, Sandra W. et al, 137
Jaeckle, Richard S., 874
Jaensch, E., 592
Jaggi, Bikki, 138
Janisse, Michel P., 209
Jarrell, Theodore W., 293
Jason, Kathryn M., 684
Jason, Leonard A., 139
Jefferson, James W., 875
Jellestad, Finn K., 294
Jensen, Hans H., 399
Jensen, Per B., 358
Jewett, D. L., 29
Jodelet, Francois, 140
Johannessen, Jan N. et al, 227
Johansson, Barbro B. et al, 359
Johnson, D. L., 121
Johnson, F. Reed, 876
Johnson, Gail V., 685
Johnson, James H., 321
Johnston, Graham A., 762
Jonderko, G. et al, 515
Jones, John W., 141

AUTHOR INDEX

Jope, Richard S., 685, 928
Jørgensen, Merete, 945
Joseph, Stephen V., 109
Joy, R. M., 295
Joy, Robert M., 296
Juntunen, Juhani, 332, 333, 361, 362, 369
Juntunen, Juhani et al, 360

Kaiser, T. Earl, 280
Kajiwara, Yuji, 683
Kallman, M. J., 308
Kamel, M., 168
Kamilov, I. K., 311
Kane, D. N., 142
Kantor, Mark A., 845
Kaplan, Ervin, 159
Kark, R. A., 746
Karns, Daryl R., 228
Karpinski, K. F., 737
Karskela, V., 352
Kaste, Markku, 362
Katritzki, G., 348
Kavale, Kenneth A., 791
Keeney, Ralph L., 30
Keith, James O., 297
Kelkar, S. A., 516
Kelly, Teresa C., 474
Kendall, Ronald J., 281
Kennedy, R. S., 143
Kessler, Josef, 298
Khachaturian, Zaven S., 753
Khuffash, Faisal A., 499
Kimler, Bruce F., 947
Kimmel, Carole A., 31, 263
Ki Moon Bang, 334
Kinch, Denise, 511
King, G. A., 686
Kinsbourne, Marcel, 833
Kinzett, N. G., 493, 494, 495
Kirk, N. S., 32
Kirkconnell, Shirley C., 517
Kirouac, Gilles, 927
Kiss, Anna, 939
Kjellstrand, Per, 411
Klawans, Harold L., 775
Kleeman, Walter B., 33
Klein, Stephen B., 687, 688
Kleinhesselink, Randall R., 172
Klotz, M. L., 891
Knafle, June D., 518
Knapczyk, Dennis R., 815
Knave, Bengt, 144, 201
Koëter, Herman B., 905, 912
Köhler, Ch., 286
Kohler, G.-K., 877
Koltes, Karen H., 689
Koltun, Arnold, 483
Kontrová, Jana, 71
Koob, George F., 906
Korgeski, Gregory P., 145, 252
Korol, B. A., 744
Korpela, Marja, 937
Kožená, L., 340, 341
Kracke, Kevin R., 519
Kraemer, Ursala, 600
Krafft, Kathleen M., 486
Krall, Vita, 576
Krall, Vita et al, 520
Krämer, G., 473
Krekule, P., 354
Kresse, M., 348
Krigman, Martin R., 643
Kronus, Carol L., 146
Kruesi, Marcus, 588
Krulik, R., 690, 691
Kulig, Beverly M., 938
Kumar, P., 56
Kumar, R., 508
Kuntz, L. A., 143
Kurlychek, Robert T., 147
Kurtz, Perry J., 299
Kutscher, Charles L., 692
Kutscher, Cheryl S., 692
Kutscher, Nancy L., 692

Lacher, Thomas E., 281
Lachman, Barry S., 258
Lacroix, Roger, 278
Lacz, Joseph P., 693
Lalonde, Monique, 126
Lamon, Joel M., 756

Landa, Beth, 490
Landis, Theodor, 521
Landrigan, Philip J., 34, 148
Lang, H. A., 352
Langdon, F. J., 35
Langolf, Gary D., 587
Lansdown, Richard, 602
Lanthorn, Thomas, 694
Larsby, B., 363
Larson, Gerald E., 569, 593
Larson, K., 581
Larson, Marilyn B., 215
Laties, Victor G., 441, 450, 695, 853
Latto, Richard, 863
Laughlin, Nellie K., 717, 719
Laughton, Watson, 696
Laursen, Peter, 878
Law, H. G., 94
Lawrence, P. L., 705
Lawson, Billie Z., 149
Lazar, Alexandru, 150
Lazar, Joel M., 465
Leal, B. Z., 282
LeBoutillier, Janelle C., 607
Lehotzky, Kornelia, 300, 939
Lehotzky, Kornelia et al, 301
Lehr, Paul R., 618
Leleux, N., 485
Lenaerts, Claudia, 941
Leon, Gloria R., 252
le Quesne, Pamela M., 36
Leslie, Dennis C., 162
Lester, David, 151
Lester, M. L., 208, 595
Lester, Michael L., 522, 816
Levenson, Hanna, 152, 153, 154
Levin, Edward D., 697, 698, 699, 700, 701, 702, 940
Levin, Harvey S., 253, 255
Levine, Adeline G., 200
Levine, Tina E., 703
Levitan, Herbert, 839
Levitan, Herbert et al, 846
Leviton, Alan, 470, 471, 921
Levy, Charles J., 254
Levy, Florence, 817
Levy, René H., 412
Lewin, Roger, 244
Lewis, M. F., 305, 306
Lewis, Mark F., 307
Lewis, Mark H., 792
Lewis, Paul D., 459
Lewis, Stephen J., 229
Lilienthal, Hellmuth, 704, 720, 941
Linaweaver, P. G., 859
Lindgren, May, 934
Lindström, Kari, 37, 38, 335, 364, 365
Lindstrom, Kari, 366
Lindvall, Thomas, 7, 86, 87, 855, 858, 879
Lin-Fu, Jane S., 523
Link, Bruce, 157
Linnville, Steven E., 717, 719
Lipková, Valéria, 71
Lipman, J. J., 705
Lipsey, Mark W., 128
Liška, Jozef, 71
Livesey, D. J., 706
Livesey, P. J., 614, 615, 616, 706
Ljungberg, Tomas, 731
Llera, Juan-Carlos, 647
Lockard, Joan S., 412
Lockwood, A. P., 224
Lodge, David, 762
Löfgren, Lennart, 953
Long, Charles J., 860
López-Ibor, J. J., 818, 819
Lorentzen, Per, 367
Lorenzana-Jimenez, Marte, 413
Lorton, Dianne, 707, 708
Loseke, N., 485
Louis-Ferdinand, Robert T., 741, 742
Lowensohn, Brent A., 39
Lowenstein, L. F., 451
Lown, Bradley, 745
Lowndes, Herbert E., 269
Lucchi, L., 739
Lucchi, L. et al, 709
Luisto, Marjaana, 349
Luken, Ralph A., 876
Lundh, B., 883

Luria, S. M., 880
Lyes, M., 224
Lyngbye, Troels, 942
Lyon, Steve, 768

Mac Isaac, David S., 524
Mackay, Colin, 155
MacPhail, Robert C., 310
MacPhee, Donald, 243
Mactutus, Charles F., 302, 621, 769, 907
Madden, Nancy A., 525, 526
Madnawat, A. V., 40
Maggiotto, Michael A., 156
Maghazaji, H. I., 527
Magliano, C., 182
Magnier, Monique, 917
Magos, Laszlo, 710
Mailman, Richard B., 643, 792
Mailman, Richard B. et al, 847
Maizlish, Neil A., 368
Malecki, Richard A., 229
Mamsen, Pia, 358
Mantere, P., 528
Marban-Mendoza, Nahum, 303
Marchok, Patricia L., 751
Margolis, F. L., 76
Markesberry, William R., 193
Markowitsch, Hans J., 298
Markowitz, Jeffrey S., 157
Markowska, Alicja, 294
Marlar, Rickey J., 630
Marler, Matthew R., 491
Marlowe, Mike, 452, 453, 530, 531, 532, 533, 534, 535, 536, 537, 538, 539, 546, 591
Marlowe, Mike et al, 529
Marquis, Karen L., 711
Martelin, Tuija, 119
Martin, John E., 869
Massari, V. John, 418
Massaro, Edward J., 712, 745
Massaro, Thomas F., 712
Matikainen, E., 369
Mattei, Osvaldo, 349
Mattes, Ben B., 668
Mattes, Jeffrey, 821
Mattes, Jeffrey A., 793, 820
Mattsson, J. L., 943
Mattsson, Joel L., 304
Maugh, Thomas H., 158
Maurissen, Jacques P., 41
Maximilian, V. Alexander et al, 370
Mayfield, Sandra A., 540
Mayo, Lieser M., 396
Mayron, Lewis M., 159
Mayron, Lewis W., 42
Mayton, Daniel M., 160
Mazis, Michael B., 161, 162
McAlaster, R., 208, 595
McCabe, Philip M., 293
McCracken, James T., 541
McCunney, Robert J., 43
McDonald, Brian E., 944
McFarland, Dennis J., 713
McGann, Barbara, 483
McGeer, E. G., 728
McGeer, Edith G., 728
McIntire, Roger W., 908, 915
McKinley, Michael P., 179
McLamb, Ronnie L., 769
McLeod, W. R., 163
McMichael, A. J., 961
McMichael, William H. et al, 715
McNally, Michael R., 353
Meigs, J. Wister, 590
Mele, Paul C., 714
Meller, Emanuel, 380
Mendez, Carlos, 778
Mendez, V., 402
Mendez, Victor, 403
Menon, N. K., 746
Merigan, William H., 853, 908, 915
Merigan, William H. et al, 715
Mertens, H. W., 305, 306
Mertens, Henry W., 307
Michaelson, I. Arthur, 670, 673, 716
Mick, David L., 253
Middleton, Paulette, 198
Mihevic, Patricia M., 870, 881
Mikkelsen, Sigurd, 945
Milar, Christopher R., 542, 544
Milar, Christopher R. et al, 543

Millar, Ian B., 602
Miller, Bruce L., 164
Miller, Diane B., 245
Miller, Gregory D., 712
Miller, John E., 893
Miller, Terry P., 545
Min, Sung Kil, 882
Mindus, Per, 144, 201
Minkova, N., 78
Mitchell, J. A., 308
Miya, T. S., 748
Miyake, Hirotsugu, 414
Mohan, Philip J., 506
Molfese, Dennis L., 717, 719
Molik, Beate, 704
Monroe-Lord, L., 816
Montgomery, Mark R., 906
Mookherjee, S., 438
Moon, Charles, 537, 539, 546
Moon, Charles E., 538
Moore, M. R., 547, 649, 650, 651
Moore, Michael R. et al, 548
Mordelet-Dambrine, Madeleine, 917
Moreau, T., 475
Moreau, Thierry, 246
Morgan, Ben B., 1
Morgan, Donald P., 255
Morgan, G., 508
Morgan, Martha E., 667
Morgan, Newlin T., 53
Morganti, John, 745
Morison, Rufus, 309
Morrison, John H., 718
Morrow, Lisa A., 187, 381
Morrow-Tlucak, Mary, 491
Morse, Philip A., 717, 719
Moser, G., 165
Moser, Virginia C., 310, 415, 416, 417
Mosher, Barbara S., 479
Mottet, N. Karle, 275, 933
Mullenix, Phyllis, 909
Muller, Keith E., 856, 873
Munoz, Carmen, 720
Murao, Koji, 683
Murawski, Benjamin J., 339
Murdock, Larry L., 290
Murphy, Arthur L., 688
Murphy, Michael, 497
Murphy, Sheldon D., 320, 326, 944
Murthy, R. C., 608
Mushak, Paul, 544, 573
Muzrabekov, Sh. M., 311
Mytilineou, Catherine, 222

Nadzhimutdinov, K. N., 311
Naim, Michael, 848
Nasrallah, Henry A., 874
Nation, Jack R., 623, 721, 722, 723, 724
Nausieda, Paul A., 775
Navarro, P. Larrain, 166
Needleman, Herbert, 470, 921
Needleman, Herbert L., 454, 471, 472, 549, 550, 551, 552, 554, 555, 556, 557
Needleman, Herbert L. et al, 553
Nelkin, Dorothy, 167
Nelson, B. K., 418, 419
Nelson, Benjamin K., 420
Nelson, C. J., 13, 263
Nelson, Jeffrey L., 421, 422
Netterstrøm, Bo, 878
Neuschwander, J., 581
Newland, M. Christopher, 946
Newman, Elisa B., 805
Ng, Wendy W., 946
Nielsen, J. A., 902
Nielsen, Niels O., 371
Nielsen, Per, 371
Nielsén, Sören, 89
Nigg, Joanne M., 16
Niklowitz, Werner J., 725
Nishida, Hirobumi, 372
Nolan, Kevin R., 558
Noland, Elizabeth A., 726
Norén, J. G., 501
Norton, Stata, 903, 909, 947
Nowak, Robert T., 230
Null, David H., 727
Nurminen, Markku, 119

AUTHOR INDEX

Oakey, Richard, 211
Ödkvist, L. M., 342, 363
Ödkvist, L. M. et al, 373, 374
Oelke, Dieter, 660
O'Flynn, R. R., 948
Oglesby, D. M., 220
O'Hara. David M., 479
Ohara, Ikuo, 848, 849
Ohlin, P., 883
Ohlson, Carl-Göran, 953
Ohsumi, Noboru, 203
Okasha, Ahmed, 168
O'Kusky, J. R., 728
O'Kusky, John R., 729, 730
Oler, Jacqueline, 597
Olson, Birgitta A., 375
Olson, Kirsten L., 312
Olton, David S., 718
Olvey, K. M., 843
Ørbæk,Palle, 934
Ørbæk,Palle et al, 376
Orlebeke, J. F., 57
O'Rourke, Michael, 497
Orr, Robert H., 169, 170
O'Shaughnessy, Donald, 226
O'Shea, James A., 822
Oskarsson, Agneta, 731
Osman, N. M., 168
Otsuka, Shin-ichiro, 849
Otto, D., 559
Otto, D. A., 884
Otto, D. et al, 560
Otto, David A., 44, 54, 171, 857
Overmann, Stephen R., 732
Ozemek, H. S., 220

Padich, Robert, 733, 785
Palanichamy, S., 268
Pallak, Michael S., 172
Panem, Sandra, 11
Papaioannou, Rhoda, 589
Parker, Donald C., 173
Parker, Howard A., 45, 174
Parker, Howard B., 231
Parker, Linda A., 233
Parkes, M., 564
Parkinson, David K., 187
Partanen, Timo, 361
Paterson, Anna T., 770
Patton, Jim H., 734
Paul, Howard S., 571
Paulsen, Karen, 313, 314
Pearce, Jennifer, 579
Pedersen, Darhl M., 175
Pedersen, Grethe, 358
Peele, David B., 315, 393
Perez, Edgardo L., 885
Perino, Joseph, 561, 562, 563
Perlman, Daniel, 209
Perry, Raymond P., 209
Perry, Ronald W., 45, 174
Peters, David A., 292
Petersen, Uwe, 377
Peterson, Rebecca L., 176
Petit, Ted L., 605, 606, 607
Petzold, J., 877
Pfeiffer, Carl C., 588, 589
Pfister, William R., 317
Pfister, William R. et al, 316
Pihl, R. O., 564
Pihl, Robert O., 757
Piikivi, Leena, 949, 950
Pilisuk, Marc, 250, 951
Pleva, Jaro, 455
Plevova, J., 910
Podell, Richard N., 794
Poje, Gerald V., 232
Pollack, Ellen H., 318
Pontecorvo, Michael J., 398
Porter, John J., 313, 314
Porter, Seymour F., 822
Poul, Jean-Michel, 952
Powell, Kelly, 750
Pradhan, S. N., 405
Praed, Jeffrey E., 400
Prah, James D., 856, 857, 884
Prelipceanu, D., 886
Preston, Valerie, 177
Prinz, Ronald J., 823
Prokeš, J., 690, 691
Proshansky, Harold M., 46, 47
Prosser, T. D., 748

Protess, David L., 178
Prusiner, Stanley, 179
Pryor, Gordon T., 409, 423, 424, 425, 426, 427, 428, 432
Pueschel, Siegfried M., 565
Pujara, K. K., 566
Putz, Vernon R., 887
Putz-Anderson, Vernon, 378
Pym, Denis, 48

Quah, Ruth F., 590
Quimby, Kelvin L. et al, 911

Rabideau, Gerald F., 49
Rabinowitz, Michael, 471
Radke, James M., 730
Rafales, Lee S. et al, 735
Raghavan, M. V., 566
Raiten, Daniel J., 567
Rakow, Steven J., 50
Rank, Jette, 429
Rapoport, Judith L., 812
Rapp, Doris J., 824
Rasmussen, Peder, 501
Ratcliffe, J. M., 568
Rath, J., 220
Rea, Thomas M., 430
Reams, Steven H., 861
Reavey, Philip C., 499
Rebert, Charles S., 409, 423, 424, 425, 428, 431, 432
Rees, David C., 433, 434, 435
Reischl, Peter, 319
Reisen, C. A., 850
Reisen, Carol A., 851
Reiter, L., 559
Reiter, Lawrence W., 322
Revusky, Sam, 233
Rice, Deborah C., 736, 737
Richardson, John H., 688
Richer, Connie A., 738
Rimland, Bernard, 569, 593, 795, 796
Rippere, Vicky, 825
Rius, R. A., 739
Rivera, Maria, 157
Roberts, Eugene, 180
Roberts, William A., 823
Robertson, R. F., 914
Robins, Eli, 773
Robinson, George, 171
Roche, S. et al, 888
Rodier, Patricia M., 905, 912
Rodnitzky, Robert L., 253, 255
Rodriguez, Gary P., 181
Rodriguez-Gamazo, M., 819
Rodriquez, Ward, 786
Roginski, Edward T., 740
Rolfe, Ursula, 462
Romanski, Lizabeth M., 293
Roney, Paul L., 320
Rose, Terry, 826
Rosecrans, John A., 321
Rosellini, Robert A., 277
Rosen, Jeffrey B., 741, 742
Rosengarten, Helene, 380
Rosenthal, E., 678
Rosenthal, Eugene, 743
Roshon, Melinda S., 827
Ross, Sherman, 10
Ross, W. Donald, 570, 571, 572
Rothblat, L. A., 850
Rotrosen, John, 102
Rotton, James, 184, 185, 186, 828
Rotton, James et al, 183
Routh, Donald K., 573
Royalty, Joel, 744
Rubin, Robert J., 906
Ruch, Marcella W., 829
Rummo, Judith H., 574
Rummo, Nicholas, 889
Rump, E. E., 96
Ruppert, Patricia H., 322
Russell, Roger W., 51, 52
Russo, Dennis C., 496, 525, 526
Ruth, Richard I., 575
Ryan, Christopher M., 187, 381

Sachs, Henrietta K., 576
Sadovnikova, L. D., 256
Saito, Kazuo, 437, 959

Sakaguchi, T., 920
Salas, Manuel, 413
Sallade, Jacqueline B., 830
Salvaterra, Paul, 745
Salvatore, Santo, 890
Salzinger, Kurt, 234
Sanderson, Blythe A., 760
Sandman, Peter M., 891
Sandmark, Björn, 953
Sǎndulescu, Georgeta et al, 257
Sanes, Jerome N., 53
Sarlanis, Kiriako, 889
Sauerhoff, Mitchell W., 716
Sauter, Diana L., 188
Sawchenko, Paul, 696
Saxby, P., 956
Saxena, V. B., 384
Saxena, Vinod B., 56, 955
Scanland, Vera B., 478
Scevola, M., 182
Schaller, Karl-Heinz, 596
Schalock, Robert L., 746
Schantz, Susan L., 702
Schaumburg, H. H., 866
Schaumburg, Herbert H., 54, 336
Schauss, Alexander G., 577
Schiffman, Susan S., 189
Schmidt, Hans, 410
Schmidt, James C., 640, 747
Schneider, Kenneth C., 190
Schneider, Mary L., 702
Schnell, R. C., 748
Schnorr, Janet K., 323
Schoenheit, Carolyn M., 400
Schoental, R., 191
Schoenthaler, Stephen J., 831
Schön, H., 764
Schottenfeld, Richard S., 382, 578
Schreiner, Gerd, 661, 749
Schroeder, Stephen R., 544
Schrot, J., 913, 914
Schulz, David W., 774
Schum, Timothy R., 258
Schütz, Andrejs, 962
Schwark, Wayne S., 750
Schwartz, Arthur S., 751
Schwartz, Pamela M., 20
Scott, Nancy E., 954
Selbst, Steven M., 579
Selikoff, Irving J., 25
Sembrat, Melanie, 692
Senewiratne, B., 259
Seppäläinen, Anna M., 383
Serby, Michael, 102
Seth, Prahlad K., 330
Settle, Robert B., 162
Setzer, J. V., 419
Setzer, James V., 378
Shaffer, Howard J., 192
Shaheen, Sandra J., 580
Shapiro, Martin M., 752
Sharma, Raghubir P., 324
Shearer, T. R., 581
Shechter, Mordechai, 219
Shek, Judy W., 776
Shepherd, Michael, 55
Sherman, A. D., 436
Shield, Lloyd K., 193
Shih, Tsung-ming, 753
Sholiton, Marilyn C., 571, 572
Shor, Ronald E., 194
Shrum, John W., 325
Siegfried, William D., 206
Silbergeld, Ellen K., 235, 456, 457, 718, 754, 755, 756
Silva, Phil A., 582
Silverman, A. Paul, 236
Silverman, Marvin, 885
Simmel, Edward C., 265
Simon, F., 218
Simpson, Ronald D., 125
Simpson-Housley, P., 166
Simson, Richard, 3
Sine, Larry F., 583
Singer, George, 52
Singer, Raymond, 954
Singh, Jaya, 56, 384, 955
Singhal, Radhey L., 292
Sinha, S. N., 40
Skerfving, Staffan, 962
Slangen, J. L., 57
Smirnov, V. K., 58

Smith, Marcia D., 915
Smith, Marjorie, 584
Smith, Marjorie et al, 585
Smith, Mark J., 757
Smith, Michael J., 195
Smith, Philip J., 59, 586, 587
Smith, Richard M., 325
Smith, Robert F., 916
Smith, W. Lynn, 892
Snodgrass, Earl W., 813
Snowdon, Charles T., 758, 759, 760
Snyder, Solomon H., 196
Sobotka, Thomas J., 761
Sohler, Arthur, 588, 589
Soler, Edgardo, 185
Solomon, Henry, 100
Sorenson, Sally S., 431, 432
Soria, J., 819
Sparber, S. B., 678
Sparber, Sheldon B., 681
Spence, Ian, 762
Spencer, Peter S., 336
Spring, Carl, 832
Spyker, Joan M., 458
Staatz, Christina G., 273
Ståhle, Lars, 731
Stamper, Colleen R., 326
Stanczak, Daniel E., 860
Stark, Alice D., 590
Steen, J. A., 305, 306
Steen, Jo A., 307
Stefanko, Michael, 936
Stegner, Steven E., 653, 654
Stein, Elliot A., 327
Steinberg, Marshall, 60
Steinberg, William, 197
Steinbusch, H. V., 286
Steiner, John, 570
Stellern, John, 531, 537, 539, 546, 591
Sterling, Harold, 832
Sterman, Arnold, 260
Stevensson, Leif T., 879
Stewart, Thomas R., 198
Stiles, Martha C., 250
Stineman, Carl H., 763
Stock, Alfred, 592
Stollery, Brian T., 385
Stone, James M., 640
Stone, Jimmy D., 199
Stone, Russell A., 200
Strahilevitz, Aharona, 893
Strahilevitz, Meir, 893
Struempler, Richard E., 593
Struwe, Göran, 144, 201, 386
Stupfel, Maurice, 917
Sturm, Randall, 467
Sturman, John A., 776
Succop, Paul A., 486
Summers, David M., 202
Suter, Kurt E., 660, 661, 764
Sutterlin, A. M., 237
Suzuki, Tatsuzo, 203
Svendsgaard, David J., 484
Svenson, Ola, 854
Svensson, Leif 1., 894
Swanson, James M., 833
Swanson, Joan R., 387
Swartzwelder, H. S. et al, 765
Swyt, Carol, 498
Szeberenyi, Judit M., 939

Takahashi, Kazuko, 203
Takeda, Tsuneichi, 132
Tamaki, Yoshitaka, 238
Tanaka, K., 920
Tanaka, Yoshiharu, 849
Tapia, C., 204
Tariot, Pierre N., 388
Taylor, Betty, 723, 724
Taylor, D. H. et al, 766
Taylor, Douglas H., 726
Taylor, Eric, 205
Taylor, G. T., 744
Taylor, J. D., 398
Taylor, S. Martin, 177
Tedeschi, Richard G., 206
Tenkanen, Leena, 349
Terry, Robert D., 207
Tham, R., 363
Thambipillai, Shanthi, 259
Thatcher, R. W., 208, 595, 816

AUTHOR INDEX

Thatcher, R. W. et al, 594
Thatcher, Robert W., 522
Thomas, J. R., 913, 914
Thompson, Christopher, 956
Thor, Donald H., 675, 676, 677
Thorley, Geoff, 797
Thorley, Geoffrey, 834
Thorne, B. Michael, 768
Thorne, B. Michael et al, 767
Thümler, R., 473
Thurber, Andrea B., 426
Tikofsky, Ronald S., 828
Tilson, H. A., 289, 619
Tilson, Hugh A., 61, 302, 321, 621, 769, 774
Tinklenberg, Jared R., 545
Tofanelli, Ruth A., 813
Tokarek, Theresa, 785
Tola, Sakari, 361, 364
Tolonen, Matti, 119
Tondat, Lynn M., 852
Torres Cházaro, Octavio, 394
Tossman, Ulf, 731
Trabucchi, Marco, 739
Treanor, J. J., 895
Triebig, Gerhard, 596
Trigg, Linda J., 209
Trites, Ronald L., 798
Tritschler, J. M., 752
Truitt, Edward B., 902
Tryphonas, Helen, 798
Tupper, Charles R., 957
Turbiaux, Marcel, 389
Tureen, Robert, 570
Turman, Mary W., 835
Tvedt, Bjørn, 210

Ulbrich, Beate, 661, 749
Ulm, Ronald A., 752
Ungvary, G., 939
Uphouse, Lynda, 328

Urbanowicz, Marie-Anne, 602
Uyeno, Edward T., 426
Uzzell, Barbara P., 597

Valciukas, José A., 62
Valciukas, José A. et al, 598
Valentine, John H., 211
Van den Bercken, Joep, 264
Van der Zalm, Johan M., 264
Vanier, Dinoo J., 120
Varma, Andre, 260
Vasilescu, I. P., 212
Vea, E. V., 329
Vermeersch, Joyce, 832
Vetrano, K., 777
Vicente, Peter J., 896
Vickers, Colin, 770
Vimpani, G. V., 961
Vinař, O., 390
Vincent, Steven R., 730
Vitulli, William F., 771
Viveiros, Donna M., 852
Vogel, Richard A., 918
von Restorff, W., 897
von Stultz, Jeannine, 724
Vorhees, Charles V., 63, 772, 802
Vuchetich, J., 701
Vyner, Henry M., 958

Wada, Hiromi, 437, 959
Wahlström, J., 501
Wakefield, James A., 831
Walbran, Bonnie B., 773
Walczak, C., 327
Wald, Peter, 868
Waldron, H. A., 599
Walker, Mildred M., 799
Wall, Geoffrey, 213
Walsh, T. J., 619
Walsh, Thomas J., 774

Walther, Bernt, 294
Wandersman, Abraham, 107
Ward, Christopher D., 214
Ward, Jerry, 786
Washburn, M., 327
Wasyliw, Orest E., 64
Waternaux, Christine, 470, 921
Watkinson, William P., 932
Webb, Dianne B., 960
Wegert, S., 701
Wei, Eddie, 727
Weigel, Russell H., 65
Weiner, William J., 775
Weingartner, Herbert, 812
Weinstein, Neil D., 891
Weisman, Joan M., 261
Weiss, Bernard, 66, 67, 441, 800, 836
Weiss, Bernard et al, 837
Welch, Ken, 530
Wellman, Paul J., 724
Wender, Esther H., 801
Wendling, Robert, 246
Wennberg, Arne, 386
Westacott, George, 138
Westling, H., 883
White, Mary C., 215
White, Roberta F., 339, 391
White, Roberta G., 466
Whitman, Barbara, 462
Wickström, G., 365
Wiens, Arthur N., 345
Wigg, N. R., 961
Wilkes, R. L., 143
Willers, Stefan, 962
Williams, Daniel C., 194
Williams, J. Ivan, 838
Williams, R. J., 108
Williams, Sheila, 582
Wilson, M. C., 308
Wimer, Richard E., 216
Wimolwattanapun, S., 438

Winder, Christopher, 459
Winneke, G., 492
Winneke, Gerhard, 392, 600, 704, 720, 941
Wisniewski, Henryk M., 776
Wolf, Abraham W., 490, 491
Wolf, Carlos L., 648
Wolford, Rodney, 215
Wolkoff, F. Dmitri, 234
Wolpert, Edward A., 217
Woolston, Vernon L., 65
Wootten, V., 777
Wright, A. A., 665
Wright, Geoffrey R., 898
Wright, I., 218
Wright, Logan, 114
Wulff, V. J., 778

Yamada, Hiroaki, 372
Yamamoto, Bryan K., 779
Yamins, Janice G., 601
Yanagihara, Richard, 498
Yeager, David W., 725
Yesavage, Jerome A., 248, 545
Yim, George K., 317
Yokel, Robert A., 780
Young, Alice M., 742
Young, Robert W., 239
Yule, William, 602

Zaidi, Nikhat F., 330
Zeidner, Moshe, 219
Zeller, W. Patrick et al, 899
Zenick, H., 781
Zenick, Harold, 422, 733, 782, 783, 784, 785, 786
Zenick H., 624
Zuckerman, Craig H., 603

APPENDIX

Search Strategy Used to Retrieve References for the Bibliography

Alain Y. Dessaint, PhD

Any bibliographic research, whether online or manual, seeks to maximize two parameters: recall (retrieved references as a percentage of the total "universe" of relevant references) and precision (relevant references as a percentage of total retrieved references). Recall can be measured only approximately, because usually, for any but the simplest, most precise subject areas, the searcher does not know the total number of references that exist (like the stars, there is probably always one more out there). Comparisons can be made between different types of searches and between different searchers to reach an approximation of the total. Precision can best be measured by the end user, who, after consulting the original document, makes a determination as to whether it is relevant or not. Generally, an online search by an intermediary searcher (i.e., not the end user) has a precision of about 60% (Saracevik & Kantor, 1988).

Interest in the behavioral, psychological, and sociocultural aspects of environmental toxins is a relatively recent trend. References on this topic are difficult to retrieve using the "controlled vocabulary" of the *Thesaurus of Psychological Index Terms* (Fifth Edition; American Psychological Association, 1988). These *Thesaurus* terms tend to be too broad. Free-text searching by specific toxins is time consuming and also results in many "false drops" (nonrelevant references; e.g., searching *aluminum* retrieves an article on aluminum can pickers).

A balance must be struck, therefore, between comprehensiveness and relevance, between recall and precision. An attempt to get all references on a subject will result in many false drops. An attempt to limit the search solely to relevant documents will result in missing many others. In the search used to retrieve documents for this bibliography, we opted for high recall at the cost of some precision. A high percentage of nonrelevant documents were retrieved, and these were deleted after we read the abstracts. (Coincidentally, therefore, this search is a good argument for using a database that provides reliable and informative abstracts.)

The first step in constructing the search was to search the PsycINFO *Thesaurus* for appropriate index terms (or "descriptors"). Specific terms such as *lead poisoning* or *mercury poisoning* were clearly relevant, and cross-references ("broader terms," "narrower terms," "related terms") led to more descriptors that could be used. Some broad terms, such as *neurotoxins*, *toxicity*, and *poisons*, would retrieve very large numbers of records (as indicated in the *Thesaurus* "posting notes"). In an attempt to eliminate false drops, we first tried to limit retrieval of records that contained both one of these descriptors and one of a set of *environment* descriptors (viz., *environment, environmental effects, environmental stress, environmental psychology*, and *ecological factors*). However, a test search with and without the *environment* descriptors indicated that this approach eliminated many experimental articles investigating the effects of neurotoxins or poisons, without reference to environmental impact. Since these articles were clearly relevant, we abandoned this tactic.

After examining the false drops retrieved in our test search, we decided that eliminating articles that also contained one of a set of *drug* or *alcohol* descriptors would help precision. Using *not drug?* or *not alcohol?* (where *?* indicates truncation) eliminated articles that were indexed under any term beginning with *drug-* or *alcohol-* (including *alcoholic psychosis, alcoholism, alcohols, drug abuse, drug addiction, drug overdoses, drug usage,* and *drugs*).

Similarly, we limited the retrieval obtained using *solvents* by eliminating records also indexed under *inhalant abuse*.

Next, we added relevant terms not found in the *Thesaurus* and searched for these in all parts of a record (not just the descriptor field). Some terms did not result in new retrievals because the documents had already been retrieved by one of the more general *Thesaurus* terms: for example, carbon disulfide (retrieved by using *poisons* or *neurotoxins*), polychlorinated biphenyls (*poisons* or *toxicity*), carbaryl (*insecticides*), chlordecone (*insecticides* or *neurotoxins*), carbon tetrachloride (*neurotoxins*), sulfur dioxide (*pollution*), kepone (*toxicity*), benzene and xylene (*solvents*), and methyl mercury (*mercury*). Other terms, however, did result in new documents being retrieved, and these were therefore added to the search strategy: for example, asbestos (which one might have expected to be indexed under *metallic elements*, but was not), trichloroethylene and toluene (which should have been indexed under *solvents*, but sometimes were not), and toxic oil syndrome.

The final search strategy, executed on DIALOG, after these trials and errors, was as follows:

?s (toxic?/de not toxicomania/de) or (poisons or teratogens or neurotoxins or occupational exposure or pollution or carcinogens)/de
        [/de limits the search to the descriptor field]
        [? indicates truncation]
        [creates set labeled S1]

?s S1 not (ibotenic( )acid/ti,id or kainic( )acid/ti,id or lesions/de or drug?/de or alcohol?/de)
        [excludes these categories from Set 1]
        [( ) indicates that the two terms must occur together]
        [creates set labeled S2]

?s insecticides or DDT (insecticide) or dieldrin or parathion or solvents/de or carbon( ) tetrachloride or formaldehyde or toluene
        [creates set labeled S3]

?s S3 not (inhalant( )abus?/de,ti,id or glue( )sniffing/de,ti,id or solvent( )abus?/ti,id or self( ) poison?/ti,id)
        [creates set labeled S4]

?s (metallic elements or cobalt or copper or lead (metal) or lead poisoning or mercury (metal) or mercury poisoning or carbon monoxide or carbon monoxide poisoning)/de
        [creates set labeled S5]

?s aluminum or arsenic or asbestos or cadmium or manganese or thallium or tin or food additives or toxic( )oil( )syndrome or ethylene( )dibromide or hydrogen( ) sulfide or halothane or trichloroethylene
    [creates set labeled S6]

?s S2 or S4 or S5 or S6
    [eliminates duplicates retrieved by more than one set of index terms and creates set labeled S7]

?s S7/1973:1989   [limits search to documents added to PsycINFO between 1973 and 1989]

SEARCH TIP

To retrieve Environmental Toxins records that were added to PsycINFO after April 1989, use the above strategy through S7, then:

?s S7 and ud=8905:9999

REFERENCE

Saracevik, Tefko & Kantor, Paul. (1988). A study of information seeking and retrieving: II. Users, questions and effectiveness. *Journal of the American Society for Information Science*, 39, 177-196.